Statistics for Advanced Practice Nurses and Health Professionals

Manfred Stommel, PhD, is a professor in the College of Nursing, Michigan State University. Dr. Stommel's recent research program has centered on the body mass index (BMI), its measurement in surveys, as well as antecedents and consequences of variations in the BMI. In addition, he has focused on the mortality and morbidity impacts of obesity and physical activity among different population groups. As the 2008/2009 Academy Health Senior Service Fellow at the CDC/National Center for Health Statistics, he specialized in the analysis of federal health surveys, such as the National Health Interview Survey (NHIS) and the National Health and Nutrition Examination Survey (NHANES) linked to the National Death Index. Dr. Stommel has published over 100 peer-reviewed papers and a book on clinical research methods. He is a regular reviewer for numerous medical and nursing research journals.

Katherine J. Dontje, PhD, FNP-BC, is director of the graduate clinical programs and assistant professor/nurse practitioner in the College of Nursing, Michigan State University. Dr. Dontje teaches in the doctorate of nursing practice and masters programs. She has an active clinical practice encompassing the full scope of primary care. Dr. Dontje has been principal investigator (PI) or co-PI on 12 research projects, including a W.K. Kellogg Foundation-funded project on university-based nurse-managed care and a Robert Wood Johnson Foundation-funded project on the quality of outcomes from three models of nurse-led primary care. She is presently a member of an interdisciplinary research team focusing on patient and provider aspects of the electronic health record. She has published numerous peer-reviewed articles on informatics and evidence-based practice for patients in primary care. Dr. Dontje has presented at regional, national, and international conferences. She has received numerous honors and awards, is a member of American Nurses Association (ANA), American Association of Nurse Practitioners (AANP), Midwest Nursing Research Society (MNRS), Sigma Theta Tau International (STTI), and the Michigan Council of Nurse Practitioners, and has served in leadership capacity for many of them. She serves as a reviewer for *Computers, Informatics, Nursing* and *The Journal for Nurse Practitioners*.

Statistics for Advanced Practice Nurses and Health Professionals

Manfred Stommel, PhD
Katherine J. Dontje, PhD, FNP-BC

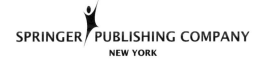

SPRINGER PUBLISHING COMPANY
NEW YORK

Springer Publishing Company, LLC
11 West 42nd Street
New York, NY 10036
www.springerpub.com

Acquisitions Editor: Margaret Zuccarini
Composition: Exeter Premedia Services Private Ltd.

ISBN: 978-0-8261-9824-2
e-book ISBN: 978-0-8261-9825-9

Data sets for SPSS, SAS, STATA, and Excel are available at www.springerpub.com/stommel .supplements

14 15 16 17 / 5 4 3 2 1

The author and the publisher of this Work have made every effort to use sources believed to be reliable to provide information that is accurate and compatible with the standards generally accepted at the time of publication. Because medical science is continually advancing, our knowledge base continues to expand. Therefore, as new information becomes available, changes in procedures become necessary. We recommend that the reader always consult current research and specific institutional policies before performing any clinical procedure. The author and publisher shall not be liable for any special, consequential, or exemplary damages resulting, in whole or in part, from the readers' use of, or reliance on, the information contained in this book. The publisher has no responsibility for the persistence or accuracy of URLs for external or third-party Internet websites referred to in this publication and does not guarantee that any content on such websites is, or will remain, accurate or appropriate.

Library of Congress Cataloging-in-Publication Data
Stommel, Manfred, author.
Statistics for advanced practice nurses and health professionals / Manfred Stommel, Katherine J. Dontje.
    p. ; cm.
  Includes bibliographical references.
  ISBN 978-0-8261-9824-2—ISBN 978-0-8261-9825-9 (e-book)
  I. Dontje, Katherine J., author.   II. Title.
  [DNLM: 1. Statistics as Topic—Nurses' Instruction.   2. Clinical Nursing Research—methods.
  3. Nurse Practitioners. WA 950]
  RT68
  610.73072′7—dc23
                                                                              2014002661

Printed in the United States of America by McNaughton & Gunn.

Contents

Preface

This book has been written with a view of what the future practice of graduates from Doctor of Nursing Practice (DNP) programs and other advanced health care providers looks like. In particular, graduates of DNP programs and other health care providers need to be advocates of using the best research evidence available to facilitate both practice and system changes. National organizations of many health professionals have emphasized the importance of using the best evidence to improve health care of individuals, decrease the cost of care, and prevent errors across health care systems. All of this requires a solid grasp of statistical reasoning, which underlies much of the empirical information presented in research journals. In this book, our aim is to provide the reader with more than an introductory level comprehension of statistics. In particular, our emphasis is on *understanding* the most commonly encountered statistical models in the research journals. We believe that the "cookbook approach" to statistics, consisting of the memorization of formulas and rules, is not really helpful, as the correct interpretation of statistical tests and models requires an understanding of the underlying logic of the models employed.

The information provided in this book is divided into five parts, covering basic statistical reasoning and four different classes of statistical models. Part I covers the principles of statistical inference in clinical trials and observational studies, reasons for why we use statistical testing, and how we use it in the context of different research designs, as well as an overview of the basic descriptive statistics. Part II discusses statistical models used with continuous and interval-level outcome variables, which include *t*-tests, linear regression, analysis of variance, and some extensions of these models. Part III addresses statistical tests and models appropriate for categorical outcome variables. Part IV explores the use of time-to-event or survival analysis, which are often used in clinical research. Part V provides an overview of measurement models with an emphasis on reliability and validity of self-report and medical test data. In all chapters, we used examples relevant to clinical practice to provide information on how to use and interpret each of the statistical analysis models introduced. Exercise questions at the end of each chapter, and selected answers at the end of the book, serve the purpose of deepening the understanding. The book can be used as a stand-alone text for those readers primarily interested in understanding the models, but we offer some data sets in SPSS, STATA, SAS, and Excel formats on an accompanying website (www.springerpub .com/stommel.supplements) for those who want to engage in applied analysis themselves. The website also contains additional exercise questions and solutions.

The health care provider of the future needs to understand how to read statistical research and evaluate the quality of the research. Given the ever-increasing sophistication of statistical analyses in health care journals, it is important that clinicians acquire a level of understanding that enables them to interpret the results of research studies correctly and translate this information into practice. Readers of this book will be able to accomplish these tasks as well as to choose appropriate statistical methods for their own translational research. At least, readers should be able to recognize when more sophisticated analyses are necessary, and should have sufficient understanding of statistical reasoning to engage and converse with a statistical expert when needed. One important aspect of the translation model is to apply the best evidence available about clinical conditions in real-life clinical settings. The statistical methods described in this book will help health care providers to evaluate outcomes of quality improvement projects and system changes to determine the effectiveness of the evidence within their own clinical population.

Finally, we sincerely hope that readers find the information in this book useful and actually grow excited about the contributions that statistics can make to health care. Statistical reasoning provides a different way of looking at the world, which is particularly helpful when thinking about the health of populations or the evaluation of health care systems. In short, we believe that the study of statistics does not only consist of the acquisition of techniques and tools, however necessary, but opens up new ways of thinking about health-related problems. If we succeed in conveying both the ideas and our enthusiasm for statistical analysis, we shall have accomplished our goals.

Manfred Stommel, PhD
Katherine J. Dontje, PhD, FNP-BC

Acknowledgments

Textbooks do not get written by the authors alone, they also require support from many other persons. First, we would like to acknowledge Margaret Zuccarini at Springer Publishing Company, LLC, whose mix of flexibility and encouragement was just the right medicine to keep the authors on track. Dr. Stommel would also like to express his thanks to Dean Mary Mundt for her support and patience during the long period of textbook writing. Last, but not least, Dr. Stommel expresses his deep gratitude to his wife, Dr. Petra von Heimburg, for enduring many lost evenings, when he was "holed up" in the office. Dr. Dontje would like to acknowledge the encouragement of Dr. Barbara Given over the years and of Dr. Teresa Wehrwein throughout this project.

PART I. FOUNDATIONS FOR STATISTICAL THINKING

CHAPTER 1

Introduction: The Role of Statistics in Research and Clinical Practice

Many students in clinically oriented degree programs wonder why they are required to take statistics courses. There are several ways to answer this question, but it is probably best to start with a clinical example.

Suppose that you have a patient who has coronary artery disease and occasional episodes of angina, but only when exercising heavily. The patient comes to you and asks whether he should have a cardiac catheterization and possible stents put in with the procedure. How would you go about evaluating this? There are, of course, numerous different opinions on the subject, and the patient has friends who are encouraging him to get the procedure, as these friends had four to five stents implanted and reportedly are doing well. You search the literature and find that, for stable coronary artery disease, there are three main choices of treatment (medical therapy, angioplasty, or bypass surgery); however, the statistics indicate that, among stable angina cases, none of these have any significantly greater long-term benefit in terms of length of life or recurrence of heart attacks over the other (Boden et al., 2007; Hueb et al., 2004). As you review the studies, you are confronted with a variety of statistics, but how do you explain these convincingly to your patient, when "common sense" appears to suggest that opening up an artery should "save his life"?

Probably the first thing to emphasize would be that it is not enough to cite a few individual cases for whom a particular clinical intervention appears to have been successful. One reason we cannot rely on results from individual cases is that what works in one case may or may not work in another case. Human beings almost always show a range of responses to a given nursing or medical intervention. Thus the question arises: How do we then decide which treatment or intervention is better or worse? It turns out that statistics alone cannot answer this question either. The inference that an intervention is causally effective is also based on the quality of the research design of the intervention study. But statistical considerations are an essential aspect of how to design an effective intervention study that can answer the desired question.

Given the almost infinite variability of human responses to clinical treatments and interventions, we need a method by which we can separate "accidental" individual variability from *systematic*, treatment-related effects. As we will see, statistical models can be used to estimate *average* effects of interventions as well as provide information on the amount of uncertainty or relative certainty that must be attached to these estimates.

We use statistics not only in the evaluation of clinical interventions or treatments but also to generalize from the evidence obtained in a study sample to the target populations of interest. For example, data from the National Health Interview Survey (NHIS) conducted by the National Center for Health Statistics (NCHS) linked to the National Death Index have been employed to estimate the effects of adherence to the 2008 Physical Activity Guidelines (Centers for Disease Control and Prevention [CDC]) on the subsequent mortality risk of adult U.S. residents (Schoenborn & Stommel, 2011). In such studies, we use sample data to draw inferences about health conditions in larger target populations. While the aim is to describe patterns of mortality, morbidity, and health behaviors in the target population, we use surveys that employ random/probability sampling designs that, in some sense, "represent" or "reflect" the characteristics of the target population with sufficiently high accuracy.

Statistics are, in fact, all-pervasive in today's health care systems. We use it to evaluate the performance of medical interventions, the effectiveness of screening programs, to gauge quality improvement projects in health care delivery, to assess the performance of nursing students on the NCLEX or certification exams, to establish critical test scores that should trigger nursing or medical interventions, and so forth. Statistical evidence plays a major role in judging not only the quality of care delivered, but also its cost effectiveness. Statistics are also an important tool for providers and public health officials, as they engage in assessments of how well they are doing compared to other health delivery organizations, or compared to benchmarks derived from nationwide or statewide studies. Last, but not least, the evidence to support and evaluate clinical practice guidelines or guidelines for healthy behaviors (e.g., the CDC 2008 Physical Activity Guidelines) is grounded in statistical information.

By contrast, consider personal experience. In a way, all of us are "reckless generalizers" in our personal lives. We all believe we have an idea of what "human nature" is like, even though we get to know well only a few dozen individuals in a lifetime (and they are decidedly not a representative cross-section of the human race!). Similarly, from the very limited experience we have as patients with our primary care providers, dentists, or nurses, we draw inferences about their quality as providers. Suppose a patient with a diphtheria infection is misdiagnosed by her provider as having mononucleosis (easy to do in the initial phases of these diseases) and receives the wrong treatment, should she conclude that the provider is "incompetent?" Suppose you have evidence that the provider in question made such a diagnostic mistake only once in 25 years of practice, while another provider accumulated a long list of complaints for misdiagnoses. As this example shows, we cannot make credible inferences based on a single event; we need large amounts of data to discover a *pattern* of behavior. Hence, we need statistics. It allows us to distinguish among isolated events ("outliers"), systematic patterns of events (average differences or "effects"), and events whose occurrence cannot be predicted ("random errors"). All of this information is needed to evaluate outcomes of interest to health care providers.

Let us look at this a bit further. Not only are no two individuals exactly alike in terms of their biological characteristics and life experiences; as living organisms they are also subject to continual change over time. For example, as every nurse knows, people's "true" diastolic blood pressure (DBP) fluctuates, even during short time periods, before and after a meal, and so forth. On top of that, there are measurement errors associated with any clinical measure you can think of: For instance, blood pressure (BP) measures vary depending on whether the cuff is applied to the right or left arm, whether the cuff is more or less pressurized, whether the patient has more or less muscle tissue, and so forth. Similarly, any body temperature measure varies based on where the thermometer is applied (under the armpit, the tongue, etc.), and any nurse, who has ever tried to establish the height of an infant, knows that it is impossible to get the "true" value. In short, uncertainty is part of everything we do, whether to estimate the likely survival of a patient with a recent Stage 4 lung cancer diagnosis or the recovery time after a triple bypass operation. Thus, we need to have realistic estimates of the uncertainty attached to our predictions, so that we can make rational decisions about which clinical interventions are better or worse. Statistical methods do just that. You might say statistics is the branch of mathematics that puts uncertainty (and probability) at the center of its models. It allows us to estimate the risks we engage in when we make informed decisions. It is for that reason that statistics has become a central part of clinical reality.

Finally, there is also a very pragmatic reason why providers have to become savvier in the evaluation of statistical information. On a daily basis, many of our patients follow mass media reports on health-related topics or search the Internet to get information about a disease or illness they might have or a medical treatment that they believe they might need. Such reports very often cite statistics from clinical trials or epidemiological studies. Certainly, advertisements for pharmaceutical drugs or claims on highway posters that this or that hospital is in the "top 100" for knee surgery, and so forth, all tend to cite statistics that may or may not be relevant to the claims involved.

For users of statistics, the most important issue has become how to evaluate all this statistical information and how to make intelligent choices based on it. For current and future clinicians, an additional problem is that the statistical information in medical and nursing research journals is becoming ever more sophisticated: just witness a special issue of *Nursing Research* (Volume 61(3), 2012) entirely devoted to newer statistical models used by nursing researchers. Yet knowing more about statistics is essential for clinicians to understand and interpret clinically relevant evidence. While today's clinicians do need a solid conceptual grounding in major statistical concepts, they do not need to know the particular mathematical structures of the major estimation techniques, for example, least squares, maximum likelihood, or partial likelihood estimation that underlie many statistical models (all of which require some knowledge of calculus). Instead, clinicians do need to understand the basic *logic* of statistical estimation, basic probability concepts, and how inferential statistical decisions are made. To draw correct inferences from statistical information also includes awareness that statistics are an integral part of the research design of a study. To take just one example: how one interprets the outcome of a *t*-test differs, depending on whether or not the data come from an experimental study with random assignment, a survey based on random sampling, or whether the data are cross-sectional or longitudinal. Thus, statistical evidence cannot be interpreted without knowing something about the study design context, the sampling design, as well as how measurement error can affect the results.

When an advertisement claims that a certain drug reduces bleeding by 35%, one should immediately ask how that figure was established. Without context, such a number is virtually impossible to interpret. What is the reference group compared to which the 35% reduction was observed? How large a sample of men/women was studied? Was the sample representative of the U.S. population at large or only of certain segments, for example, only women, only Whites, only persons younger than 40 or older than 65, or persons with a particular disease, and so forth? Were there measurement problems? Could the study show a causal connection between the drug or treatment and the outcome? Are there alternative treatments that are even better? Does the treatment work only under certain conditions, and so forth? Many of these questions involve statistical reasoning and statistical methods; so it is no accident that statistics has become a major component of the education and training of future clinicians.

This book is intended as a textbook for graduate nursing students and others who are preparing for advanced clinical practice roles. As it is addressed to clinicians, we present the major statistical models most often encountered in nursing, medical, and epidemiological research. Past statistics textbooks for nursing students have almost exclusively focused on statistical models derived from psychometrics and educational research, but have neglected models that should be of primary interest to advanced practice nurses, such as life table and survival analysis as well as the evaluation of diagnostic and screening tests. This book is intended to close this gap without sacrificing the more traditional topics from psychometrics (e.g., reliability and factor analysis), which continue to be relevant, particularly for behaviorally oriented nursing research. The overall goal of this book is to provide the learner with a larger range of statistical models and concepts, which are used in clinical research and as a basis for evidence-based clinical practice. This includes skills in "mining" data sets that are needed for the clinical management of patient populations.

Despite our goal of providing the reader with an introduction to more complicated statistical models than the *t*-test, analysis of variance (ANOVA), and linear regression, the presentation of the material does not require any calculus or matrix algebra, but relies on some knowledge of college algebra. Because students may have forgotten how to read and use exponential and logarithmic functions, a brief refresher has been provided in Appendix H to facilitate the discussion of logistic and survival regression models. On the whole, the emphasis in this book is on verbal explanations, and the use of worked out examples to explain the more complicated ideas of statistical inference. However, statistics is an inherently mathematical subject and it cannot be learned by completely shying away from mathematics. Neither can the science of nursing research be understood without mathematics (Henly, 2012). Some statistical formulas (e.g., standard deviations, covariance/correlations, odds ratios) are essential in understanding the material. Thus, they are not only introduced, but also accompanied by detailed verbal explanations. In addition, exercise questions at the end of each chapter (selected answers are provided in Appendix J) will provide opportunities to become familiar and comfortable with using such formulas and interpreting them correctly.

Our experience in teaching statistics for nurses at the graduate level shows that some students are apprehensive about taking a statistics course. We believe that part of the reason for this is that too many students were taught introductory statistics with an emphasis on memorizing formulas, but never really understood what the subject was about and how it relates to clinical practice. The information you will find in this book is designed to give you a solid understanding of the statistical methods we introduce. We believe that memorizing formulas alone does not really give you an understanding of the value of statistical analysis, and besides, formulas will be forgotten as soon as the course is over. In this book you will have the opportunity to learn about statistical reasoning and how it can provide the clinician with the contextual information necessary to make clinical decisions in particular instances. However, that requires understanding the conceptual basis for statistical methods, which, incidentally, also provides a much better aid to memory.

In sum, we hope we have made a convincing case for why statistics should be part of any clinician's tool kit, but more than that: We think of the subject of statistics as an exciting field that can transform the way you look at health care and clinical practice. If we succeed in changing students' outlook on statistics, it is our experience that it changes their outlook on clinical practice forever.

REFERENCES

Boden, W. E., O'Rourke, R. A., Teo, K. K., Hartigan, P. M., Maron, D. J., Kostuk, W. J., . . . Weintraub, W. S.; COURAGE Trial Research Group. (2007). Optimal medical therapy with or without PCI for stable coronary disease. *The New England Journal of Medicine, 356*(15), 1503–1516.

Centers for Disease Control and Prevention. (2008). *Physical Activity Guidelines Advisory Committee Report, 2008.* Washington, DC: USDHHS.

Henly, S. J. (2012). Strength in numbers: Mathematics and nursing research. *Nursing Research, 61*(4), 241.

Hueb, W., Soares, P. R., Gersh, B. J., César, L. A., Luz, P. L., Puig, L. B., . . . Ramires, J. A. (2004). The Medicine, Angioplasty, or Surgery Study (MASS-II): A randomized, controlled clinical trial of three therapeutic strategies for multivessel coronary artery disease: One-year results. *Journal of the American College of Cardiology, 43*(10), 1743–1751.

Schoenborn, C. A., & Stommel, M. (2011). Adherence to the 2008 adult physical activity guidelines and mortality risk. *American Journal of Preventive Medicine, 40*(5), 514–521.

CHAPTER 2

Properties of Variables: Levels of Measurement

Before discussing levels of measurement in more detail, we start with a small data set such as you might encounter in a clinical setting. Table 2.1 shows an excerpt from a data file containing information on 10 study participants who were patients at several rural clinics.[1] The codebook in Table 2.2 provides additional information on how to read the numbers in Table 2.1. Note that information in quantitative data files, like the one presented here, is usually organized in spreadsheet format, using rows and columns.

In this format, the rows represent **cases**[2] and the columns represent **variables**. For instance, look at the column labeled "ID." Each row of this column contains the identification number of a particular subject. In the column labeled "Age" we see different entries in each row, reflecting the age (in years) of each of the subjects denoted in the ID column. Now look at the column labeled "Sex." From the codebook in Table 2.2 we learn that the number "1" of the variable "Sex" refers to women and the number "2" to men. As this column contains at least two distinct values, the entries in the column represent a **variable** in this data set.

The concept of a **variable** is fundamental to quantitative research and plays a central role in statistics. In the most general sense, variables are the *measured representations* of the concepts we are interested in. As clinicians we might talk about concepts like "depression" or "hypertension," but after we collect information about these concepts, they become variables in our data sets. For example, the systolic and diastolic blood pressure (BP) readings constitute variables in the data set; so do the scores that survey participants receive based on their responses to a measurement tool like the Center for Epidemiologic Studies-Depression Scale (CES-D). As the name "variable" implies, the scores *vary across subjects*, that is, as we go up and down a given column, we see several distinct **values**, which would be the individual

---

[1] Dates and other information were changed for confidentiality reasons.
[2] "Cases" may be defined as different individuals, different emergency department visits, billing records, and so forth; in longitudinal studies with repeated measures of subjects, each row may represent observations of an individual subject taken at a single time point, and so forth.

TABLE 2.1 Example of Quantitative Data File

ID	SITE	DATE	AGE	SEX	SYSBP	DIABP	CES-D	SRHEALTH
1	8	10/06/2006	21	1	110	76	9	4
2	2	10/14/2005	46	2	123	81	0	4
3	8	07/26/2006	34	1	119	82	14	4
4	6	02/09/2006	28	2	132	87	22	3
5	3	10/27/2005	55	2	141	94	11	3
6	4	09/23/2005	49	1	137	89	32	3
7	1	11/11/2005	51	2	150	108	6	2
8	2	09/25/2005	32	1	118	79	2	4
9	6	02/09/2006	40	1	123	83	15	4
10	6	09/12/2005	45	1	129	91	9	3

scores of the CES-D assigned to each of the patients in the study sample.[3] In short, a variable comprises the actual measurement outcomes or the scores that represent the concept in a study.

If in a particular study there is no variation among the scores in a column—let us say that all studied individuals are female and the only code in the column for "Sex" is "1"—then the numbers in the column would represent a **constant** in this study and data set. By contrast, a variable must take on at least two values for it to vary. For example, the variable *sex* normally consists of the two categories: female or male, here represented by the codes 1 and 2.

As, in the most general sense, *statistical analysis shows how the variation in one or more variables is linked to the variation in other variables*, constants in a data set are of no use other than describing a characteristic of the total study sample. For instance, if in a particular study all participants are female, then we could no longer analyze how sex is related to some outcome of interest, because there is no variation in sex.

TABLE 2.2 Codebook for Data in Table 2.1

VARIABLE	VARIABLE LABELS	VARIABLE CODES
ID	Subject identification no.	1–10
Site	Clinical site no.	1–8
Date	Date of clinic visit	MM/DD/YYYY
Age	Age (in years) at visit	Range: 21–55
Sex	Respondent's sex	1 = female, 2 = male
SysBP	Systolic blood pressure	Recorded in mmHg
DiaBP	Diastolic blood pressure	Recorded in mmHg
CES-D	Center for Epidemiologic Studies-Depression Scale	Possible score range: 0–60
SRHealth	Self-rated health scale	1 = poor, 2 = fair, 3 = good, 4 = excellent

---

[3] Note that scores may not only vary among different subjects, but they may also vary within subjects over time, as when we take repeated BP measures on the same subject. As we will see later, the distinction between within-subjects variation and between-subjects variation is fundamental to many statistical models.

LEVELS OF MEASUREMENT

When we analyze data, we must make assumptions about the **measurement levels** of the variables involved. According to a classic paper by Stevens (1946), we generally distinguish four levels of measurement: (a) **nominal** or **categorical**, (b) **ordinal**, (c) **interval**, and (d) **ratio** levels. As we will see, the determination of levels of measurement is important because it affects what kinds of mathematical operations involving a particular variable are appropriate.

Whether or not to speak of a **nominal** level of "measurement" is, in some ways, questionable. The creation of a nominal variable only requires us to use mutually exclusive categories into which we sort our objects or characteristics of study participants. Examples of nominal variables would be sex (female vs. male), blood types (A, B, O), or marital status. Such variables have categories that have no obvious ordering, which means that the assignment of numerical values to these categories is inherently arbitrary. For instance, let us consider the assignment of numerical values to the categories of the variable "marital status" (see Box 2.1).

BOX 2.1	EXAMPLES OF ALTERNATIVE CODING SCHEMES FOR THE VARIABLE "MARITAL STATUS"

Coding Scheme 1: 1 = married, 2 = single/never married, 3 = divorced, 4 = widowed

Coding Scheme 2: 1 = divorced, 2 = married, 3 = widowed, 4 = single/never married

Coding Scheme 3: 1 = single/never married, 1 = married, 3 = widowed, 4 = divorced

(There are $4 \times 3 \times 2 \times 1 = 24$ different coding schemes/sequences possible for this four-category variable.)

The main principle to remember here is that each different coding scheme is equally defensible and equally valid. This is so because the numbers serve just as labels or "names" (that is why it is called a "nominal" level of measurement) of the categories, and the measurement operation really consists only of grouping subjects into mutually exclusive categories: you may be either married or single, but you cannot be both at the same time. As the value labels are arbitrary, we cannot involve them directly in mathematical operations; for instance, it would be nonsensical to speak of the "average marital status" in a study sample as being "2.4." The same can be said about blood types: They may be listed in any order, with the categories denoting differences, without ranking them as "better" or "worse." We can, of course, count the number of cases in a study sample that fall into each of the categories defined by a nominal variable. As we will see, appropriate statistical tests for such nominal variables are all based on such counting operations.

With an **ordinal** level of measurement, the numerical values assigned to the categories of a variable are no longer completely arbitrary: the values assigned to the categories must form a rank order, indicating more or less of the attribute being measured. For instance, in Table 2.1 we can see the scores associated with the responses of 10 patients to a question asking them to rate their own health on a four-point scale: 4 = excellent, 3 = good, 2 = fair, 1 = poor. Here we have a variable, whose categories form a rank order. It would have been perfectly fine to assign the values 19 = excellent, 8 = good, 5 = fair, and 2 = poor, as such an assignment would preserve the rank order: $19 > 8 > 5 > 2$. In both the original data set and the alternative assignment of numerical values to the categories, the information contained in the assigned values is that of a rank order: the second highest values refer in both cases to "good," the lowest value to "poor." Thus, as long as the rank order is not changed, any numerical scheme that preserves this rank order would be acceptable. However, the *distances between the categories are not defined*: a respondent would say that "good" health is better than "fair" health, but he or she would find it impossible to say that "excellent" health differs from "good" health as much as "fair" health differs from "poor" health.

Clinical judgments often result in ordinal scales. A prominent example would be the Apgar[4] score (Casey, McIntire, & Leveno, 2001) to evaluate the health and progress of a newly born baby. Pain scales like the visual analog scale (Hawker Mian, Kendzerska, & French, 2011) are another example of an ordinal scale frequently encountered in clinical settings.

Interval-level measures are less common in health- and illness-related data, except for the classic example of temperature. Both the Fahrenheit and Celsius scales are widely used, and they are perfectly equivalent as expressed in the equation $°F = 9/5°C + 32$. Yet both scales have zero points defined on the basis of an essentially arbitrary external criterion. (For Celsius, it is the temperature at which water at sea level freezes; for Fahrenheit, it is the temperature at which brine—a mixture of water and ammonium chloride—freezes.) While the scales define distances, for example, in the Celsius scale, the difference between the temperature at which water boils and at which it freezes is divided into 100 equal degrees, they cannot be used to construct ratios. For example, it would *not* be legitimate to say that 20°C is "twice as warm" as 10°C. You can see that by converting the degrees Celsius into degrees Fahrenheit: Using the conversion formula ($°F = 9/5°C + 32$), for 20°C we get 68°F, as 9/5 (20) + 32 = 58; and for 10°C we get 50°F, as 9/5 (10) + 32 = 50. Thus, expressed in degrees Fahrenheit, the two temperatures are $°F = 68$ and $°F = 50$, but the ratio of 68/50 is no longer equal to 2.

In addition to temperature, population-normed test scores are often interval-level variables. For instance, in standard IQ tests, the mean population score within an age group is arbitrarily set to 100, and any individual score is considered in relation to this population norm (Becker, 2003). Such scales do not have natural zero points, and so it would be inadmissible to consider a person with an IQ score of 160 "twice as intelligent" than a person with an IQ score of deviation 80. Pulse oximetry readings (Barker, 2002) are also interval measures, as they do not have a natural zero point (at least not in a living person). With interval measures, it is possible to calculate statistics like means, variances, and standard deviations because they only require that distances between values are well defined.

Ratio-level measures are quite common in clinical settings and research: Height and weight, time from surgery to recovery, gestational age, and so forth are all ratio-level measures familiar to clinicians. They have natural zero points and all basic arithmetic operations (addition, subtraction, multiplication, and division) can be performed on the values of ratio scales. For instance, you can say that a person weighing 270 pounds is three times heavier than a person weighing 90 pounds.

STATISTICS AND LEVELS OF MEASUREMENT

It should be noted that many of the ratio- and interval-level measures are also **continuous** variables, even though in practice, such variables are recorded in **discrete** values. A continuous variable is one that can take on any value on the real number scale. Thus we could, in principle, record a person's age in minutes or even seconds, even though empirically such precise measures would be impossible to come by. They would also be unnecessary, as there is no reason to believe that such fine gradations in the age variable would have any substantive value. Still, it is worth noting that in many statistical models we assume that the underlying

---

[4]Named after Dr. Virginia Apgar, the word is also an acronym for: appearance, pulse, grimace, activity, respiration.

variables are continuous, even though the actual measurements are discrete, that is, they have a certain degree of granularity, as when we measure age in terms of years among adults.

Even though we have divided variables into four measurement levels, in many ways the most important distinction is that between the first two types of variables (nominal/categorical and ordinal) and the latter two (interval and ratio variables). These two groups of variables are also referred to as **qualitative** versus **quantitative** variables; or as **nonmetric** versus **metric** variables. As we will see, statistical measures and tests appropriate for nominal and ordinal data, usually called **nonparametric** statistics, differ from measures and tests appropriate for interval- and ratio-level data, which are also known as **parametric** statistics.

Finally, it is worth noting that the distinction among variables with different levels of measurement is by no means absolute. In fact, we often convert variables with a higher level of measurement to ones with a lower level of measurement. One important clinical application is the use of **threshold values** instead of the information from the full metric measures. For instance, low birth weight (LBW) is defined as a birth weight of less than 2,500 grams. The resulting categorical variable of low versus normal birth weight, which might be coded 1 and 0, should be considered an ordinal-level variable even though the distinction between ordinal and nominal is not important, when only two categories are involved.[5] Other examples of employing threshold values in clinical practice (and also clinical research) would be using cut-off points on diagnostic or screening tests such as tests for the detection of diabetes (Zhang et al., 2005). Threshold values for continuous scale measures are important in clinical practice, because they are often used to trigger treatment recommendations or actions. On the other hand, to condense continuous scale measures into two or a few categories entails discarding a lot of information on individual variability.

SUMMARY

The appropriateness of any statistical model depends on the degree to which the data meet the assumptions of the model. Data are made up of variables, which, in turn, may represent different levels of measurement. The categorization of variables according to their levels of measurement is important because it determines what kinds of mathematical operations are legitimate when involving particular variables in statistical analysis. The broadest distinction among statistical models is that between parametric and nonparametric statistics. For most purposes, variables measured at the interval level or higher can be analyzed using parametric statistics. However, in multivariate analysis of health care data, that is, statistical analysis that involves more than two variables simultaneously, we often find a mixture of categorical and continuous variables. As we will see later in this book, *the choice of appropriate statistical models is largely governed by the properties of the dependent or outcome variables.*

EXERCISES

1. Determine the level of measurement for the following variables:
   (a) Pap smear results
   (b) Body mass index
   (c) Food groups
   (d) Biopsy results from breast tissue
   (e) Food preferences
   (f) Religious affiliation

---

[5] Inconsistencies in rank order can only emerge, if there are at least three categories involved.

2. Convert the diastolic blood pressure (DBP) scores in Table 2.1 into rank orders, assigning the rank 1 to the highest score (108) and rank 10 to the lowest score (76). Then compute the mean rank-order scores for men and women; also compute the mean *original* DBP scores for men and women. Do these two summary measures give you essentially the same information?

3. Is it legitimate to say that a baby with an Apgar score of 10 is twice as healthy as a baby with an Apgar score of 5? Why or why not?

4. List three applications in which threshold scores of continuous scale measures are used to trigger clinical actions.

5. The four levels of measurement (nominal, ordinal, interval, ratio) can themselves be rank-ordered according to a list of criteria, which shows each "higher" level of measurement possessing additional measurement properties that the "lower" level lacks. List the criteria appropriate for each level of measurement.

REFERENCES

Barker, S. J. (2002). "Motion-resistant" pulse oximetry: A comparison of new and old models. *Anesthesia & Analgesia, 95*(4), 967–972.

Becker, K. A. (2003). *History of the Stanford-Binet Intelligence scales: Content and psychometrics* (Stanford-Binet Intelligence Scales, 5th ed., Assessment Service Bulletin No. 1). Itasca, IL: Riverside.

Casey, B. M., McIntire, D. D., & Leveno, K. J. (2001). The continuing value of the Apgar score for the assessment of newborn infants. *The New England Journal of Medicine, 344*(7), 467–471.

Hawker, G. A., Mian, S., Kendzerska, T., & French, M. (2011). Measures of adult pain. *Arthritis Care & Research, 63*(S11), S240–S252.

Stevens, S. S. (1946). On the theory of scales of measurement. *Science, 103*(2684), 677–680.

Zhang, P., Engelgau, M. M., Valdez, R., Cadwell, B., Benjamin, S. M., & Narayan, K. M. (2005). Efficient cutoff points for three screening tests for detecting undiagnosed diabetes and pre-diabetes: An economic analysis. *Diabetes Care, 28*(6), 1321–1325.

CHAPTER 3

Descriptive Univariate Statistics

In Chapter 2, we introduced the concepts of **variables** and **levels of measurement**. In this chapter, we are concerned with describing the numerical distributions that characterize variables in a particular study sample. More precisely, we are concerned with **univariate descriptive statistics**. Statistics are summary measures that describe and condense information contained in the distributions of values on single or multiple variables. If a statistic refers only to the *description of study sample data*, it is called a **descriptive** statistic. If the statistic is used to characterize *a larger target population*, or if the intent is to generalize *beyond* the sample data, then we are dealing with **inferential** statistics.

Statistics are also often divided into **univariate**, **bivariate**, or **multivariate** statistics, depending on whether they describe data distributions for a single variable (univariate), two variables (bivariate), or multiple variables (multivariate). In this chapter, we are focusing on **univariate descriptive statistics**. Before one engages in more complex statistical modeling and statistical inference, it is always a good idea to inspect the study data at hand carefully, because errors in analysis are more easily detected if one "knows" the data and has acquired an "instinctive feel" for them.

THE FREQUENCY DISTRIBUTION

The simplest way to summarize information on a variable is to represent the distribution of values or categories in a **frequency distribution**. For instance, Table 3.1 shows data from a nutrition study (Baker et al., 2007), in which 869 mothers were observed feeding their toddlers. The table shows how the observers rated the amount of TV watching during mealtime, choosing one of four predetermined categories.[1]

As the name tells us, a frequency distribution associates *mutually exclusive* categories, which might be labeled using a verbal or numerical code, with the frequency of their occurrence. For instance, in Table 3.1, we can see that 19 study participants chose the rating "often," which has been assigned the numerical code "3" in this data set. The table also provides information on the percentages of study participants who chose each category/rating, as well as the cumulative percentages. The latter are counted from either the bottom or the top, given

---

[1]The four-point response scale constitutes an ordinal rating scale, as the quantities of TV watching are not determined in precise numerical time units.

TABLE 3.1 TV-Watching Patterns During Mealtime: Observer Ratings

TV IS ON/WATCHED . . .	CODE	FREQUENCY	PERCENTAGE	CUMULATIVE PERCENTAGE
Not at all	(1)	462	53.2	53.2
Occasionally	(2)	28	3.2	56.4
Often	(3)	19	2.2	58.6
Always/throughout the meal	(4)	360	41.4	100.0
Total		869	100.0	

the percentage of cases that fall into the current category plus all categories below (or above) in the distribution. For instance, in Table 3.1 we see that 56.4% of the observers responded that TV was either not watched at all or only occasionally during mealtime. Overall, it is relatively easy to see that most mothers in the study sample either do not watch TV at all during mealtime (53.2%) or they watch it throughout (41.4%). This **bimodal** distribution, that is, a distribution with two peaks or modal categories, is even easier to see in a **bar graph** (see Figure 3.1).

All the information contained in the bar graph is already contained in the frequency distribution, but graphs often provide an easy way of seeing the pattern instantly. In the frequency distribution, values (which denote the categories of the variable) are paired with their frequency of occurrence in the data. In the bar graph, the height of the bar indicates the absolute frequency or, in this case, the relative frequency (= percentage) of cases that fall into each of the categories.

Yet another graph that can easily convey the distribution of a variable with few categories is the **pie chart** (Figure 3.2). The pie chart should include all categories of a variable, so that each slice represents the magnitude of a particular category relative to the total.

So far, the examples involved variables with a few **discrete** categories. Frequency distributions as well as pie charts and bar graphs become unwieldy if the number of categories exceeds 15 to 20. With truly **continuous** variables, like systolic blood pressure (SBP), it is often necessary to group the actual values into larger categories as shown in Table 3.2. The table

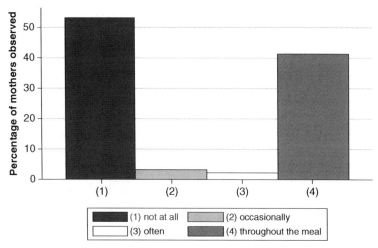

FIGURE 3.1 TV-Watching Patterns During Mealtime: Observer Ratings (Percentage of Mothers Observed to Watch TV During Mealtime).

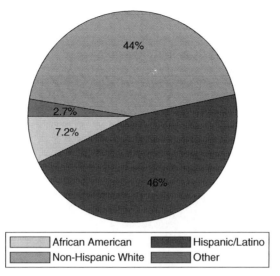

African American   Hispanic/Latino
Non-Hispanic White   Other

FIGURE 3.2 Race/Ethnicity of Mothers: Percentage Distribution Among 869 Subjects.

shows the distribution of SBP among 7,529 participants in the 2009–2010 National Health and Nutrition Examination Survey (NHANES).[2] In this table, the intervals below 172 mmHg are all of width 10 (e.g., 122–131), but the highest two categories are of width 20 (172–191) and width 51 (182–232). While this choice of intervals accommodates the sparsely populated extreme categories and saves a lot of space in the presentation of the frequency distribution, it can be misleading to the casual observer. In general, it is preferable to use categories of a single width in a frequency distribution of grouped data, unless extreme **outliers** (rare values at the high or low end of the distribution) make this difficult.

TABLE 3.2 Distribution of SBP Among 7,529 U.S. Adult Residents

SBP CATEGORIES (in mmHG)	FREQUENCY	PERCENTAGE	CUMULATIVE PERCENTAGE
72–81	12	0.2	0.2
82–91	199	2.6	2.8
92–101	868	11.5	14.3
102–111	1,636	21.7	36.0
112–121	1,809	24.0	60.1
122–131	1,315	17.5	77.6
132–141	792	10.5	88.1
142–151	421	5.6	93.7
152–161	235	3.1	96.8
162–171	127	1.7	98.5
172–191	87	1.1	99.6
182–232	28	0.4	100.0
Total	7,529	100.0	

[2]The table does *not* provide population estimates for U.S. residents, but only shows the distribution among individual participants in the mobile examinations of the NHANES.

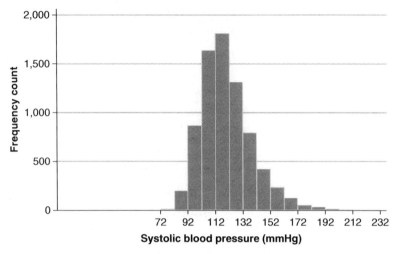

FIGURE 3.3 Systolic Blood Pressure Readings Among 7,529 Adults: 2009–2010 NHANES Participants in Mobile Examinations.

SBP is a ratio-level, quantitative variable. Such variables are often displayed graphically in the form of a **histogram**. The histogram is similar to a bar graph in that the heights of the histogram bars indicate either absolute or relative frequency (percentage) of occurrence. However, as in the frequency distribution of Table 3.2, the histogram combines values into intervals, which are designed to give the "best" representation of the overall shape of a distribution.[3] Figure 3.3 shows the histogram for the data in Table 3.2, except that the histogram does not combine the extreme categories with mmHg greater than 171 into larger intervals. On the other hand, the price to be paid is that the small frequencies in the extreme intervals make the bars almost invisible in height. Nonetheless, the histogram conveys at a glance the essential shape of the distribution: The SBP readings among 7,529 NHANES participants in the mobile examinations form a **unimodal** distribution that is **skewed** to the right. That is, this distribution shows a single peak (= the mode), with the largest number of participants having an SBP between 121 and 132, and it has a longer tail on the right or at the upper values.

In addition to skewness, single or multiple peaks, frequency distributions have other characteristics, such as extreme **outliers**, that may make it more difficult to summarize the information in a single statistic. How summary measures are affected by the characteristics of a frequency distribution will be shown in the following sections.

MEASURES OF CENTRAL TENDENCY

Frequency distributions can provide a lot of information about a variable, but they become cumbersome instruments when we deal with many variables and want to make comparisons involving many groups. Thus, in most instances, we use summary measures that represent the distribution of values at a glance. Most important are the measures of central tendency. The purpose of a measure of central tendency is to indicate, using a single number, where the *bulk* of the cases are located.[4] We commonly use three different measures of central tendency, the **mode**, the **median**, and the **mean**.

---

[3]Statistical software like STATA, SPSS, or SAS use algorithms to "optimize" the graphical display of histograms, but the interval choices can be overridden by the user.
[4]We discuss to what extent this is possible in this chapter.

DEFINITION OF THE MODE

The mode is the most frequently occurring value in a frequency distribution.

The mode is simply the most commonly occurring value in a frequency distribution of a variable. For instance, in Table 3.1 the most frequently occurring value is the value 1, which is the numerical code for the category "not at all." In Table 3.2 the most frequently occurring SBP readings lie within the category "112 to 121 mmHg." The mode is an appropriate measure of central tendency for all kinds of variables: nominal/categorical, ordinal, interval/ratio, as counting cases for each category does not involve any assumption about the measurement properties of the variables involved. Yet it is worth pointing out that the mode is quite an imperfect measure of central tendency, if a distribution is *not* unimodal or highly skewed. For instance, the frequency distribution in Table 3.1 is bimodal, having two high-frequency categories at the opposite end of the rating scale. Thus, while it is true that 53.2% of the ratings involved the "not at all" category, 41.4% of the ratings were in the "always" category. Clearly, in this situation, the mode is an imperfect measure of central tendency. Occasionally, a frequency distribution may not have a unique mode if there are two or more categories that occur with the same frequency. On the other hand, the mode is not a bad measure of central tendency for the frequency distribution in Table 3.2. Over 60% of all SBP readings have values between 102 and 131, that is, they fall into the modal category and the two adjacent categories. The reason for the representativeness of the mode is that the frequency distribution in Table 3.2 is unimodal and has only a moderately skewed distribution.

DEFINITION OF THE MEDIAN

After rank-ordering all observations or cases in a distribution from those with the lowest values or scores to those with the highest, we obtain the median observation by counting $(n + 1)/2$ from either the bottom or the top of the rank-ordered distribution.

   If the number of observations is uneven, the median value is the score of the $(n + 1)/2$th observation. If the distribution has an even number of observations, the median is the arithmetic mean of the two observations above and below $(n + 1)/2$.

The **median** is the 50th percentile of a distribution or, what amounts to the same, the median is the value that divides a distribution into two halves: below the median there are the 50% with the lower scores and above the median there are the 50% with the higher scores. As this definition implies, the values or scores that make up a variable must at least be capable of being rank-ordered, otherwise talking of "lower" or "higher" scores makes no sense. Thus, it would not be sensible to talk of the "median marital status," as the scores assigned to a nominal variable like marital status, for example, 1 = married, 2 = single, and so forth, are completely arbitrary. By contrast, any ordinal rating scale, interval- or ratio-level variable yields scores that can be rank-ordered from lowest to highest values.

As a consequence, we can obtain a median value for such variables. Consider the two small frequency distributions of pulse oximetry scores in Table 3.3. Let us first look at the sample with 11 observations. We can write out the oximetry values or percentages in rank

TABLE 3.3 Two Distributions of Pulse Oximetry Readings

PERCENTAGE OF ARTERIAL HEMOGLOBIN	SAMPLE OF 11 OBSERVATIONS: FREQUENCY	SAMPLE OF 10 OBSERVATIONS: FREQUENCY
90		1
92	1	
93	1	
95	2	1
96	4	3
97	2	4
98	1	
99		1

order from lowest to highest percentage, repeating each value as indicated by the frequency in Table 3.3:

92   93   95   95   96   96   96   96   97   97   98

There are $n = 11$ observations; thus the median observation is the sixth observation: $(n + 1)/2 = (11 + 1)/2 = 6$. That observation has an oximetry score of 96.

Now consider the second frequency distribution with 10 observations:

90   95   96   96   96   (96.5)   97   97   97   97   99

Note that the median value of 96.5 is not part of the distribution itself. Rather, with 10 observations, the median observation would be the 5.5th observation: $(n + 1)/2 = (10 + 1)/2 = 5.5$. As the 5.5th observation does not exist, we assign the arithmetic mean for the two adjacent values of 96 and 97 as the median value: $(96 + 97)/2 = 96.5$. This value meets our definition of the median, as it divides the distribution into two halves, such that 50% of the scores are at or above and 50% are at or below the median value.

The median may be employed appropriately as a measure of central tendency for variables with ordinal *or higher levels of measurement*, that is, interval- and ratio-level variables. As we will see after discussing the mean, the median is not sensitive to outlier value, which makes it often a preferred measure of central tendency.

The most common measure of central tendency is the **mean**. Strictly speaking, a mean requires that the variable for which it is computed is measured at the interval level of measurement, because adding scores and dividing them by the number of scores assumes that the distances between the scores are defined. Going back to the oximetry readings shown in Table 3.3, we find the mean for the sample of 11 observations to be:

$$\bar{x} = \frac{90 + 93 + 95 + 95 + 96 + 96 + 96 + 96 + 97 + 97 + 98}{11} = 95.5$$

The mean for the sample of 10 observations is:

$$\bar{x} = \frac{90 + 95 + 96 + 96 + 96 + 97 + 97 + 97 + 97 + 99}{10} = 96$$

DEFINITION OF THE MEAN

The mean is defined as follows:

$$\bar{x} = \frac{1}{n}\sum_{1}^{n} x_i$$

In words: the mean is defined as the sum of all observations for a particular variable divided by the number of observations.

Comment: We use the symbol $\bar{x}$ (read: "x bar") for the mean. This symbol is customarily used to denote the *sample* mean. Later, we encounter the Greek letter μ as the symbol for the *population* mean.

The summation operator $\sum$ indicates that the x values, ranging from the first to the nth value in the data should be summed. Thus, a more elaborate algebraic expression for the shorthand above would be:

$$\bar{x} = \frac{x_1 + x_2 + \cdots + x_n}{n}$$

One of the advantages of the mean as a measure of central tendency is that it takes into account information from all observations. As it turns out, that is also its disadvantage. Recall that the median only involves rank-ordering of all values, but the actual median is either the exact value of the $(n + 1)/2$th observation or it is the mean of the values of the $n/2$th observation and the $(n/2 + 1)$th observation. The *size* of the extremely high or low values does not enter at all into the determination of the median. By contrast, the mean is sensitive to outliers, that is, extremely high and low values, particularly in a small data set. Consider the following age distribution in a small sample of 10 patients:

18   19   20   20   24   28   28   29   29   85

It is easy to see that the median is equal to 26, as it falls halfway between 24 and 28. Yet the mean of this distribution is 30. As the data show, all but one patient is younger than 30, yet the mean indicates an "average" age of 30. In this situation, the median is clearly a better measure of "central tendency," as it gives a better indication of the age of most of the patients in the sample. While the sensitivity of the mean to a few outliers lessens with increasing sample size, the mean can still be a misleading measure of central tendency in highly skewed distributions. Relatively few billionaires and millionaires can substantially skew the "average" income; this is one reason why the Census Bureau often uses medians to describe the "average" U.S. income. It is also a reason why we should avoid the term "average" in the context of describing a central tendency. The term is ambiguous, and may refer to either the mean or the median.

MEASURES OF DISPERSION

As important as measures of central tendency are, measures of dispersion are arguably even more important in characterizing a distribution of a variable.[5] First and foremost, the dispersion or spread of a distribution tells us something about individual differences, about the

---

[5]Measures of dispersion/variation play a central role in statistical estimation and inference.

inevitable variation in scores that results, whenever we measure attributes of individuals, such as height, or characteristics of organizations, such as the number of beds in a hospital or annual nursing school budgets. By far the three most common measures of dispersion are the **range**, the **interquartile range** (IQR), and the **standard deviation** (including its square, the **variance**).

All of these measures are applicable to quantitative variables, that is, variables with interval- and ratio-level measurement properties, but the standard deviation and variance may be questionable when applied to ordinal-level variables, as they assume that the distances between scale points are reflected in the actual scores. Note that none of these measures can be applied to nominal-level variables, as the scores assigned to categories of nominal variables are arbitrary, which implies that it does not make any sense to talk about "highest" and "lowest" scores.

DEFINITION OF THE RANGE

The range is the difference between the highest and lowest score of a particular variable:

Range = maximum score − minimum score

The **range** is the simplest of all measures of dispersion. We obtain it by subtracting the lowest from the highest score. For instance, in the SBP data shown in Table 3.2, the largest observed score is 232 and the lowest is 72; thus, the range is 232 − 72 = 160. The range is an important metric characterizing a distribution, because it is a measure of the largest observed distance between points on a variable, which, by definition, is occupied by the most extreme values. This is, of course, also the weakness of the range, because it is a measure of dispersion that relies only on two values and disregards the rest. For instance, among the 7,529 NHANES subjects, more than 99% had SBP values between 82 and 171, indicating considerably less variation than the range measure would indicate. To get a handle on how *typical* or rare the extreme values of a distribution are, we need a better measure of dispersion.

DEFINITION OF THE INTERQUARTILE RANGE (IQR)

The IQR is defined as the distance between the values or scores occupying the lower and upper quartiles.

The lower quartile is found after rank-ordering all observations from lowest to highest values and selecting the $(n + 1)(\frac{1}{4})$th observation; the value or score of this observation divides the distribution into the lower 25% versus the higher 75% of values.

The upper quartile is the value of the $(n + 1)(\frac{3}{4})$th observation; the value or score of this observation divides the distribution into the lower 75% versus the higher 25% of values.

IQR = 75th percentile score − 25th percentile score

The IQR provides us with more information on the distribution of a variable. The IQR refers to the middle 50% of a distribution. It is centered on the median. That is, the interval between the lower limit of the IQR and the median contains 25% of the observations, and the interval between the upper limit of the IQR and the median contains another 25% of the observations.

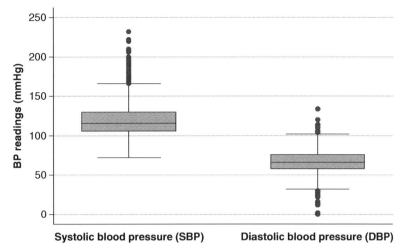

FIGURE 3.4 Box-and-Whisker Plot: Systolic and Diastolic Blood Pressure Among 7,529 Participants of 2009–2010 NHANES.

We again consider the 11 observations of oximetry values in Table 3.3, rank-ordered from lowest to highest value. The median of this distribution is 96:

92   93   95   95   96   96   96   96   97   97   98

There are $n = 11$ observations; thus the lower quartile observation is the third observation: $(n + 1)(\frac{1}{4}) = (11 + 1)/2 = 3$. That observation has an oximetry score of 95. The upper quartile observation is $(n + 1)(\frac{3}{4}) = (11 + 1)(\frac{3}{4}) = 36/4 = 9$, which has an oximetry score of 97. If the lower and upper quartiles fall between two observations, the difference between the two adjacent values is usually apportioned by adding 0.75 times the distance to the lower values of the lower quartile and 0.25 times the distance to the lower value of the upper quartile, but other rules exist as well.

Having defined the range and the IQR, we are now in a position to construct a box-and-whisker plot, which nicely summarizes a distribution using five to seven numbers. Figure 3.4 provides a display of a box-and-whisker plot.

First, concentrate on the graph for the SBP in Figure 3.4. It depicts the box-and-whisker plot for the data displayed in the frequency distribution of Table 3.2. The median value (50th percentile) for this SBP distribution is 116, depicted in the graph by the line within the box. The upper limit of the IQR (75th percentile) is 130, and is depicted in the graph by the upper border line of the box. The lower limit of the IQR (25th percentile) is at 106, and is depicted in the graph by the lower border line of the box. Thus, the box contains the middle 50% of the SBP distribution: IQR = 130 − 106 = 24. The whiskers (also known as Tukey[6] hinges) are constructed by adding 1.5 × IQR to the 75th percentile value and subtracting 1.5 × IQR from the 25th percentile value. Thus we get the following value for the upper whisker: 130 + 1.5 × 24 = 130 + 36 = 166; the lower whisker is drawn at SBP = 106 − 36 = 70. Any SBP value above the upper whisker or below the lower whisker would be considered an outlier. As the frequency distribution in Table 3.2 shows, the lowest recorded SBP value is 72; thus it is located above the lower whisker, but the distribution has outliers on the upper side with a maximum recorded value of 232. In the example of the diastolic blood

---

[6]Tukey (1977).

pressure (DBP) distribution depicted in Figure 3.4, we have a median value of 66, a 75th percentile of 76, a 25th percentile of 58, and an IQR of $76 - 58 = 18$. The upper whisker is drawn at DBP $= 76 + 1.5 \times 18 = 103$ and the lower whisker is drawn at $58 - 1.5 \times 18 = 31$. There are outliers at both the upper and lower tails of the distribution with extreme values of zero (probably a recording error) and 134 as the largest recorded value.

Box-and-whisker plots offer a convenient graphical depiction of a frequency distribution. In Figure 3.4, it is immediately apparent that the distribution of DBP values is more or less symmetric, whereas the SBP values are skewed toward the upper tail. We also see that most of the DBP values are confined within a narrower range than the SBP values: the IQRs are 18 (DBP) versus 24 (SBP) and the *ranges of the whiskers* are 45 (DBP) versus 96 (SBP).

SEVEN (OR FIVE) NUMBER SUMMARY OF BOX-AND-WHISKER PLOTS

Box-and-whisker plots are based on seven (sometimes five) numbers that offer a good description of unimodal frequency distributions:

Maximum Value
(75th Percentile Score + 1.5 × IQR)
75th Percentile Score
Median
25th Percentile Score
(25th Percentile Score − 1.5 × IQR)
Maximum Value

Sometimes, the whiskers (in parentheses) are omitted from the box plots resulting in a basic five-number summary to characterize a frequency distribution.

While box plots convey important information about a frequency distribution, by far the most important measure of the spread of a distribution of a quantitative variable is the **standard deviation**. As the definition of the standard deviation (and its square, the **variance**) shows, the standard deviation is a summary statistic that takes every value of a variable distribution into account. (By contrast, the range and the IQR each only rely on two numbers in the data.) The standard deviation thus provides a single index number, which can be interpreted as a measure of the *average distribution of values around the mean* of the distribution. Even though the computation of a standard deviation is straightforward, it becomes quickly unwieldy and time consuming, even if one deals with only moderately large study samples. Of course, we use computers for this purpose, but it is instructive to work through a simple example to understand what the formulas represent. Table 3.4 shows again a distribution of pulse oximetry readings (variable X), but to simplify manual calculations, the data involve only five readings from five persons.

MEASURES OF THE SHAPE OF FREQUENCY DISTRIBUTIONS

For interval- and ratio-level variables, one can also compute measures of **skewness**, or "lopsidedness" versus symmetry, and **kurtosis**, or peakedness versus spread of a distribution. The use of such measures is most appropriate for unimodal distributions, that is, frequency distributions with a single peak.

TABLE 3.4 Computation of Sample Standard Deviation for Five Pulse Oximetry Readings (X = Percentage of Arterial Hemoglobin)

(1)	(2)	(3)	(4)
ID index (i = 1 to 5)	X_i	$X_i - \bar{X}$	$(X_i - \bar{X})^2$
1	92	92 − 94 = −2	$(-2)^2 = 4$
2	93	93 − 94 = −1	$(-1)^2 = 1$
3	94	94 − 94 = 0	$0^2 = 0$
4	95	95 − 94 = 1	$1^2 = 1$
5	96	96 − 94 = 2	$2^2 = 4$

$$\bar{x} = \sum \frac{X_i}{n} = \frac{(92+93+94+95+96)}{5} = 94 \qquad s_x^2 = \sum \frac{(X_i - \bar{X})^2}{4} = \frac{(4+1+0+1+4)}{4} = 2.5$$

$$s_x = \sqrt{s_x^2} = \sqrt{2.5} = 1.58$$

Notes:

1. Column (2) of Table 3.4 contains the deviations of each X-value from the mean. By necessity, the sum of the deviations from the mean equals zero.
2. The squared deviations from the mean in column (4) are either positive or zero: they cannot be negative. Likewise, both the variance and the standard deviation are equal to or greater than zero: $s_x^2 \geq 0$ and $s_x \geq 0$.
3. The standard deviation is a summary statistic that measures the spread of values around the mean in the original measurement units. By contrast, the variance is a measure of the average *squared* deviations from the mean.
4. Like the mean, both the standard deviation and the variance can be strongly influenced by outliers, particularly in small samples. For instance, if we replace the lowest value in the above example (92) with 72, we get a variance of 102.5 and a standard deviation of 10.1.

DEFINITIONS OF THE STANDARD DEVIATION AND VARIANCE

The sample standard deviation of a variable x, denoted either as s_x (or SD_x), is defined as follows:

$$s_x = \sqrt{\sum \frac{(x_i - \bar{x})^2}{n-1}}$$

In words: the standard deviation is the square root of the variance s_x^2 and is a measure of the average deviation of the values of a variable x from its mean $\bar{x}$.

Its square is the variance (the expression under the square root), which is the average squared deviation:

$$s_x^2 = \sum \frac{(x_i - \bar{x})^2}{n-1}$$

Comment: Notice that the denominator of the sample standard deviation (and variance) equals $n-1$ and not n. We divide the sample value by $n-1$ (known as the "degrees of freedom"), because there is a mathematical proof (see Appendix A for further explanation) that dividing the sample variance by $n-1$ gives us an unbiased estimate of the population standard deviation. The population variance uses N as its denominator and is usually symbolized by the Greek letter σ_x^2 (small sigma) instead of s.

$$\sigma_x^2 = \sum \frac{(x_i - \mu_x)^2}{N}$$

The definition/formula of the skewness statistic shows that the numerator, containing the deviations of individual values from the mean, is raised to the third power. Thus, a preponderance of large positive deviations, raised to the third power, would lead to a skewness value that exceeds zero, indicating a tendency toward a right-hand longer tail.[7] A preponderance of large negative deviations from the mean raised to the third power would imply a distribution with a longer left-hand tail. A skewness value of zero indicates perfect symmetry around the mean.

DEFINITIONS OF SAMPLE SKEWNESS AND KURTOSIS

The sample skewness of a variable x is defined as follows:

$$Skewness = \frac{\frac{1}{n}\sum(x_i - \bar{x})^3}{(s_x)^3}$$

In words: the skewness is defined as the ratio of the "third moment" divided by the standard deviation, s_x, raised to the third power. The third moment is a measure analogous to the variance, but the sum of the deviations from the mean is raised to the third power.

The sample kurtosis of a variable x is defined as follows:

$$Kurtosis = \frac{\frac{1}{n}\sum(x_i - \bar{x})^4}{s_x^2}$$

In words: the kurtosis is defined as the ratio of the "fourth moment" divided by the variance, s_x^2. The fourth moment is a measure analogous to the variance, but the sum of the deviations from the mean is raised to the fourth power.

The definition/formula for the kurtosis statistic shows that, in the numerator, both positive and negative deviations from the mean are raised to the fourth power. This means that the larger the deviations from the mean in either direction, the larger the kurtosis value. Thus, larger kurtosis values indicate a distribution with a wider spread or thicker tails as well as a sharper, thinned-out peak, and smaller kurtosis values indicate a distribution with a narrower spread, thinner tails, and a more rounded peak.

As we will see in Chapter 5, both skewness and kurtosis can be employed to examine how closely a given frequency distribution resembles the normal distribution.

For a graphical illustration of skewness and kurtosis, take a look at Figures 3.5 and 3.6. In Figure 3.5, we see two distributions of baby-weight data (both samples of size 800) that differ primarily in terms of their skewness. The left distribution is almost symmetric and resembles the shape of a normal distribution (skewness value: 0.1), and the right distribution has a substantial right-leaning tail (skewness value: 1.1).

The skewness of a distribution can also be inferred from the relative values of the mode, median, and mean. We already saw that the mean is sensitive to extreme values or outliers.

---

[7]Recall that a squared number is always positive, for example, $(-2)^2 = (2)^2 = 4$, but a number raised to the third power changes its sign with the base number, for example, $(-2)^3 = -8$, $(2)^3 = 8$; in addition, as the base number increases, the number raised to the third power increases exponentially; thus, large positive or negative outliers would have a big effect on the skewness statistic, for example, $(-3)^3 = -27$, $(5)^3 = 125$, and so forth.

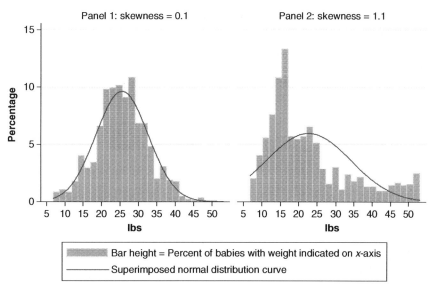

FIGURE 3.5 Two Distributions of Baby Weights (lbs): Lower (Panel 1) Versus Higher (Panel 2) Skewness.

This also influences the magnitude of the mean relative to the median and mode. As a general principle, the following relationships hold:

mode = median = mode (if distribution is symmetric, e.g., normal distribution);

mode < median < mean (if distribution is skewed to the right; panel 2, Figure 3.5);

mode > median > mean (if distribution is skewed to the left).

Figure 3.6 shows a left-hand distribution similar to that in Figure 3.5, but this time the emphasis is on the kurtosis value of 3.3 (a normal curve has a kurtosis value of 3.0). In the

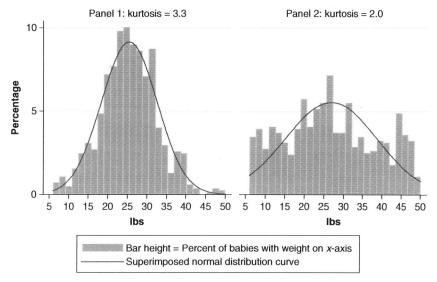

FIGURE 3.6 Two Distributions of Baby Weights (lbs): Higher (Panel 1) Versus Lower (Panel 2) Kurtosis.

right-hand panel, you can see an altered distribution with a kurtosis value of 2.0. It is flatter than the normal curve and both tails of the distribution are thicker, meaning they contain a larger proportion of cases than what would be expected, if the distribution were normal.

SUMMARY

1. In general, before summary statistics are computed, it pays to look at the frequency distribution as well as bar charts or histograms and, specifically, look for outliers and bimodal or multimodal distributions. The latter may lead one to question the appropriateness of certain measures of central tendency or dispersion.

2. As a general rule, you can always use a measure/statistic that is appropriate for a lower level of measurement and compute it for a variable with a higher level of measurement. There are sometimes good reasons to do so. This is so because the appropriateness of a measure of central tendency or dispersion does not only depend on the level of measurement of a variable but also the shape of its frequency distribution. As we have seen, ordinal measures like medians and the IQR are not sensitive to outliers (because, strictly speaking, an outlier requires the assumption of distance!), whereas interval/ratio-level measures are. Thus medians and the IQR are often used to characterize quantitative variables, even though means and standard deviations can be computed.

3. For all of these univariate statistics, we can also estimate the parallel population statistics; but that requires an understanding of statistical inference and the probability models on which it is based, a topic to which we turn in the next chapter.

EXERCISES

1. The following data show 10 primary care patient depression scores based on the Center for Epidemiologic Studies-Depression questionnaire instrument, which produces standardized scores for depressive symptomatology: 5, 7, 8, 9, 11, 12, 13, 16, 18, 22. Using a hand calculator
   (a) Compute the mean.
   (b) Compute the median.
   (c) Compute the standard deviation.
   (d) Compute the IQR.
   (e) Replace the highest value—22—with a new highest value—38, and repeat the computations in (a) to (d).
   (f) What did you notice, when comparing the results using 22 as the most extreme score versus using 38 as the most extreme score?

2. Suppose you have three distributions of DBP scores, each with a mean of 87:
   Distribution A: 80, 82, 84, 86, 88, 90, 92, 94
   Distribution B: 78, 80, 82, 84, 90, 92, 94, 96
   Distribution C: 78, 79, 80, 81, 82, 98, 99, 99
   (a) Rank-order the standard deviations of the three distributions by magnitude before actually calculating them; then provide your reasoning for the chosen rank order.
   (b) Based on visual inspection, which of the three distributions is skewed? Provide the reasoning for your answer.

3. Total blood cholesterol (TBC) is measured in terms of milligram per deciliter (mg/dL). Suppose, you read about a study sample in which the standard deviation of TBC is 40 and the IQR is 30. What is the likely reason for this difference?

4. Suppose the mean age of a sample of eight patients is 40, with ages ranging from 20 to 60. Is it possible (yes or no) that
   (a) The standard deviation of age in this sample equals zero?
   (b) The standard deviation of age equals 30?

   Provide reasoning for your answers.

REFERENCES

Baker, S., Horodynski, M. A., Coleman, G., Auld, G., Klein, A., Contreras, D., . . . Chapman, P. (2007 March–2012 February). *Healthy toddlers and strong families through a positive feeding environment.* USDA-NRI Cooperative State, Research, Education, and Extension Service. Retrieved from http://www.reeis.usda.gov/web/crisprojectpages/0209564-healthy-toddlers-and-strong-families-through-a-positive-feeding-environment.html

Tukey, J. W. (1977). *Exploratory data analysis.* Reading, MA: Addison-Wesley.

CHAPTER 4

Probabilities

So far, we have discussed descriptive statistics, that is, statistics that are used to summarize the information contained in the (sample) data at hand. However, in clinical research we are almost always interested in making inferences beyond the study sample at hand. When you read about a study conducted at a particular hospital or clinic, you are usually not interested in the individual study participants themselves (as they are not your patients), but you read the study in order to learn about an intervention or observation that may be relevant to your patients. In other words, you are interested in drawing inferences beyond the particular study sample at hand, which means you are interested in *generalizing* beyond the data of the study report. How can this be done?

PROBABILITY

If we want to draw inferences beyond the data at hand, we need to know how well the sample data "reflect" the target universe we are interested in. For example, if a drug trial shows that an antihypertensive drug is effective among 90% of the study participants, we need to know how likely it is that this success rate can be repeated with a different sample of patients. As we already discussed in Chapter 1, variability in individual human beings is substantial; that fact alone should caution us that the results from any single study, however well executed, will reflect idiosyncrasies unique to the study participants. Furthermore, there are many other sources of variability and error. For instance, it is almost impossible to avoid all measurement errors: Just think of measuring a patient's blood pressure; it can vary depending on equipment, correct size of a pressure cuff, positioning of patient, patient anxiety, or activities such as recent smoking or drinking of caffeine. So it is unlikely that we would have obtained exactly the same results if patient observations had been made at different times, if a different sample of study participants had been chosen, or different measurement techniques or tests had been employed. Because of this inherent **randomness** of all data, we need a **probability model** that allows us to make decisions about how likely or unlikely particular sample observations are, given the prevalence of such observations in the relevant target population.

┌───┐
│   **DEFINITION OF RANDOMNESS AND PROBABILITY**   │
├───┤
│   We call an event "random," if an *individual* outcome of this event cannot be predicted. │
│   However, we may well be able to predict the *proportion* of times that a certain outcome │
│   will occur "in the long run." (*Note*: probabilities vary between 0 and 1.) │
│   When we talk about the "probability" of an event, we refer to a statement about how likely │
│   it is (what are the chances?) that the event will occur, given our current state of knowledge. │
└───┘

Probabilities can be stated with or without conditions attached to them. For instance, we may want to know the chances that a U.S. resident will be infected with the flu during the period from January to April in a particular year. Or we may want to know a conditional probability: Given that a person has received a flu vaccine in October or November, what are the chances that this person will come down with severe flu symptoms between January and April? How would one answer such a question?

In principle, when it comes to calculating probabilities, we have two ways of doing it:

1. We sometimes use past empirical evidence to estimate the probability of an event occurring in the future. (Notice that the legitimacy of such an inference depends on the *assumption* that the process that produced the event in the past has not changed and will hold at least in the near future.)

2. Alternatively, we can use a priori reasoning and mathematics to come up with an answer based on a few assumptions and rigorous derivations.

Probabilities Based on Past Empirical Evidence

Suppose a couple wanted to know *before a pregnancy has commenced* what the probability is of having a boy. Consulting a U.S. Vital Statistics report (www.cdc.gov/nchs/data/nvsr/nvsr53/nvsr53_20.pdf), you would find that in 2002 the sex ratio for firstborn children was 1,048.[1] This tells us that, for every 1,000 girls born in the United States, there were 1,048 boys born. We can convert this into a **probability**: The probability of having a boy is: $P(\text{Boy}) = 1,048/2,048 = .512$.[2] As the historical data show, a similar sex ratio is observable in many countries, but it has recently declined somewhat. Thus, if all we know is that a U.S. woman is about to become pregnant, it is a reasonable guess to say that the probability that she will bear a boy is $P(\text{Boy}) = .512$ and the probability that she will have a girl is $P(\text{Girl}) = 1 - P(\text{Boy}) = 1 - .512 = .488$.

As it turns out, these probabilities do vary a little bit with birth order: The sex ratio declines somewhat if a woman bears multiple children, for example, from 1,055 for a first child to 1,040 for a third child. If we convert the last two sex-ratio numbers into probabilities, we get so-called **conditional probabilities**: The probability of having a boy, *given* that it is a firstborn child, can be written as: $P(\text{Boy}|\text{1st born}) = 1,055/2,055 = .513$; the probability of having a boy, given that it is a thirdborn child can be written as: $P(\text{Boy}|\text{3rd born}) = 1,040/2,040 = .510$. The sex ratio varies also a little bit by race/ethnicity, with non-Hispanic Whites having a slightly higher sex ratio

---

[1] The sex ratio is defined as the number of male births divided by the number of female births multiplied by 1,000.

[2] As we have a ratio of 1,048 boys to 1,000 girls, the proportion of boys among all births is 1,048/(1,048 + 1,000).

(1,054) than non-Hispanic Blacks (1,032). Overall though, given the fairly stable sex ratios across different groups, we cannot improve our estimates substantially knowing the birth order or the race of the mother. In more technical language: In this case, the conditional probabilities are fairly similar to the overall or **unconditional probability** of a male or female child being born.

There is also very little evidence that the sex of prior babies to the *same* mother (say, the first two births were girls) changes the probability of a particular sex in subsequent births: The sex ratio for the third child born to the same woman, given that the first two births were boys, remains at 1,040.

Probability Estimates Based on Mathematical (a Priori) Reasoning

Suppose you randomly select a sample of four hospital patients from a total "population"[3] of eight hospital patients with the following characteristics: Five of these patients have heart disease (HD) and three have cancer (CNC). What is the probability that all the patients in your sample of four have HD? We can reason as follows.

If we *randomly* draw the first patient from the hospital population using a *simple random sampling* procedure, wherein each patient has the *same* chance of being selected into the sample, the chances are $5/8 = 0.625$ that the first patient has HD. After the selection of the first patient with HD, there remain four HD and three CNC patients in the population. That means that the chances of selecting again an HD patient from the remaining population are $4/7 = 0.571$. With the remaining population now having three HD and three CNC patients, the chances of selecting a third HD patient from that population are $3/6 = 0.5$. Finally the probability of selecting yet another HD patient from the remaining population is $2/5 = .4$. What we have done here is to use a sampling process known as **sampling without replacement**: After each selection, the probability calculations were exclusively based on the distribution of cases *remaining* in the population, and are not influenced by any of the prior selections. Thus, we can use the multiplication rule of probabilities: When two or more events are *independent* of each other, we can multiply their probabilities to obtain an overall probability for all of the events occurring together. Here we want to know the probability of selecting a sample of four HD patients from a population of five HD and three CNC patients. The answer is that $P(4HD) = (5/8) \times (4/7) \times (3/6) \times (2/5) = .071$ or 7.1%.

As this example shows, we often can calculate the *expected* probabilities of events occurring, if we can make reasonable assumptions about the process that generated the data. These assumptions are incorporated into our **probability model**. Here we used simple random sampling without replacement from a larger population. The full probability model would enumerate all possible sample outcomes (or "**events**") and would attach a probability value to each of these outcomes. Together, the probabilities of all possible outcomes add up to 1, because it is certain that one of the outcome events will occur. For instance, in addition to the event described above (all four sample members have HD), there are other outcome possibilities (such as the first three randomly chosen members having CNC). Using our probability model, we can make decisions about how likely or unlikely certain sample observations are.

DEFINITION OF SAMPLE SPACE AND PROBABILITY MODEL

The set of all possible outcomes or events constitutes the sample space. The probability model specifies the probabilities attached to each possible event in the sample space.

---

[3]The small numbers are for illustrative purposes only.

Elementary Probability Rules

As we have already seen, a probability is a number between (and including) 0 and 1. More formally, we can write about the probability of an event A:

$$0 \leq P(A) \leq 1$$

The sum of the probabilities of all possible events in the sample space (S) equals 1. $P(S) = P(A) + P(B) + \cdots + P(Z) = 1$, if events A, B, …, Z are mutually exclusive (disjoint) and account for all possible outcomes or events. The probability of an event not occurring equals 1 – the probability of the event occurring: $P(\sim A) = 1 - P(A)$.

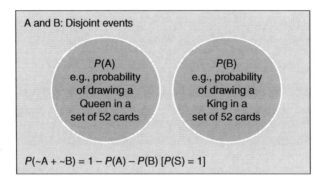

In order to discuss further probability rules, we must first consider if the events of interest are **independent** or not.

DEFINITION OF INDEPENDENCE

Two (or more) events are considered independent if the probability of event A remains the same, regardless of the occurrence of event B.

Consider the following examples: Suppose the probability that a U.S. resident in the age group 50 to 59 gets the flu, $P(F)$, in a given year is .06 or 6%. This probability is about the same for men and women: $P(F|f) = P(F|m)$. Thus, the event "catching the flu and developing flu symptoms" is independent of gender in this age group. Another way of looking at this is: Knowing that an adult between 50 and 59 years of age is male or female does not improve our prediction of who will catch the flu in a given year. Now suppose that parents of school children (PSC) are three times more likely to get the flu in a given year than other adults of the same age who do not live with children in school: $P(F|PSC) = .09$ and $P(F|\sim PSC) = .03$, then parental status and the probability of catching the flu in a given year would be related; they would not be independent of each other.

If two or more events are **independent**, then we can ascertain the probability of their joint occurrence using the **multiplication rule**:

$$P(A \text{ and } B \text{ and } C) = P(A) \times P(B) \times P(C)$$

$P(A \text{ and } B \text{ and } C)$ refers to the joint occurrence of events A and B and C. Earlier, we saw that the probability that a pregnant American woman will have a girl is .488. As the probability of having a girl for one woman (A) is independent of the probability of having a girl for another woman (B), we can calculate the probability that three randomly chosen pregnant women all have a girl using the multiplication rule: $P(A) \times P(B) \times P(C) = .488 \times .488 \times .488 = .488^3 = .116$. The chance that three randomly chosen pregnant women all give birth to a girl is less than 12%! For five women, that chance is less than 3%.

Many events are *not* independent, that is, the probability of their occurrence changes, given that some other event or condition has already occurred. We already alluded to this dependence in the example of parental status and the probability of catching the flu. A classic example of conditional probability is the change in the mortality risk conditional upon age. For instance, the unconditional probability of dying from HD in the United States during 2009 was .001952 (CDC Vital & Mortality Statistics).[4] In other words, among the estimated 307,007,000 U.S. residents in 2009, some 599,413 individuals (195.2 per 100,000) died of HDs. The data also show that the conditional probability of dying from HD, given that a U.S. resident was between 45 and 64 years old, was 82.8 deaths per 100,000 and 431.7 per 100,000 for a U.S. resident between 65 and 74 years of age.

CONDITIONAL (AGE-BASED) PROBABILITIES OF DYING FROM HEART DISEASE IN U.S. RESIDENT POPULATION OF 2009

AGE GROUPS	U.S. POPULATION	$P(A)$	DEATHS FROM HEART DISEASES	$P(A$ and $B)$	$P(B|A)$
45–64	44,592,000	.14525	36,922	.0001203	.000828
65–74	20,792,000	.06772	89,759	.0002924	.004318
Total	307,007,000	1.00000	599,413	.0019524	.001952

In 2009, the Census Bureau estimate of the total U.S. resident population was 307,007,000, with 44,592,000 persons between the ages of 45 and 64. If one had drawn a person randomly from among all U.S. residents of 2009, the probability of such a person being 45 to 64 years old would be $P(A_1) = .145$, as 14.5% of the 2009 U.S. resident population was in that age group (A_1). The joint probability of a person in that age group (45–64) dying from HD was: $P(A_1$ and $B) = .0001203$ ($= 36,922/307,007,000$). As we know the overall probability of event A and the joint probability of events A_1 and B, we can obtain the conditional probability of the event B, given that A is true:

$$P(B|A_1) = P(A_1 \text{ and } B)/P(A_1) = .0001203/.14525 = .00828$$

Labeling the "event" that a person of age 65 to 74 as A_2, we obtain the conditional probability of dying from an HD in that age group as:

$$P(B|A_2) = P(A_2 \text{ and } B)/P(A_2) = .0002924/.06772 = .00438$$

Formally, conditional probabilities can be computed as follows:

$$P(B|A) = P(A \text{ and } B)/P(A),$$

where $P(B|A)$ is the probability that an event B occurs, given that event A has occurred, $P(A$ and $B)$ is the probability of the joint event (A and B), and $P(A)$ is the probability of

---

[4]Because the probabilities (or proportions) of people dying from a specific disease tend to be small, the convention is to report the number of deaths per 100,000. In this case, this would be 195.2 deaths per 100,000 U.S. residents.

34 I. FOUNDATIONS FOR STATISTICAL THINKING

event A. In our example, the event A refers to being a member of a specific age group and the event B refers to deaths from HDs.

Two more basic probability rules need to be considered here, the addition and the general multiplication rules. The **addition rule** can be formally stated as follows:

$$P(A \text{ or } B) = P(A) + P(B) - P(A \text{ and } B)$$

Suppose, the probability of suffering hypertension is $P(A) = .3$, the probability of having arthritis is $P(B) = .05$, while the joint probability of having both hypertension and arthritis is $P(A \text{ and } B) = .025$. From this it follows that the probability of having hypertension *or* arthritis is $P(A \text{ or } B) = .3 + .05 - .025 = .325$. Notice, we subtract the joint probability $P(A \text{ and } B)$ from the sum of the probabilities of hypertension and arthritis, because the two probabilities overlap, that is, they involve, in part, the same individuals. In the case of two **disjoint events** (see above), the addition rule simplifies to: $P(A \text{ or } B) = P(A) + P(B)$, **if** $P(B|A) = P(A|B) = 0$. If, in our example, no person with hypertension has arthritis $[P(A|B) = 0]$ and no person with arthritis has hypertension $[P(B|A) = 0]$, then we can simply add the two unconditional probabilities to get the joint probability.

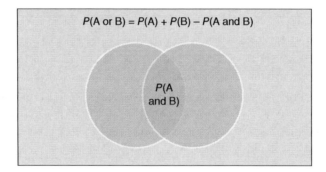

Finally, we consider the **general multiplication rule**. It can be stated as follows:

$$P(A \text{ and } B) = P(A)P(B|A)$$

Earlier we showed that the conditional probability of dying from HD, given that a U.S. resident was between 45 and 64 years old, was $P(B|A) = .000828$, while the probability of being between 45 and 54 years old in 2009 was $P(A) = .14525$. Thus the probability of a death from HD among persons aged 45 to 64 was $P(A \text{ and } B) = .000828 \times .14525 = .0001203$.

Notice that the general multiplication rule simplifies to the special multiplication rule in the case of independent events, as independence implies that $P(B|A) = P(B)$. If the probability of dying from HD were the same regardless of age, then all conditional probabilities $P(B|A_i)$ would be equal to the unconditional probability $P(B)$ and the general multiplication rule simplifies to the special multiplication rule for independent events:

$$P(A \text{ and } B) = P(A)P(B|A) = P(A) \times P(B)$$

Bayes' Theorem

When we employ screening tests, such as mammography or the prostate-specific antigen test, we judge their effectiveness using information about the accuracy of the tests as well as the incidence of the disease in the target population. The accuracy of a screening test is usually summarized in two numbers: its sensitivity and its specificity.

Sensitivity is defined as the proportion of *positive* results, *given* that the tested person has the disease. This is a conditional probability of having a positive test result, given the person has cancer (C), which can be expressed more formally as: $P(+|C)$. Based on information from the National Cancer Institute (NCI, 2013), the overall sensitivity of mammography is approximately 79% (it is lower in younger women aged <49 and higher in older women). Thus, we write: $P(+|C) = .79$.

Specificity can be expressed as the probability of a *negative* test result, *given* that the tested person is free of the disease: $P(-|{\sim}C)$.[5] The average specificity for mammography is approximately 90% (again, it is lower in younger and higher in older women). More formally, $P(-|{\sim}C) = .90$.

Based on the Surveillance Epidemiology and End Results data of the Centers for Disease Control and Prevention (SEER, 2013), the prevalence of breast cancers among women aged 40 to 49 was 904 per 100,000. Thus, the probability that a woman in this age group has breast cancer is $P(C) = .00904$. What we want to know about the screening test is, of course, this: What is the probability that a woman, whose test comes back positive, actually has breast cancer: $P(C|+)$? Bayes' Theorem provides the answer:

BAYES' THEOREM

$$P(C|+) = \frac{P(+|C) \times P(C)}{[P(+|C) \times P(C) + P(+|{\sim}C) \times P({\sim}C)]},$$

where $P(C)$ = the probability of having breast cancer, $P({\sim}C)$ = the probability of not having breast cancer, $P(+|C)$ = the probability of a positive mammography among women who have breast cancer, and $P(+|{\sim}C)$ = the probability of a positive mammography among tested women who do not have breast cancer.

This formula looks forbidding, but we can decompose it step by step:

1. In the numerator on the right-hand side, we have: $P(+|C) \times P(C)$, that is, the conditional probability of a positive test result, given that a woman is between 40 and 49 years old, which is multiplied by the prevalence of cancer in that age group. As $P(+|C) = .79$ and $P(C) = .00904$, we get .00714 for the proportion of women with positive mammography tests. In other words, if mammography is performed on 100,000 women in this age group, some 714 of these women would have a positive test result *and* would have the cancer ("true positives").

2. The denominator contains two expressions, with the first being the same as the numerator. The second expression after the plus sign, $P(+|{\sim}C) \times P({\sim}C)$, is the product of two terms: the conditional probability of a positive test, *given* that the tested person does *not* have cancer, $P(+|{\sim}C)$, times the probability that a woman aged 40 to 44 does not have cancer, $P({\sim}C)$. We already know the specificity of the average mammography test: $P(-|{\sim}C) = .90$. As among all tested women, who do

---

[5]The symbol "~" stands for "not" and "~C" refers to "not having cancer."

TABLE 4.1 Example of Mammography Screening Test Results for Women Aged 40 to 49

MAMMOGRAPHY	TRUE STATE OF AFFAIRS		TOTAL
	HAS BEAST CANCER	NO BREAST CANCER	
Positive	714	9910	10,624
Negative	190	89,186	89,376
Total	904	99,096	100,000

not have breast cancer, the test result from a mammography is either negative or positive, $P(+|\sim C)$ must be $1 - P(-|\sim C)$, which is $1.00 - .90 = .10$ in this example. Thus, 10% of the women, who do not have breast cancer, will have a positive mammography. Finally, as we know the prevalence of breast cancer among women aged 40 to 49 to be $P(C) = .00904$, $P(\sim C)$ must be equal to $1 - P(C)$ or $1 - .00904 = .99096$. In short, among 100,000 women aged 40 to 49, 99,096 would not have breast cancer. However, as the mammography test has a specificity of 0.90, it will return 10% positive test results among these 99,096 women *without* breast cancer, which amounts to 9,910 *false positive* test results. Now, we can see that Bayes' Theorem gives us the desired answer:

$$P(C|+) = \frac{P(+|C) \times P(C)}{[P(+|C) \times P(C) + P(+|\sim C) \times P(\sim C)]}$$

$$= \frac{0.79 \times 0.00904}{[0.79 \times 0.00904 + 0.10 \times 0.99096]} = 0.067$$

In short, if a woman aged 40 to 49 receives a positive mammography result, the probability that she actually has breast cancer is only 6.7%. If you go back to the formula of Bayes' Theorem, you will see that it is a ratio of two probabilities: the probability of having a positive mammography if you have breast cancer, over the probability that all tested women have a positive mammography regardless of whether they have the disease or not. In other words, it is the ratio of true positives over all positive test results. This can be seen even better in the following 2×2 table that shows the mammography data standardized to 100,000.

Table 4.1 shows that out of 100,000 women between 40 and 49 years screened for breast cancer, we can expect a total of 10,624 positive test results. Of these, 714 would be true positive, which amounts to 6.7%. This number is also known as the positive predictive value (PPV). What Bayes' Theorem allows us to do is to convert anterior probabilities, for example, the probabilities of having positive test results given the presence or absence of disease, into posterior probabilities, that is, the probabilities of having a disease given a positive test result.

SUMMARY

In this chapter, we have discussed basic probability rules and some principal approaches to estimating probabilities. In the following chapter, we put some of this reasoning to use when we discuss one of the most fundamental concepts in statistical inference: the sampling distribution. As we will see, sampling distributions are probability distributions that enumerate all the different ways in which a study sample could be selected from a target population or all the different ways in which study participants could be randomly assigned to treatment or control groups. It is this information against which we judge how likely or unlikely certain study outcomes are as a result of mere chance events, such as random sampling. This will give us a basis for deciding whether or not study results should be taken seriously.

EXERCISES

1. A box contains 50 balls, 30 of which are red and 20 of which are white.
   (a) What is the probability of drawing 5 red balls on 5 draws, if you draw each ball separately and replace it (put it back into the box) every time after the drawing?
   (b) What is the probability of drawing 5 red balls on 5 draws, if you do not replace the balls, but draw the balls successively without replacement?

2. Suppose, in the U.S. population, 15% of adults are "heavy drinkers" (more than 3 drinks daily for men, more than 2 drinks daily for women). Suppose also that 10% of such heavy drinkers develop liver cirrhosis over a lifetime, while only 1% of the other adults (including moderate drinkers and abstainers) develop liver cirrhosis over a lifetime. What would be the probability that any U.S. adult develops liver cirrhosis over a lifetime?

3. Three persons each throw a die independently. What are the chances that:
   (a) All three persons throw a 5?
   (b) Only two out of three persons throw a 5?
   (c) Only one person throws a 5?
   (d) Nobody throws a 5?
   (e) Two persons throw a 5 and one person throws a 6?

4. Suppose, the probability of catching the flu in a given year is .06 and the probability of experiencing pollen allergies in a given year is .3. Does it follow that the probability of experiencing both the flu and the pollen allergies is $P(F) \times P(P) = .06 \times .3 = .018$ or 1.8%?

5. Suppose, the probability of hypertension among underweight persons (body mass index [BMI] < 18.5) equals .025, among normal weight persons (18.5 ≤ BMI < 25) it is .05, among overweight persons (25 ≤ BMI < 30) it equals .15, and among obese people (30 ≤ BMI) it is equal to .35. What, if anything, can we conclude about the overall probability that a person is hypertensive?

6. A screening test has a sensitivity of 0.95 and a specificity of 0.98. The disease the screening test is used to test for has a population prevalence of 500 in 100,000 or 0.005. What is the probability that a person who tests positive on this screening test actually has the disease?

7. Suppose, the probability of having a stroke in a given year among older adults (80+) is .02, the probability of spending at least one night in a hospital is .2, and the conditional probability of ending up in the hospital, given that an older adult had a stroke, is .8.
   (a) What is the probability of an older adult to have a stroke and end up in a hospital overnight?
   (b) What is the probability of an older adult to not have a stroke and end up in a hospital overnight?

(c) What is the probability of an older adult to either have a stroke or end up in a hospital, but not both?

(d) What is the probability of an older adult to neither have a stroke nor end up in a hospital overnight?

REFERENCES

National Cancer Institute (NCI). (2013). *Breast cancer screening concepts.* Retrieved January 18, 2013, from http://www.cancer.gov/cancertopics/pdq/screening/breast/healthprofessional/page4

SEER. (2013). *Cancer of the breast (invasive): United States cancer prevalence estimates.* Retrieved January 20, 2013, from http://seer.cancer.gov/csr/1975_2009_pops09/browse_csr.php?sectionSEL=4&pageSEL=sect_04_table.25.html

Logic of Statistical Inference: The Sampling Distribution and Significance Tests

STATISTICAL INFERENCE AFTER RANDOM SAMPLING OR RANDOM ASSIGNMENT

As mentioned in the last chapter, using mathematical probability models to draw inferences from samples about populations can only be done, if the sample selection is based on some type of probability or random selection procedure. Depending on the complexity of the sampling plan and the particular statistical estimator[1] in question, the mathematics of statistical inference can be quite involved. However, the basic principles are not that complicated. Furthermore, understanding the underlying logic of statistical inference is essential for interpreting statistical output that is intended to provide information about particular target *populations* on the basis of observed *sample* values. Likewise, statistical output that reports on the results of a clinical intervention study, that is, a clinical trial, entails inferences that go beyond the particular data set. As it turns out, the statistical concepts involved are the same, whether we draw inferences after random sampling from a larger target population or random assignment in a clinical trial. This should not be surprising, as both procedures are based on the random selection of subjects, cases, or observations from a larger "population" of subjects, cases, or observations.

It is worth noting, though, that the purpose of statistical inference is different in the two situations. When we draw a random sample from a larger target population, we are usually concerned with the question of how well the sample represents this larger population. When we conduct a clinical trial, we select subjects from the study sample comprising all enrolled individuals and assign them randomly to intervention and control groups. The purpose of such random assignment is to create comparison groups with similar background characteristics so that we can draw *causal* inferences about the effectiveness of an intervention. The key concept that provides the link between the sample data and the target population or the link between a particular random assignment and inferences about the causal effectiveness of an intervention is that of the **sampling distribution**.

---

[1] A statistical estimator is a formula used to estimate a population parameter based on observed sample values. For example, we use the sample mean (the sample statistic) to estimate the population mean (the population parameter). A particular sample value for the estimator is called a sample *estimate*.

THE SAMPLING DISTRIBUTION

One of the most fundamental concepts in all of statistics is the **sampling distribution**. It is the sampling distribution of a test statistic that bridges the divide between particular sample data on the one hand and generalizable estimates on the other. Given its importance, we demonstrate how a sampling distribution can be derived in the case of a very simple random assignment process. This will shed light on the concept of a sampling distribution and show you how this concept is intimately connected to other fundamental statistical concepts such as **significance testing** and **confidence intervals**.

For the purposes of this discussion, we offer a somewhat unrealistic example of a physical activity intervention designed to lower blood pressure (BP) among eight hypertensive individuals. Table 5.1 shows the diastolic blood pressure (DBP) of these hypertensive individuals *before* any intervention takes place. In the simplest case of a clinical trial, we would randomly assign four of these subjects to an intervention group that participates in the physical activity intervention, while the remaining four subjects would be enrolled in a control group, which may involve some kind of group activity that is not physically demanding. As it turns out, there are 70 *distinct* ways of assigning four out of eight subjects to two groups (intervention and control).[2]

Let us take a look at a few particular random assignments. Suppose our random assignment results in selecting individuals A, C, D, and E into the intervention group. This implies that individuals B, F, G, and H end up in the control group. In that case, the mean DBP score, before any intervention is undertaken, would be equal to (103 + 101 + 100 + 98)/4 = 100.5 in the intervention group and (102 + 97 + 96 + 95)/4 = 97.5 in the control group. Thus, this particular random assignment outcome would result in a mean DBP *difference* between the intervention and control groups of 3 (=100.5 − 97.5) *before* the intervention takes place. Of course, the random assignment process could just as likely have selected individuals C, E, F, and H into the intervention group and individuals A, B, D, and G into the control group. In that case, the mean DBP difference between the intervention and control groups, before

TABLE 5.1 Diastolic Blood Pressure (DBP) Among Eight Hypertensive Individuals

INDIVIDUAL	DBP
A	103
B	102
C	101
D	100
E	98
F	97
G	96
H	95

[2]The number of distinct combinations can be computed using the following formula: $n!/(n_1!n_2!)$, where n stands for the total sample size, n_1 for the number of subjects in one of the comparison groups, say the intervention group, and n_2 stands for the number of subjects in the other (control) group. The symbol "!" is read as "factorial" and is expressed as the following product: $n \times (n-1) \times (n-2) \times \cdots \times 2 \times 1$. For the data in Table 5.1, the formula amounts to: $8!/(4!4!) = (8 \times 7 \times 6 \times 5 \times 4 \times 3 \times 2 \times 1)/(4 \times 3 \times 2 \times 1 \times 4 \times 3 \times 2 \times 1) = 40{,}320/(24 \times 24) = 70$.

TABLE 5.2 Frequency Distribution of Mean Differences Resulting From 70 Possible Random Assignments of Eight Hypertensive Individuals (Data in Table 5.1)

Mean difference	−5.0	−4.0	−3.5	−3.0	−2.5	− 2	−1.5	−1	−0.5	0	0.5	1.0	1.5	2.0	2.5	3.0	3.5	4.0	5.0
Frequency	1	1	2	3	4	4	4	6	6	8	6	6	4	4	4	3	2	1	1

the intervention takes place, would be $97.75 − 100.25 = −2.5$. As there are 70 distinct ways of assigning these 8 individuals to two groups with 4 members each, the random assignment process can maximally result in 70 distinct mean differences. However, some of the random assignments, though involving different sets of individuals, yield the same mean difference. As it turns out, for the data in Table 5.1, there are only 19 distinct mean differences that would be generated with the 70 distinct random assignments. We can present the results in a frequency distribution (Table 5.2).

If we divide the occurrence of each unique mean difference by the number of all possible unique random assignments, we get a probability distribution as depicted in Figure 5.1. This probability distribution is the **sampling distribution of the mean difference** in DBP resulting from random assignment alone.

It is worth looking at Figure 5.1 in more detail. We have already seen that there are 70 distinct ways of assigning 4 out of 8 individuals to an intervention group and the other 4 to a control group. If the random assignment process is truly unbiased, then each of the 70 distinct ways of selecting individuals into the intervention or control group is equally likely. Suppose, we select individuals A, B, C, and D into the intervention group and individuals E, F, G, and H into the control group. From the data given in Table 5.1 it can easily be calculated that this random split would result in an intervention group mean DBP of 101.5 and a control group mean DBP reading of 96.5.

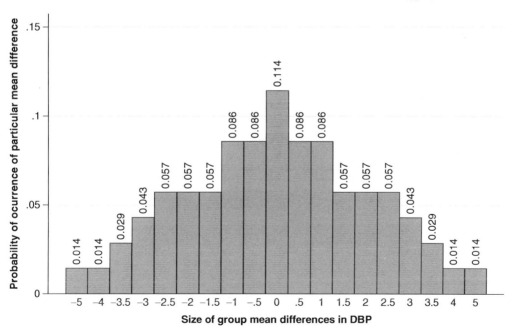

FIGURE 5.1 Sampling Distribution of Mean Differences for Table 5.1 Data Based on All Distinct (70) Random Splits of 8 Subjects Into 2 Groups of 4.

In short, this particular random assignment outcome would have resulted in a mean DBP difference of +5. For these data, no other assignment combination would result in a mean DBP difference of +5. As there are 70 possible distinct ways of assigning the 8 individuals to the two groups, the probability of this particular outcome occurring by chance, that is, by random assignment, is 1/70 or .014. In Figure 5.1, the number at the top of the bar associated with the mean difference of +5 is .014, indicating the probability that this outcome occurs by chance.

Now look at the mean DBP difference of −3. There are three distinct combinations of selecting individuals into the intervention and control groups that would result in a mean DBP difference of −3.[3] Thus, the probability of a mean difference of −3 resulting from random assignment would be equal to 3/70 = .043. Now we can see why the sampling distribution is considered a *probability distribution*: Each distinct outcome, which in this example is any of the mean differences shown in Figure 5.1, has a certain "chance of occurring." That "chance of occurrence" or "probability" is simply the proportion of times the assignment process produces this particular outcome *among all possible outcomes*.

What is the value of this information for making inferences in an experimental intervention study (clinical trial) with random assignment? The sampling distribution shows us *all* the possible mean differences between treatment and control groups that *can* result from mere random assignment. In addition, the sampling distribution provides information on the probability with which each of these outcomes occurs. It is this information against which we judge the "significance" of our results after the intervention. Suppose that, after random assignment, subjects in the treatment group are exposed to a physical activity intervention and subjects in the control group are not (they may be exposed to a social activity intervention). After the intervention is completed, subjects in both the treatment and control groups are again compared with respect to their mean DBP scores. Let us assume that, after the intervention, the mean DBP score in the treatment group equals 92 mmHg, and 96 mmHg in the control group.[4] If the study is well controlled and no other systematic differences in exposure occur between the intervention and control groups, we now have a relevant decision criterion in our hands.

From the sampling distribution, we know that a mean DBP difference between the intervention and control group of −4 or even more extreme occurs in only 2/70 or 2.9% of all possible random assignments. Conversely, 97.1% of all random assignments would have produced a mean difference in DBP *above* −4. Now we have a choice: Do we consider this evidence strong enough to conclude that the intervention produced the difference of −4? In this example, we would have 97.1% confidence that the intervention is effective, as only 2.9% of all random assignments could have produced the observed difference between intervention and control groups. However, a 2.9% risk (probability) remains that our inference concerning the effectiveness of the intervention is wrong. This risk, or *the probability of wrongly concluding that an intervention is effective when in fact mere random assignment produced the results*, is also known as the **Type I error**.

In short, the reasoning behind our inference concerning the effectiveness of an intervention in a randomized study can be summarized as follows:

1. Subjects are **randomly assigned** to various treatment and control conditions. (In the simplest case, there is one intervention/treatment group and one placebo/control

---

[3]The combinations for intervention–control groups are: DEFH–ABCG, CEGH–ABDF, BFGH–ACDE.
[4]In behavioral studies, one can often observe a "placebo effect": Just the knowledge of subjects that they are participating in a physical activity trial with the aim of lowering their BP, may induce many individuals to watch their diet and improve their exercise. But this self-induced improvement should have the same average effect in either comparison group.

group, but in many trials there are more comparison groups, as when we vary the "dosage" or intensity of an intervention.)

2. A **test statistic** is selected for the outcome variable(s) of interest. (In the current example, the test statistic is the mean difference in the DBP scores between the intervention and control groups.)

3. After random assignment, it is possible to construct a **sampling distribution of the test statistic**. That is, for each possible unique outcome of the test statistic generated by the chance assignment, the sampling distribution shows us the associated probability of its occurrence. (As the sampling distribution encompasses *all possible* outcomes from the random assignment process, the sum of the probabilities of all unique outcomes adds up to 1.)

4. If the random assignment process is unbiased, we can formulate the so-called **null hypothesis** about what we expect the *mean* test statistic to be in the absence of any intervention effect. (For example, in the case of a *mean difference* between the intervention and control group, some random assignments will result in a larger intervention than control group mean; other random assignments will result in a smaller intervention than control group mean. For all possible random assignments of subjects to an intervention and a control group, the *average* difference between the two groups would be expected to equal zero.)

5. In the next step, the test statistic computed on the data *observed after the intervention* is compared to the sampling distribution of the test statistic that would prevail if the null hypothesis were true. (Recall that, if the null hypothesis is true, the data are generated by random assignment alone and the intervention itself has no effect.) Thus, we can determine how probable or likely the observed (postintervention) test statistic would be under the null hypothesis.

6. Finally, we must have a criterion for deciding at what point we consider an outcome to be "unlikely" to have been produced by mere random assignment. This cut-off point is called the **significance level** and is usually denoted by the Greek letter α (alpha). If the significance level is set at, say, 0.05 or 0.01, we would then conclude that the intervention is effective (there is a "statistically significant effect"), if the probability of the observed outcome (or p-value) falls below this significance level. On the other hand, if we find that the observed difference might well have been the result of mere random assignment (say, $p > .35$), then we would have very little confidence in the effectiveness of the intervention.

The logic of random assignment fits very nicely with the statistical models used to analyze data from experimental studies or clinical trials. The value of the sampling distribution is that it gives us a context in which to interpret a particular sample result, as it answers the question of how likely or unlikely a specific result would have occurred by chance alone. It is important to understand, though, that for the correct estimation of the probabilities we need to know the *shape* of the sampling distribution of a particular test statistic. That is not always easy. In principle, we could generate sampling distributions of test statistics empirically, as we have done here. That becomes more tedious and time-consuming as sample sizes increase.[5] In addition, when we generate random samples from an original target population,

---

[5]Even a very modest sample of 30 subjects can be split into 2 groups of 15 in over 155 million ways.

say, all patients who stayed overnight in a Michigan hospital during a given year, we cannot resample from this target population, as it would be prohibitively expensive.[6] However, there is an alternative.

In most instances of statistical inference, we can employ *idealized* mathematical descriptions of the sampling distributions, some of which, like the *t*-, *f*-, normal, and chi-square distributions are the basis for the most common statistical tests found in the literature. Of course, the use of these idealized, theoretical sampling distributions should depend on the degree to which the data meet the underlying assumptions. How we determine whether particular variables in a data set meet the assumptions of the statistical models employed will be a recurrent theme in the chapters to follow. For now, we focus on understanding one very important mathematical (sampling) distribution, the *normal* or *Gaussian*[7] *distribution*.

THE NORMAL DISTRIBUTION

The **normal distribution** is one of the most important theoretical distributions used in statistical inference. The formula for the normal curve, which describes the shape of the function containing the area of the normal density distribution, looks somewhat forbidding:

$$y = \frac{1}{\sigma\sqrt{2\pi}}e^{\frac{(x-\mu)^2}{2\sigma^2}}$$

However, it is actually fairly easy to work with the normal distribution. At first, we should note that the normal distribution involves a family of distributions, whose members are characterized just by two numbers: the mean of the distribution (μ)[8] and its standard deviation (σ)[9]. Every other symbol in the formula, for example, π and e, just stands for a particular fixed number that is shared by all normal curves.[10] Figure 5.2 shows two normal distributions with different means and different standard deviations. The left distribution is normal with $\mu = 0$ and $\sigma = 2$ [also written as: $N(0, 2)$], and the right distribution is normal with $\mu = 10$ and $\sigma = 3$ [also written as: $N(10, 3)$]. As one can easily see, normal distributions are completely symmetric around the mean, with the area under the curve both to the right and left of the mean comprising 50% of the total area. Consequently, the mean of a normal distribution is also its median, as it divides the distribution into its upper and lower 50%. As can be seen from the height of the curve in the graph as well, the mode, which is the most frequent value of a distribution, also equals the mean and median in a normal distribution.

As the essential characteristics of all normal curves are the same, it is easier to work just with the *standard normal curve*, which has a mean of zero and a standard deviation of one [$N(0, 1)$]. Any normal distribution can always be transformed into a *standard normal distribution* by using the following transformation: $z = (x - \mu)/\sigma$. That is, if we take each value of a nonstandard normal distribution, subtract its mean, and divide by its standard deviation, we obtain $N(0, 1)$.

---

[6]Resampling from an already collected *sample* data set is, of course, possible with modern high-speed computers. This technique is increasingly employed to obtain approximate empirical constructions of sampling distributions that are mathematically intractable (a process known as bootstrapping).

[7]Named after Karl Friedrich Gauss (1777–1855), who offered the first complete mathematical description of this distribution.

[8]Recall from Chapter 3 that the Greek letter μ is the symbol for the *population* mean.

[9]The Greek letter σ is the symbol for the *population* standard deviation.

[10]$\pi = 3.1416$; $e = 2.7183$.

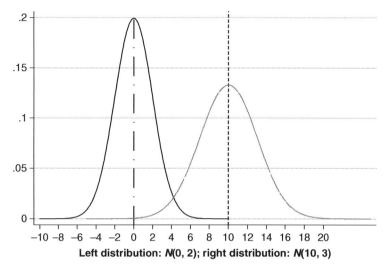

Left distribution: *N*(0, 2); right distribution: *N*(10, 3)

FIGURE 5.2 Comparison of Two Normal Distributions.

Figure 5.3 displays a standard normal curve. By definition, if we subtract the mean from a distribution, then the transformed distribution has a mean of 0; in addition, if we divide a distribution by its standard deviation, then the transformed distribution has a standard deviation of 1. That is why the standard normal distribution is written as $N(0, 1)$. The graph in Figure 5.3 divides the area under the curve into three zones. The area between $\pm 1\sigma$ (short dashed vertical lines) encompasses 68% of the total area, the area between $\pm 1.96\sigma$ (dot-dashed vertical lines) encompasses 95% of the total area, and the area between $\pm 2.58\sigma$ (long dashed vertical lines) accounts for 99% of the total area. It follows that the areas *outside* the limits of $\pm 1\sigma$, $\pm 1.96\sigma$, and $\pm 2.58\sigma$ must be equal to 32%, 5%, and 1%, respectively. The important part to notice is that this property of the standard normal curve, for example, that the area inside -1.96 and $+1.96$ standard deviation units accounts for 95% of the total area and the area outside these limits accounts for 5% of the total area, holds for all normal curves, regardless of the particular

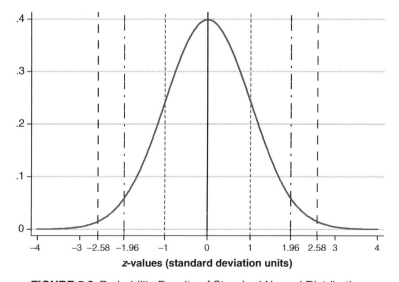

z-values (standard deviation units)

FIGURE 5.3 Probability Density of Standard Normal Distribution.

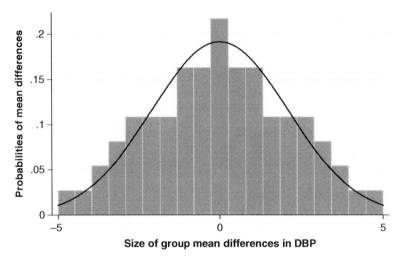

FIGURE 5.4 Sampling Distribution of Mean Differences With Normal Curve: 70 Distinct Splits of 8 Subjects Into 2 Groups With Normal Curve Superimposed.

values of their means or standard deviations. Thus, if we know that a sampling distribution is shaped approximately like the normal distribution, then we can use the normal distribution to estimate the probability that values in the distribution exceed a certain number. We already know some of the z-values and their associated probability values (p-values). For instance, the probability that a randomly drawn number from a normal distribution exceeds +1.96 standard units is 2.5%.[11] As the table in Appendix B shows, the probability that a randomly drawn number from a normal distribution exceeds 2.32 standard units is .0102 or about 1.0%. While integral calculus is employed to compute the exact sizes of areas under the normal curve, we can use the convenience of either statistical software or printed tabulations (as in Appendix B) to tell us the probabilities associated with particular ranges of the z-values.

How useful is the normal distribution for statistical inference? That depends on whether or not we can assume that the sampling distribution of a test statistic actually follows the normal distribution, at least in an approximate way. Let us go back to the sampling distribution in Figure 5.1, but this time we superimpose a normal curve, as shown in Figure 5.4. Given that Figure 5.4 displays the sampling distribution of mean differences between two groups of a very small sample ($n = 8$), it is remarkable how close this distribution comes to the normal distribution. (In part, this is due to the fact that the underlying "population" distribution is at least symmetric, even though it follows the shape of a uniform distribution,[12] not a normal distribution.)

Concerning the symmetry and approximate normal shape of this sampling distribution, it needs to be emphasized that, with very small samples ($N < 30$), sampling distributions of means are only symmetric, if the underlying population distribution is also symmetric. However, as samples grow in size, the sampling distributions of sample *means* and of sample *mean differences* become more and more symmetric, even if the underlying population distribution is not symmetric. What is more, the sampling distributions of mean and mean differences approach the shape of the normal distribution, when $N > 120$. This process is

---

[11] Recall that 5% of the area lies outside −1.96 and +1.96; thus with a symmetric distribution, 2.5% of the area lies either below −1.96 or above +1.96.

[12] Table 5.1 shows that each of the eight individuals has a different DBP; thus each DBP value occurs with a probability of 1/8, which makes the distribution "uniform."

codified in the **Central Limit Theorem**.[13] Its significance is that sampling distributions of means and mean differences take on the shape of a normal distribution in large samples, *even if the underlying population distribution has a different shape*. While the example in Figure 5.4 shows a sampling distribution derived from a very small sample, this tendency toward "normality" is already visible.

Suppose we use the normal distribution to determine the likelihood that certain mean differences in DBP between intervention and control groups for the data in Table 5.1 occur by chance alone. We know the exact probabilities from Figure 5.1. We saw that, for this *sampling distribution*, a mean difference of (−4) or more extreme occurs by chance in 2.9% of all random assignments.[14] Now, let us use the normal distribution as an approximation. In order to convert the distribution in Figure 5.4 to a standard normal distribution, we employ the z-transformation. We already know that this particular sampling distribution has a mean of $\mu = 0$, but we also need an estimate of the standard deviation of this sampling distribution (σ).[15] Recall that this sampling distribution of mean differences consists of 19 distinct mean differences, which occur with the frequencies as indicated in Table 5.2. Thus, we can use the standard deviation formula of Chapter 3 to compute the standard deviation for the sampling distribution in Figure 5.1: It is 1.79. With this information in hand, we can now convert the mean difference of −4 into a z-score:

$$z = \frac{x - \mu}{\sigma} = \frac{-4 - 0}{2.085} = -1.92$$

On the normal curve, the area to the left of −1.92 occupies approximately 2.74% of the total area. In short, despite the very small sample used, our answer is already similar to the exact calculations that are the basis for Figure 5.1.

SIGNIFICANCE TESTING

Let us go back to the problem of statistical inference after random assignment. Random assignment alone will occasionally produce large differences between an intervention and control group, even though there is no intervention effect. If we conclude in such a case that the intervention is effective, then we commit a **Type I error**. Random assignment can also result in a finding of *no* difference between the intervention and control group, *even though there is an intervention effect*. If data lead us to conclude that there is no intervention effect, even though there is one, we commit a **Type II error**. As we base our conclusions on data influenced, in part, by a random assignment process, we cannot completely avoid such erroneous inferences. The decision-making situation is shown in the graph of Figure 5.5. The figure shows two standardized sampling distributions of normal shape. (Again, as we can always convert measured scores into standardized scores using the z-transformation, we only have to consider the standard normal distribution.) The distribution on the right side (black curve) is centered on the null hypothesis value of zero. That is, it depicts the situation in a clinical trial when the null hypothesis ($H_0 = 0$) is true. Even if the antihypertension intervention is not

---

[13] For a mathematical derivation, see Bulmer (1979).

[14] We just add the probabilities of the (−4) and the (−5) mean differences, each of which occurs with a (rounded) probability of .014; actually, the probabilities are .01429, resulting in a combined probability of .02858 or .029.

[15] The standard deviation of a sampling distribution goes by the special name of the **standard error**, because it captures the average error in estimating the "true" population parameter based on sample estimates.

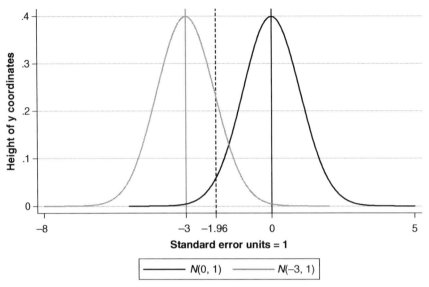

FIGURE 5.5 Comparison of Two Standard Normal Sampling Distributions Centered on Null Hypothesis Value of 0 and Research Value of –3.

effective at all, different *random* splits after random assignment would sometimes produce positive and sometimes negative differences in mean DBP. Occasionally, these differences will be large. Thus, with a large enough sample, we get a normal distribution of mean differences based on all random splits around the true null value of zero.

Now assume for the moment that the intervention is effective. Let us say our physical activity intervention reduces DBP by three standardized units. While the "true" mean difference between the intervention and control group would be –3, not all random splits will result in a difference of –3. Again, we can expect a normal distribution of all possible mean differences, this time centered on the true difference of –3 (depicted in the light gray normal curve on the left side of Figure 5.5).

Now we employ our decision criterion, according to which we either accept or reject the evidence as being strong enough to conclude that there is an intervention effect. This decision criterion is known as the **significance level** (or *α*-level). Suppose we decide, before the clinical trial commences, that we will accept the research hypothesis of an intervention effect, if we can be **95% confident** that our conclusion about the intervention effect is correct. This is the same as setting the significance level at $\alpha = 0.05$, as it amounts to accepting a probability of error of up to 5%. The error in question is the Type I error of falsely rejecting the null hypothesis and thereby implicitly accepting the research hypothesis. As in our example, the sampling distribution of the mean differences can be assumed to have a normal shape, and we know that 95% of the values of the normal distribution lie within the range of –1.96 to +1.96 **standard errors**, we can draw the desired inference. If observed mean differences are either smaller than –1.96 or larger than +1.96 standard errors,[16] then our decision criterion leads us to infer that these differences are of a magnitude that makes it *unlikely* that they are the result

---

[16]Note that we employ a so-called two-tailed test: If 5% of all *z*-values in a standard normal distribution fall outside the –1.96 and +1.96 limits, then on either side we get 2.5% below –1.96 and 2.5% above +1.96.

of mere random assignment; in fact, we can be 95% confident that such differences are "real" and not due to chance.[17]

So far, we have looked at the decision situation only from the point of view of avoiding a Type I error, the error of wrongly concluding that an intervention is not effective, when in fact it is. Suppose someone asks: Why should we tolerate a Type I error as high as 5% ($\alpha = 0.05$)? Why not make the risk smaller and shoot for $\alpha = 0.01$ or even $\alpha = 0.001$? As already mentioned, the true effect of the intervention may be to lower DBP in the intervention group by 3 standard errors, a situation that is depicted in Figure 5.5 with the (light gray) normal curve centered on the value (-3). As we employ the significance level of $\alpha = 0.05$, we would, in effect, reject the null hypothesis, whenever our data show a mean difference between the intervention and the control group that exceeds 1.96 standard errors. In Figure 5.5, a vertical dashed line is inserted at the value of $z = (-1.96)$[18] in order to demarcate the decision line: Should the outcome after the intervention show a mean difference of less than -1.96, we would come to the correct conclusion that the intervention is effective, as we reject the null hypothesis in this situation. But suppose the observed mean difference after the intervention is somewhat larger than -1.96, say -1.5, then we would conclude that this difference is not large enough to warrant the conclusion that there is an intervention effect. However, we need to ask: What is the probability of observing a mean difference *larger* than -1.96, even though the true intervention effect equals -3? As we used random assignment and BP readings are subject to random measurement error, some outcomes will be larger than (-1.96), despite the fact that the true intervention effect equals (-3). As the normal curve centered on the true difference of -3 shows, a substantial area under this normal curve is located to the right of the dashed vertical line. In other words, mere random assignment may produce a mean difference outcome larger than -1.96, even if the true difference is -3 (**Type II error**).[19] As the distance between -3 and -1.96 equals 1.04 standard units, the probability of a Type II error equals the area under the normal curve for all z-values that exceed 1.04. Appendix B tells us that this probability is .1492 ($=1 - .8508$) or about 14.9%. Thus, in 14.9% of all random assignments, we would declare the intervention to be not effective because we accept the null hypothesis whenever the outcome shows a difference above -1.96. Thus we commit the Type II error of concluding that there is no effect, when in fact there is one.

TRADE-OFFS BETWEEN TYPE I AND TYPE II ERRORS

Table 5.3 shows the decision situation when making inferences about intervention effects in clinical trials after random assignment. There are four possible outcomes:

1. The intervention is effective, and we reject the null hypothesis based on the data and the predetermined significance level. That is the correct inference, also called a "true positive."

2. The intervention is effective, but we accept the null hypothesis based on the data and the predetermined significance level. That is an incorrect inference, called the "Type II error."

---

[17]As we will discuss in the next chapter, there are sometimes good reasons to use significance levels other than 0.05 as our decision criterion.

[18]We do not show a vertical dashed line for $+1.96$, as our general expectation is that the intervention will lower DBP.

[19]The Type II error is also indicated by the Greek letter β (beta).

3. The intervention is *not* effective, and we reject the null hypothesis based on the data and the predetermined significance level. That is an incorrect inference, called a "Type I Error."

4. The intervention is *not* effective, but we accept the null hypothesis based on the data and the predetermined significance level. That is a correct inference, also called a "true negative."

TABLE 5.3 Statistical Decision Making for Significance Tests

TEST OUTCOMES		TRUE OUTCOMES	
		H_0 IS NOT TRUE, THAT IS, THE INTERVENTION *IS* EFFECTIVE	H_0 IS TRUE, THAT IS, THE INTERVENTION *IS NOT* EFFECTIVE
Conclusions based on evidence from the sampling distribution	H_0 is rejected, that is, the observed mean difference is "sufficiently rare" and thus qualifies as being "statistically significant"	Correct inference ("true positive")	Type I error (α)
	H_0 is accepted, that is, the observed mean difference could "well" have been produced by random assignment alone and thus is *not* considered "statistically significant"	Type II error (β)	Correct inference ("true negative")

Given this decision situation, it can be seen that there are trade-offs between the magnitudes of the Type I and the Type II errors. Suppose, we are not satisfied with a Type I error of $\alpha = 0.05$. We may want to have a higher level of confidence in the effectiveness of an intervention and stipulate that we desire at least 99% confidence that we draw the correct conclusion when we reject the null hypothesis. As we can see in Figure 5.3, if we reject the null hypothesis if $\alpha \leq 0.01$, then we would call a result "statistically significant" only, if the standardized mean difference score (z-value) is smaller than −2.58. In Figure 5.5, this newly chosen significance level would mean that the dashed vertical line is moved to the left, centered on the value of −2.58. While such a shift would reduce the area under the black normal curve to the left of the vertical line, it would increase the area under the light gray normal curve to the right of the dashed vertical line. In short, while this new decision criterion reduces the probability of a Type I error, it simultaneously increases the probability of a Type II error. How we should think about these trade-offs is discussed briefly in the next chapter.

SUMMARY

In this chapter, we have discussed what can be considered the most fundamental idea in all of statistics. Statistical inference requires (a) the assumption that the data at hand have been generated by a process that includes random elements, such as random assignment or random sampling; (b) that we have a probability model that describes how a statistic of interest fluctuates or varies among different data sets generated by the same process such as random assignment. Given these assumptions, we can generate sampling distributions of the statistics of interest, which allows us to test hypotheses about the magnitude of the true (population) values of these statistics.

The concepts discussed in this chapter are subject to frequent misunderstandings and confusion; so it is worthwhile to clarify a few points:

1. The **sampling distribution** should *not* be confused with the actual distribution of variables in a (sample) data set or in the population. The sampling distribution is a theoretical distribution, which shows how sample statistics, that is, statistics actually computed on a particular data sample, would vary, if the experiment were repeated (infinitely) many times or if one were to draw all possible distinct samples from a given target population. Except in limited circumstances, sampling distributions can usually not be constructed empirically.

2. The measure of *dispersion* for sampling distributions is called its **standard error**. Do not confuse the standard error of a sample statistic with either the **standard deviation** of a particular variable in a study sample (denoted by *s*) or in the target population (denoted by σ). Later in the book we see how some of these standard errors are estimated on the basis of a single study sample data set.

3. The **significance level (α-value)** should not be confused with the ***p*-value**. This is a subtle distinction. The significance level is determined in advance before any data are collected. It represents the risk of a Type I error that researchers are willing to tolerate. By contrast, the *p*-value is the probability of observing the study outcomes if the null hypothesis is true. Thus, if the observed *p*-value is smaller than the predetermined significance level, the researchers will reject the null hypothesis and assume that they observe a "real" effect.

4. The **confidence level** equals 1 minus the significance level. It is the probability that the decision to reject the null hypothesis, and thus accept the research hypothesis, is, in fact, correct. Thus a 5% significance level entails a 95% confidence level.

EXERCISES

1. Define the following three concepts: distribution of sample data; distribution of population data; sampling distribution.

2. In your words: What is the difference between a standard deviation and a standard error?

3. Suppose the study sample in Table 5.1 only contains participants B to G, with A and H dropping out before random assignment.
   (a) In how many ways can the remaining six subjects be randomly assigned to two groups consisting of three individuals each?
   (b) Construct the sampling distribution of all possible mean differences between intervention and control groups.
   (c) Compute the SE of the mean difference.
   (d) Would a mean difference of 4 be "statistically significant" at the 0.05 level?

4. Using Appendix B, find the area under the normal curve if
   (a) $-0.67 \leq Z \leq +0.67$
   (b) $Z \geq 1.04$
   (c) $Z \leq -2.33$ and $Z \geq +2.33$
   (d) $Z \leq -1.65$

5. In a study of 256 randomly sampled nursing home residents, researchers find a mean low-density lipoprotein (LDL) cholesterol level of 148 mg/dL. The sample standard deviation is 20 mg/dL. The standard error of the mean is 1.25.
   (a) Is this evidence consistent with the hypothesis that the mean population LDL cholesterol level is at least 150 mg/dL, assuming you adopt a significance level of $\alpha = 0.05$?
   (b) Is the evidence consistent with the hypothesis that the mean population cholesterol level is larger than 145?
   (c) Based on the data provided, can we say that at least 10% of the nursing home residents have LDL cholesterol levels above 181?

6. Figure 5.5 shows two normal distributions, each with standard errors of 1. If the normal distribution on the left were to be centered on the mean of -3.92, what could we say about the magnitudes of the Type I (α) and Type II (β) probabilities?

7. If the significance level for a test has been set to $\alpha \leq 05$ and the p-value associated with that test turns out to be .06, what should we conclude?

8. Which error in statistical inference do you consider to be greater, a Type I or a Type II error? Can this question be answered as a matter of general principle, or does it depend on the circumstances of a particular test?

REFERENCE

Bulmer, M. G. (1979). *Principles of statistics*. New York, NY: Dover.

CHAPTER 6

Standard Errors, Confidence Intervals, and the Power of Statistical Tests

In Chapter 5, we discussed the sampling distribution of a mean difference and noted that the shape of such a sampling distribution approaches that of the normal distribution, as long as the study sample in question is reasonably large ($n > 120$). This is the case even if the underlying population distribution is not normal. We also noted that any normal distribution is characterized by only two parameters, the values of which we need to know in order to convert it into a **standard normal distribution**: the mean μ and the standard deviation σ. Of course, μ and σ are population statistics ("parameters"), whose values are generally unknown. As to the value of the population mean, we usually hypothesize it; but in order to test whether our sample mean is consistent with our hypothesized population mean, we would need to know by how much sample means vary from one sample to the next. In short, we would need to have an estimate of the **standard error of the mean** (SEM). The same problem arises in an experimental study (clinical trial) after random assignment. If the primary test statistic is a mean difference between the intervention and control group, we would need to know by how much such mean differences vary as a result of different random assignments; that is, we would need an estimate of the **standard error of the mean difference**. Thus, even if the study sample is large enough and the sampling distribution of the test statistic takes on the shape of a normal curve, we still cannot use the normal distribution to test for a specific hypothesized mean difference unless we know the magnitude of the standard error, that is, the standard deviation of the sampling distribution.

In Chapter 5, we computed the standard error *directly*, using the data from a hypothetical sampling distribution shown in Table 5.2 and Figure 5.1. In reality, we almost never construct the actual sampling distribution of a statistic like the mean difference. It is tedious and time consuming to calculate all possible outcomes of mean differences produced through random assignment: Even in the artificially small assignment process of 8 subjects to 2 groups of 4 subjects each, we came up with 70 distinct assignments. If the sample had consisted of 20 subjects, there would have been 184,756 distinct ways of assigning them to 2 groups randomly.[1] Thus, computing standard errors directly from the sampling distribution would quickly become a taxing undertaking. In the case of random sampling from a larger target

---

[1] $20!/(10!10!) = 184,756.$

population, it would simply not be feasible—due to time and monetary constraints—to draw a sufficiently large number of samples, let alone all possible random samples, of a given size from the same target population. Thus, in most situations, there is no way of obtaining an estimate of the standard error directly from data that contain information on the sampling distribution of a particular test statistic. Instead, we are usually limited to a single data set from a given target population. However, for many test statistics, statisticians have worked out formulas for the estimation of standard errors based on particular sample data.

STANDARD ERROR OF THE MEAN (SEM)

The SEM of any variable is usually estimated based on data generated from a single random sample or after a single random assignment. Its formula is: $SEM = s/\sqrt{n}$.[2] In words, the SEM is *estimated* by computing the standard deviation of the relevant variable from the sample data and dividing it by the square root of the sample size. Most important is the fact that the SEM varies inversely with the square root of the sample size. In other words, as sample sizes increase, standard errors become smaller and smaller. This is what we should expect: The SEM is a measure of how much sample *means* of the same variable vary *across* random samples of a given size drawn from the same target population. Intuitively, it is obvious that sample means from large samples vary/fluctuate less than sample means from small samples. That is, the latter are subject to a wider "margin of error." Also note in the Definition of SEM box the effect of the finite population correction (FPC) on the standard error. As n grows larger and approaches N, $[n \rightarrow N]$, $N - n$ approaches zero. Thus, if the "sample" actually comprises the total target population, there is no longer any sampling error since we would have population data.

This inverse relationship between **sample size** and **sampling fraction** on one hand, and the size of the **standard error** on the other, holds for standard errors of *all* sample statistics, not just the SEM.[3] This implies that the precision of our estimates can be improved, if we increase the size of our study samples.[4]

DRAWING INFERENCES ABOUT POPULATION PARAMETERS: CONFIDENCE INTERVALS

In Chapter 5, we showed how to use information about the sampling distribution of a test statistic to test hypotheses concerning the effectiveness of an intervention in a random-ized clinical trial. However, in many situations, we are not just interested in the "statistical

---

[2] The rationale for the formula can be demonstrated as follows: A sample mean is really a sum of n inde-pendent random variables, that is, each of the cases whose values are used to compute the sample mean is independently and randomly selected; formally, we can rewrite: $\bar{X} = (1/n)(X_1 + X_2 + \cdots + X_n) = (1/n)$ $X_1 + (1/n)X_2 + \cdots + (1/n)X_n$. But the variance of a sum of independent random variables is the sum of their variances $(\sum s_i^2)$. Since these variables are all drawn from the same population, they all must have the same variance: $\sum s_i^2 = ns_i^2$. In addition, the variance of a variable multiplied by a constant (here: $1/n$) equals the variance of the variable times the square of its constant: $(1/n^2)s_i^2$. Since we have n variances involved in the mean, we get $n(1/n^2)s_i^2$ or $(1/n)s_i^2$. The square root of this expression is the sought after expression for the estimated standard error: $s/\sqrt{n}$.

[3] Later in this book, we encounter many other statistics like correlation coefficients, odds ratios, or regression coefficients, all of which are subject to sampling fluctuations, the magnitudes of which are estimated via their associated standard errors.

[4] Of course, that adds to the cost and time of data collection.

DEFINITION OF SEM

The SEM of a variable x is a measure of the average variation of sample means around the population mean. It is estimated as:

$$\text{SEM} = s_x/\sqrt{n},$$

where s_x stands for the sample standard deviation and n the sample size. The sample standard deviation is computed as usual:

$$s_x = \sqrt{\sum \frac{(x_i - \bar{x})^2}{n-1}}$$

Comment: The formula for SEM assumes that the study sample is only a small fraction of the target population (say, less than 5%). If the study sample comprises a larger proportion of the target population, it is necessary to multiply the SEM with an FPC factor of

$$\text{FPC} = \sqrt{\frac{N-n}{N-1}},$$

where N is the population size and n the sample size.

---

significance" of our findings. Rather, we want to have an estimate of the actual magnitude of the effect. Likewise, when health researchers sample from large target populations, they are usually interested in the *accuracy* of their estimates, that is, they want to be able to estimate the margins of error of their estimates.

As we have already emphasized,[5] *if a randomly selected study sample is reasonably large ($n \geq 120$),*[6] we can assume that the sampling distribution of a mean or a mean difference takes on the shape of the normal distribution. If we also have an estimate of the standard error, then we can use the normal distribution to estimate the probability that sample means fall within various margins of error.

Suppose we employ data from a cancer registry, which contains diagnostic information on thousands of (mostly) women with breast cancer.[7] Suppose further, we wanted to know the average age of women at the time of their breast cancer diagnosis. One way to obtain the relevant information would be to draw a random sample of size 200, compute the mean age in the study sample, and construct **confidence intervals** (CIs) for the mean as follows.

From Figure 6.1, we know that, if the sampling distribution is normally distributed, 95% (99%) of all **sample means** will lie between ±1.96 (2.58) **standard errors** of the true population mean. This fact is usually expressed in a more formal way as follows:

$$P(\mu - 1.96\,\text{SEM} < \bar{x}_i < \mu + 1.96\,\text{SEM}) = .95$$

---

[5] This is the point of the Central Limit Theorem.

[6] For samples drawn from normal populations with $n < 120$, we employ the t-distribution (see Chapter 8).

[7] See the SEER data set for more information: seer.cancer.gov/data/

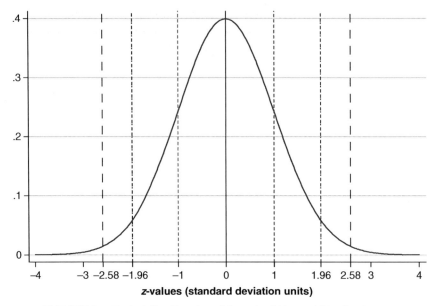

FIGURE 6.1 Probability Density of Standard Normal Distribution.

In this expression, P is short for probability, $\bar{x}_i$ refers to any sample mean from randomly drawn samples of a given size, μ refers to the true population mean, and SEM to the standard error associated with the sampling distribution of the mean. This equation simply says that 95% of all sample means of randomly drawn samples of a given size will fall within ±1.96 standard errors of the true population mean, which is the same as saying that the probability of a sample mean falling within these limits is .95.

Now let us look at the inequality inside the brackets. A few simple algebraic manipulations will get us a more interesting result still.

We start with the original inequality:

$$\mu - 1.96\ \text{SEM} < \bar{x}_i < \mu + 1.96\ \text{SEM}$$

Then we subtract μ from all three segments (which preserves the inequality):

$$-1.96\ \text{SEM} < \bar{x}_i - \mu < +1.96\ \text{SEM}$$

Then we subtract $\bar{x}_i$:

$$-\bar{x}_i - 1.96\ \text{SEM} < -\mu < -\bar{x}_i + 1.96\ \text{SEM}$$

Then we multiply by (−1):

$$\bar{x}_i + 1.96\ \text{SEM} > \mu > \bar{x}_i - 1.96\ \text{SEM}\ ^{8}$$

At first blush, this transformation may not look like much, but the end result is really remarkable and useful. If we plug this result back into our original probability equation, we get:

$$P(\bar{x}_i + 1.96\ \text{SEM} > \mu > \bar{x}_i - 1.96\ \text{SEM}) = .95$$

---

[8] You may recall the result from algebra that multiplying an inequality by a negative number reverses the inequality sign; for example, if we multiply the inequality −5 < −2 by (−1), we get 5 > 2.

In words, if we (a) take *any* random sample of sufficient size and compute a sample mean on a variable of interest, for example, the mean age at diagnosis for breast cancer patients, and (b) construct a 95% CI by way of adding or subtracting 1.96 standard errors from the sample mean, then 95% of all CIs so constructed will contain the true population mean. That is, *with a single random sample, we can have 95% confidence that the CI covers the true population mean.* Using a specific numerical example, we may find that the mean age in the sample of 200 newly diagnosed breast cancer patients is 60 and the sample standard deviation for age is 12. With this information, we can construct the 95% CI as follows:

$$P(\bar{x}_i + 1.96 \text{ SEM} > \mu > \bar{x}_i - 1.96 \text{ SEM}) = .95$$

$$P(60 + 1.96 \,[12/\sqrt{200}] > \mu > 60 + 1.96 \,[12/\sqrt{200}]) = .95$$

$$P(60 + 1.96 \,[0.85] > \mu > 60 + 1.96 \,[0.85]) = .95$$

$$P(61.67 > \mu > 58.33) = .95$$

In short, we can have 95% confidence that our CI with a lower limit of 58.33 and an upper limit of 61.67 contains the true population mean.

RELATIONSHIPS AMONG CIs, SAMPLE SIZES, AND STANDARD ERRORS

The relationships among CIs, sample sizes, and standard errors can be shown using a few hypothetical examples, as in Table 6.1. Assume that four random samples of sizes $n = 120$, 240, 480, and 960 have been drawn from the same population of newly diagnosed cancer patients. This time, researchers obtain standardized physical functioning (PF) scores from all study participants, ranging from 0 to 100.[9] For each of the four random samples drawn from the same target population, sample means and standard deviations are computed (second and third columns of Table 6.1) and used in providing the estimates for the reported standard errors and CIs.

There are a number of important observations to be made about the results in Table 6.1:

1. Sample means ($\bar{x}_i$) fluctuate/vary randomly from one sample to the next, with each sample mean being one estimate of the (usually unknown) population mean (μ).

2. Sample standard deviations (s) also fluctuate/vary randomly from one sample to the next, with each sample standard deviation being an estimate of the (usually unknown) population standard deviation (s).

3. Standard errors consistently decline in magnitude, as sample sizes increase.

4. CIs, associated with a *given* level of coverage probability, become smaller, as sample sizes increase; that is, with greater sample sizes, the accuracy of our estimates increases.

5. CIs for statistics from samples of a *given* size increase with the level of confidence required, that is, they increase with higher coverage probability. Thus, if we require greater confidence in our estimates, this comes unfortunately at the cost of lower accuracy or precision, as long as sample sizes are not changed.

---

[9] See Given, Given, Azzouz, and Stommel (2001).

TABLE 6.1 Standard Errors and Confidence Limits of Mean Physical Functioning Scores Based on Samples of Varying Size

SAMPLE SIZES (n_i)	SAMPLE MEANS $(\bar{x_i})$	SAMPLE STANDARD DEVIATIONS (s_i)	ESTIMATED STANDARD ERRORS (SE)	95% CIs (±1.96SE)	99% CIs (±2.58SE)
$n_1 = 120$	77.8	9.8	0.89	$76.06 < \mu < 79.54$	$75.50 < \mu < 80.10$
$n_2 = 240$	74.9	10.7	0.69	$73.55 < \mu < 76.25$	$73.12 < \mu < 76.68$
$n_3 = 480$	75.6	11.2	0.51	$74.60 < \mu < 76.60$	$74.28 < \mu < 76.92$
$n_4 = 960$	76.5	10.4	0.34	$75.83 < \mu < 77.17$	$75.62 < \mu < 77.38$

Finally, a note of caution: A frequent mistake in the interpretation of the SEM is to assume that it is either an estimate of the population standard deviation (σ) or the sample standard deviation (s). Neither is the case. In fact, note that standard errors are, by definition, always *smaller* than the sample standard deviations, since we divide by the square root of the sample sizes (n). By contrast, sample standard deviations give us best estimates of the population standard deviations. Most importantly, sample standard deviations do not become systematically smaller as the sample size increases, since for each 1-unit increase in denominator of the standard deviation formula we also add another deviation from the mean in the numerator. The data in Table 6.1 bear this out: There is no systematic relationship between the size of a sample and its standard deviation as well as its mean. As far as the standard deviation in the target population is concerned, it always stays the same, regardless of which samples are drawn from the target population. In sum, the SEM measures fluctuation/variation in different sample means, whereas the sample and population standard deviations are measures of the average variation in individual scores around their respective means.

EFFECT SIZES AND STATISTICAL POWER

When researchers plan for a clinical study, one of the most important questions they must answer is: How large a study sample is needed in order to show the hypothesized effect of the planned intervention? To answer this question, the researchers would need information on the relevant minimum **effect size** (ES) and they would have to decide on how much **statistical power** they would need for their intervention study.

In the previous chapter (Chapter 5), we discussed a hypothetical example of a physical activity intervention designed to lower blood pressure. In the simplest case of a randomized clinical trial, we would compare a once obtained mean systolic blood pressure (SBP) in the intervention group to that in the control group.[10] Since study participants in a clinical trial are randomly assigned to either the intervention or the control group, we would hypothesize that, before the intervention, there is no systematic mean difference in blood pressure between these comparison groups. This is our null hypothesis (H_0). By contrast, the research (or alternative) hypothesis (H_A) embodies the hoped-for ES of the intervention.

Let us say, the researchers settle on a minimum intervention ES of 4 mmHg; that is, they expect that after the intervention the mean SBP will be lower in the intervention than the control group by at least 4 mmHg. This number is not based on any statistical reasoning, but should reflect the considered judgment of the clinicians: How much of a difference should

---

[10] For a study employing multiple outcome measures of physical activity and a more complex repeated measures study design, see Buchan et al. (2011).

the intervention make for clinicians to be able to call it a "clinically meaningful effect"? It is not always easy to come up with clinically meaningful minimum ESs, but these judgments should rest on clinical experience as well as already available research that links ESs to clinical outcomes.[11] For the sake of argument, let us say that lowering the mean systolic mmHg by 4 units is clinically meaningful in terms of demonstrably lower rates of heart disease and diabetes. So we use this number in our sample size calculations, but we must convert it to a **standardized effect size**, which means we must divide the mean difference in SBP between the intervention and control groups by the standard deviation of this mean difference. Since we have two comparison groups (intervention [int] and control [ctrl]) with two estimates of the SBP standard deviation, we usually would employ a more complicated, weighted average of the standard deviation formula:

$$\sigma = \sqrt{\frac{(n_1 - 1)\, s_1^2 + (n_2 - 1)s_1^2}{n_1 + n_2 - 2}}$$

Thus the *standardized* ES for the mean difference becomes: $(\bar{x}_{int} - \bar{x}_{ctrl})/\sigma$, with σ defined as before.

Now suppose that previous studies have shown SBP sample standard deviations that vary between 6 and 10 mmHg. Given this information, we may adopt as a reasonable guess that our future study sample will have an SBP standard deviation of around 8. This would make for a **standardized effect size** of ES = 4/8 = 0.5.

Finally, we need to address the concept of **statistical power**. In Chapter 5, we discussed the Type II error in statistical inference: It refers to the probability of concluding, on the basis of available sample evidence, that an intervention is *not* effective, even if "in reality" it is. If we denote this probability as β, then we can define the power of a statistical test as $1 - \beta$. In words, the power of a statistical test is the probability that we arrive at the conclusion that an intervention is effective, when in fact it is. It seems obvious that we would want to maximize power and minimize the Type II error. Should we not design our experiments in such a way that, whenever there is an intervention effect, the resulting test confirms its existence? Unfortunately, we already know from the discussion in Chapter 5 that minimizing β (and maximizing power) involves increasing the size of α; that is, we must again consider the trade-offs between the Type I and the Type II errors.

For many studies, researchers choose conventional α-levels of 0.05 and β-levels of 0.20. This implies they are willing to accept a 5% risk that a positive inference about the effectiveness of an intervention is wrong (Type I error). At the same time, they are willing to accept a 20% risk that a negative inference about the effectiveness of an intervention is wrong (Type II error). Of course, whether these risk trade-offs are appropriate depends very much on the context of a study.[12] For instance, in the early 1990s, when no effective HIV drugs were available, the primary concern of researchers was to find any effective drug. In that situation, researchers would want to maximize the power of their tests so that whenever a drug shows promise it would be discovered as having a significant effect in a trial. This implies preferring a low probability for β, say at 0.01, with power $(1 - \beta)$ at 0.99, but accepting the risk of larger α-levels. In short, such researchers trade in a higher Type I error for the desired lower Type II

---

[11] It has become "fashionable" to group standardized ESs into arbitrary categories of "small," "medium," and "large" ESs (Cohen, 1992), but we strongly support the view that meaningful ESs in clinical research must involve clinical definitions of effectiveness.

[12] Ellis (2010).

error. On the other hand, if researchers conduct clinical trials on "me-too" drugs, for which there are widely available substitutes, their primary concern would be that the new drug is, indeed, effective; thus, they would set a very low Type I (α) risk, say 0.01, but would be willing to incur a higher Type II (β) risk. The reason is that the risk of *failing* to find a significant effect, even though the new drug is effective, is less problematic in a situation where many substitutes are available. On the other hand, in that situation, one would *not* want to run the risk of using a new drug in the belief that it is effective, even though it is not; thus, minimizing the Type I error has higher priority. In sum, while the power of a test is often set at 0.8, such decisions are subject to revisions, depending on the research project at hand.

POWER ANALYSIS AND SAMPLE SIZE

Power analysis is primarily employed for the purpose of determining necessary sample sizes before the data collection commences. It involves complicated trade-offs among four indices, such that three of the four indices determine the value of the fourth. The actual calculations involved are mathematically complex in nature and beyond the scope of this book, but there are several good software programs, both specialized stand-alone programs and subroutines of comprehensive statistical package programs.[13] To conduct a power analysis, a researcher must be able to specify the following information:

1. The significance level or willingness to commit a Type I error (α-level)

2. The desired power of the test ($1 - \beta$) or acceptable probability of finding an effect, if there is one

3. The standardized ES

4. The sample size

As mentioned, if we can determine or set the values of three of these four indices, then we get an answer to the fourth. Commonly, researchers are interested in determining sample sizes required for their studies. In those situations, they would make informed assumptions about how much of a Type I error they are willing to tolerate, how much power they desire, and the size of a clinically meaningful minimum effect, expressed as a standardized ES.

Let us start with some standard assumptions for the previous example of a physical activity intervention. We may assume that an α-level of 0.05 and power of 0.8 (i.e., $\beta = 0.2$) are adequate, while clinical experience may lead to the recommendation of a minimum standardized ES of 0.5. With these assumptions, our required sample size would be $n_1 = n_2 = 63$.[14] This means that each arm of the randomized clinical trial would need to enroll 63 subjects to meet the required assumptions.[15]

In Table 6.2, we provide sample size estimates for several combinations of α- and ($1 - \beta$)-levels, as well as for standardized ESs. For each of these indices, we offer three distinct levels in order to show the trade-offs involved between sample size and the other three indices. One important trade-off is that between minimum desired ES and sample size.

---

[13] Among the stand-alone programs are G*Power and PASS; STATA offers the "sampsi" routine.

[14] All sample size calculations, including those for Table 6.2, were performed using STATA software.

[15] Researchers customarily enroll more subjects to make up for anticipated loss to follow-up or dropouts.

TABLE 6.2 Variations in Required Sample Sizes (*n*) Depending on Three Levels of Type I Error (*α*), Power (1 − *β*), and Standardized Effect Size (ES)

α-LEVELS	POWER (1 − *β*)	STANDARDIZED ESs		
		ES = 0.2 (*n*)	ES = 0.5 (*n*)	ES = 1.0 (*n*)
0.01	0.80	584	94	24
	0.90	744	120	30
	0.95	891	143	36
0.05	0.80	393	63	16
	0.90	526	85	22
	0.95	650	104	26
0.10	0.80	310	50	13
	0.90	429	69	18
	0.95	542	87	22

The smaller the effect we want or need to discover, the larger the study samples that are required. In particular, for given levels of *α* and power, required sample sizes increase exponentially as standardized ESs become smaller. In short, if we want to discover small effects, we need very large study samples.

Required sample sizes also increase with greater desired power of the statistical tests. As the cells shaded light gray show, for given levels of *α*, and a given ES, power can only be increased at the cost of larger study samples.

Finally, required sample sizes increase when researchers want to reduce the probability of a Type I error (*α*). As the cells shaded dark gray show, for given levels of power and a given ES, reduced *α* risks can only be purchased at the cost of larger study samples.

It can be inferred from Table 6.2 that the usual trade-off between *α*-levels and power can be mitigated by raising the sample size. If it is important to increase the power while maintaining *α* and ES at a given level, this can be accomplished through greater sample size: The shaded cells in Table 6.2 show the trade-off between power and sample size for a given level of *α* and ES.

There is another situation in which power analysis is useful. Sometimes we encounter reports of intervention studies in the literature, in which the main hypothesis is not confirmed, that is, the hypothesized effect is not statistically significant. In this case, we must also ask whether the sample size was large enough so that the probability of finding the minimum ES was fairly high.[16] Suppose you read about a physical activity intervention study in which the authors could not confirm that their intervention lowers blood pressure by a standardized ES of 0.5, employing a significance level of $α < 0.05$ as their criterion for statistical significance. You also learn that the study sample involved 20 subjects in each arm of the study (intervention or control group). As it turns out, the probability that the study would produce a statistically significant intervention effect under these assumptions would only be .35. In other words, the power of the test to find a significant result was quite low at 0.35. Thus, you may well conclude that a very small sample size may have been the problem with this study.

---

[16] This is also called a post hoc power analysis.

EXERCISES

1. A researcher draws a random sample of test results from 400 patients among a total patient population of 900. The tests show a mean count of neutrophil granulocytes (white blood cells) of 80×10^8/L and a sample standard deviation of 20×10^8/L.[17]
   (a) Compute the 95% CI for the mean neutrophil granulocytes count.
   (b) Is a hypothesized population mean of 50×10^8/L consistent with the evidence?

2. Assume you have data on the mean hemoglobin levels of all patients who stayed overnight during a given year at two hospitals. A random sample ($n = 400$) of 9,000 patients at Hospital A showed a mean hemoglobin of 15 g/100 mL; a random sample ($n = 400$) of 10,000 patients at Hospital B had a mean hemoglobin level of 12 g/100 mL. The standard error for the difference in mean hemoglobin levels is 1.5 g/100 mL. Can we say that we are at least 95% confident that the patients at Hospital B had lower mean hemoglobin levels?

3. For the example in exercise 5 of Chapter 5, construct
   (a) The 95% CI for the mean low density lipoprotein (LDL) cholesterol level;
   (b) The 99% CI for the mean LDL cholesterol level.

4. In a single sentence: Why do larger study samples result in greater statistical power, all else being equal?

5. When you read in a research paper that a clinical intervention produced a "significant" effect, what exactly does that mean?

REFERENCES

Buchan, D. S., Ollis, S., Thomas, N. E., Buchanan, N., Cooper, S. M., Malina, R. M., & Baker, J. S. (2011). Physical activity interventions: Effects of duration and intensity. *Scandinavian Journal of Medicine & Science in Sports, 21*(6), e341–e350.

Cohen, J. (1992). Statistical power analysis. *Current Directions in Psychological Science, 1*(3), 98–101.

Ellis, P. D. (2010). *The essential guide to effect sizes: An introduction to statistical power, meta-analysis and the interpretation of research results.* Cambridge, UK: Cambridge University Press.

Given, B., Given, C., Azzouz, F., & Stommel, M. (2001). Physical functioning of elderly cancer patients prior to diagnosis and following initial treatment. *Nursing Research, 50*(4), 222–232.

---

[17] Alternatively, these numbers are usually written as: 8×10^9/L and a sample standard deviation of 2×10^9/L.

CHAPTER 7

Research Designs and Statistical Analysis

In Chapters 2 and 3, we considered different levels of measurement of variables and how they affect what kinds of statistics are appropriate to use when summarizing quantitative information. In Chapters 5 and 6, we discussed basic principles of statistical inference, including how sample size considerations are closely related to the question of whether statistical inference is likely to yield significant results. However, statistical considerations do not only influence measurement and sampling decisions; they are also part and parcel of decisions about research designs. Conversely, the appropriateness of specific statistical models and the interpretation of statistical information also depend on measurement, research, and sampling design decisions made before the data were gathered or generated.

As there are many excellent books available focusing primarily on research design issues, we only provide a very brief outline of research design issues and terminology (Friedman, Furberg, & DeMets, 2010; Polit & Beck, 2003; Shadish, Cook, & Campbell, 2002; Stommel & Wills, 2004). The goal is to alert you to the fact that the specific statistical models discussed in the following chapters all make assumptions about the nature of the data that are to be analyzed. As we will see, the "fit" between data and model assumptions is an important consideration in judging the appropriateness of a particular analysis.

INTERVENTION VERSUS OBSERVATIONAL STUDIES

Probably the most basic distinction in study designs is that between an **intervention** and an **observational study**. An alternative terminology frequently encountered referring to the same distinction is that between an **experimental** and a **nonexperimental** study.

Suppose you want to know about the prevalence of vitamin D deficiencies in the U.S. resident population. That information has been obtained through the National Health and Nutrition Examination Survey (NHANES) conducted by the National Center for Health Statistics (NCHS; CDC, 2012). The biannual samples of the NHANES are representative of the U.S. population and involve both survey questionnaire data and the collection of biomarkers and anthropometric information. This type of study is observational or nonexperimental, as the researchers are only interested in gathering information and not in changing or affecting some outcomes of interest.

Now suppose, you design a nutrition study with the goal of reducing incipient obesity among toddlers of low-income mothers (Horodynski & Stommel, 2005). Here the researchers are interested in producing change, in designing an intervention for a particular target population, for example, low-income mothers of toddlers, which hopefully will reduce obesity rates. This type of study is experimental: Some study participants are deliberately exposed to an intervention, and other study participants are exposed to a control group condition. If the study participants are randomly assigned to either intervention or control group conditions, we call such a study design a randomized experiment or a **randomized clinical trial**.[1]

Why is the distinction between intervention and observational studies crucially important? Suppose the NHANES survey shows that the proportion of U.S. residents with vitamin D deficiency is 35% larger among residents living in households below the federal poverty line than among residents living in households with annual income exceeding $150,000. How should we interpret this finding? Can we confidently say that lack of income is a *causal factor* contributing to vitamin D deficiency? The answer is "no," as low-income and higher-income people differ in many other ways that might be relevant here: Low-income people tend to have less education; thus their knowledge of nutrition and the effects of sun exposure may be different from that of higher-income people. In addition, low-income people tend to differ from higher-income people with respect to a host of other possibly relevant characteristics. These include age- and ethnicity-composition, gender ratios, and so forth. All of these other variables may influence nutrition patterns and thus "confound" the relationship between income and vitamin D deficiency. While there are statistical models to "control for" some of the effects of these confounding variables, we can never be sure with observational data whether we have controlled for all relevant confounders (Shadish et al., 2001; Stommel & Wills, 2004).

Now suppose that a randomized nutrition intervention study shows a difference of similar magnitude, with the intervention group having a 35% lower rate of vitamin D deficiency than the control group in a 6-month follow-up measure.[2] Note that the results from the randomized intervention study can be interpreted *causally*: If the intervention was designed specifically to target reductions in vitamin D deficiency, and the subjects exposed to the intervention are less likely to exhibit vitamin D deficiencies than the control group subjects *after* the intervention, then there is good reason to believe that the intervention made the difference. This is so, because random assignment of sufficiently large numbers of subjects to the intervention and control groups tends to create comparison groups with similar average background characteristics, thus removing systematic biases that would result from between-group differences in these background characteristics. In this particular example, random assignment of sufficiently large comparison groups should result in similar average vitamin D deficiencies between the intervention and control groups. In addition, evidence in favor of the causal effectiveness of the intervention could be strengthened further with a pretest/posttest design: Researchers may then be able to *show* that there is no systematic difference in vitamin D deficiency after the random assignment but before the intervention, while 6 months later, that is, after the intervention, vitamin deficiency rates have declined in the intervention group but not the control group.

It should be apparent now that the same statistic, say, a 35% difference in the proportion of persons with vitamin D deficiencies, must be interpreted differently, depending on whether the evidence comes from an observational or an experimental study. The reason for this is that the establishment of a cause–effect relationship between two or more variables does not only

---

[1]There are a number of good intervention study designs that do not employ random assignment. These are collectively known as quasi-experimental designs. For an excellent discussion, see Shadish et al. (2001).

[2]We assume here that both results are "statistically significant," meaning they are unlikely to be due to mere sampling fluctuation.

require that we can show that they vary together, but that we must also show that *no other variable is responsible for the effect that we are seeing* (Shadish et al., 2001; Stommel & Wills, 2004). Thus, it is always hazardous to interpret patterns of association discovered in observational studies as sufficient evidence for the existence of a cause–effect relationship: *Correlation is not sufficient evidence of causation.*

As we see in later chapters, many statistical models—for example, all the different kinds of regression models—employ an explicitly causal language, as when the analyst is asked to identify **dependent** as opposed to **independent variables**. Do not be fooled by this terminology! Just because we create a model and designate some variables as dependent or outcome variables, and others as potential independent or causal variables, does not mean we have proven the causal relationship. *Statistics alone cannot establish that the assumption of a cause–effect relationship is, in fact, correct.* In the final analysis, statistical analysis can only show that variation in presumed dependent or outcome variables is associated with variation in presumed independent variables. Causal interpretation rests on additional criteria, such as the features of the study design and the explanatory framework that links causes and effects.

ANALYSIS OF CORRELATED AND UNCORRELATED DATA

Another important distinction for statistical analysis is that between study designs that produce correlated and uncorrelated data. The distinction is not only important in terms of the interpretation of statistical information, but also affects the choice of appropriate statistical models when analyzing such data. Correlated data are an integral feature of **longitudinal, repeated-measures** studies, but also occur in some **cross-sectional** study designs.

Cross-sectional studies involve the gathering of data on study participants at a single point in time.[3] From a statistical point of view, the main feature of such data is that individual variation in characteristics, traits, or variables *across* different study participants can be assumed to be *independent* of each other. Thus, if we enroll two patients into a hypertension study, we can reasonably assume that variation in the systolic or diastolic blood pressure (BP) of the first patient does not influence, and is not correlated with, variation in the systolic and diastolic BP of the second patient.

That postulate of independence would not hold in a longitudinal study, in which we analyze repeated measures from the same subjects. Obviously, we would expect that earlier and later measurements, taken from the same individual, are correlated. If that is the case, the statistical models we employ must reflect this fact. In this book, we introduce several statistical models employed in the analysis of repeated-measures designs, as these study designs are very common in nursing and medical research. As we will see, statistical models appropriate for the analysis of data from repeated-measures studies all start with the fundamental distinction between **within-subjects** and **between-subjects variation** in scores. We generally assume that within-subjects variation results in correlated scores according to some pattern, for example, repeated BP scores on the same individual are obviously related. By contrast, between-subjects variation in scores can often, but not always, be assumed to be independent or uncorrelated.

There are some cross-sectional study designs, commonly employed in clinical studies, which also produce data that violate the independence assumption. Whenever study participants are part of relevant **clusters** or **pairs**, the analysis must take account of this feature. For

---

[3]Alternatively, some cross-sectional designs involve single measurements on study participants at varying time, but the important feature remains that for each study participant, data were collected only on a single occasion.

instance, it would not make sense to analyze data from study participants in a nutrition study, who are part of the same family and live in the same household, as if they are providing completely independent observations on nutritional intake. Likewise, the analysis of data from a study of the effects of laser surgery on correcting near-sightedness cannot assume that treatment outcomes for the two eyes of the same person are completely independent from each other.

SAMPLING DESIGNS

The interpretation of statistical information and statistical tests also depends on the sampling design employed in a study. As a general rule, statistical inference from **sample** data to target **populations** of interest is *only* feasible, *if* the sampling design involves some form of probability sampling. A probability sampling design specifies for each study participant the probability of being selected into the study sample. In the case of simple random sampling, each member of the target population has the same probability of being selected into the study sample. Statistical software packages like SAS, STATA, or SPSS usually assume, as a *default* setting, that study samples are simple random samples. However, for many practical reasons,[4] large-scale survey studies, designed to be representative of the U.S. resident population as a whole, employ complex survey designs involving both cluster and stratified sampling.[5] In such studies, the sampling ratio[6] varies, depending on where a study participant lives or which population group he or she belongs to. As a result, the estimation of standard errors and probability values associated with significance testing must be adjusted, which requires special software modifications.[7] In this book, we will not deal with data from complex survey designs. However, we think it important that the reader is aware of these complications.

SOURCES OF RANDOMNESS IN HEALTH CARE RESEARCH

Statistical models assume that the data to be analyzed are always subject to random error. That poses the question: What are the sources of this randomness?

As we have already seen, one major source of randomness in medical and nursing research is the "deliberately engineered" random assignment of study participants in clinical intervention studies to various treatment and control conditions. Here, random assignment serves the purpose of facilitating causal inferences after interventions.

As discussed in the previous section, another important source of randomness in the data we use in health care research stems from drawing random samples from larger target populations. Here, random sampling serves the purpose of drawing inferences about large target populations based on information obtained from random samples.

Yet, while randomized clinical trials or randomized intervention studies are quite common in the literature, the use of random samples for the purpose of generalizing to larger populations is far less common, except for the federal health surveys conducted by the NCHS and a few others, such as studies of health insurance claims. Despite the increased use of

---

[4] Among them is the cost of data gathering, which is substantially lower when subjects are sampled in geographic clusters; in addition, oversampling of smaller population groups, such as various minorities, allows one to make reasonably accurate inferences about these smaller groups.

[5] See the description on the NCHS website for the National Health Interview Survey and the NHANES.

[6] The sampling fraction is the ratio of sample size to population group size for a particular cluster of individuals.

[7] STATA, SPSS, and SAS-SUDAAN all allow for taking complex survey designs into account in the analysis using special subroutines.

probability sampling in health research, most clinical studies rely on convenience samples ("we take any patient we can get, who meets our eligibility criteria"), in which case one *cannot* use statistical methods to make inferences about the target populations.

There is, however, a third source of randomness in health care studies: measurement error. Anyone, who has taken BP measures on particular patients, knows that the readings of diastolic and systolic BP vary from one occasion to the next, both because a patient's actual BP varies (due to having taken a prior meal, having slept insufficiently, being nervous, etc.) and because the measurement procedure itself is error prone (using different arms, using different cuff pressure, using different instruments, etc.). In addition, even with the best quality controls, errors in data entry cannot always be avoided. Because of this lack of **reliability** in measurement, we often require several measures before we have sufficient confidence in the results. All clinical tests and data have a certain degree of unreliability (presence of measurement error), and when we employ statistical models, we must take account of this unreliability as it is a component of every individual score. In this book, we discuss a few classic statistical measurement models that incorporate the assumption of random measurement error.

Considering the major sources of random error, it should be apparent that no data are without some random error. Thus, it is always appropriate to use inferential statistical methods, even with data from a convenience sample of an observational study. However, it is important to understand what **statistical significance** and **confidence intervals** (CIs) mean under the various circumstances:

1. In a randomized experiment, the main source of random error is the random assignment process itself; thus, a "statistically significant" effect is one that is unlikely to be the result of mere random assignment.

2. In an observational study using simple or complex probability samples from a large target population, the primary source of random error is the sampling process; thus, a "statistically significant" correlation pattern is one that is unlikely to be the result of mere random sampling.

3. Finally, in an observational study based on a convenience sample, a "statistically significant" pattern is one that is unlikely to be the result of mere random measurement error. But note, in the latter case, statistical inference cannot be used to support causal conclusions, nor inferences about larger target populations.

In all of these situations, *nonsignificant* results should be treated with extreme caution: They may just indicate a nonrepeatable, inconsequential pattern and nothing more than that.

SUMMARY

The appropriateness of any statistical model depends on the degree to which the data meet the assumptions of the model. When we employ a statistical test to draw causal inferences about the effectiveness of an intervention, it is not enough that we find "significant differences" between an intervention and a control group after the intervention has taken place. The validity of the significance test in this situation is based on the assumption that study participants were randomly assigned to the various intervention and control conditions (if there are more than two groups).

When we assert that women in their 40s have a significantly greater risk of breast cancer than women in their 30s, we assume that the study data on which we based our inference involved some form of probability sampling. Without it, the statistical inference from study samples to target populations and the CIs for our estimates are not valid.

Whenever we employ statistical tests and engage in statistical inferences, we make assumptions about the nature of the data we are dealing with. Some of these assumptions are based on the study and sampling designs that were employed to generate the data. Other assumptions involve the measurement models employed. Further assumptions pertain to the actual data and their empirical distribution in the target population of interest. As we will see later, assumptions about the shape of the data can, and must, be tested to see whether the data conform to the assumptions of the model used in a particular analysis.

In the following sections of this book, we focus broadly on three classes of statistical models, distinguished for the most part in terms of the characteristics of the dependent/outcome variable(s) involved. In particular, we focus on (a) linear models, often appropriate for the analysis of continuous outcome variables (Part II, Chapters 8–14); (b) models for categorical outcome measures (Part III, Chapters 15–18); and (c) models for time-to-event-, failure-, or survival-data (Part IV, Chapters 19 and 20). We also include (d) statistical models for the evaluation of measurement properties and measurement error (Part V, Chapters 21 and 22), as measurement is an integral part of both research and clinical evaluations.

EXERCISES

1. In a nursing home, mattresses in one wing are of Brand A and in another wing are of Brand B. Data collected over a year show nursing home residents in the rooms of wing A are 40% more likely to experience bed sores than residents of the same nursing home in rooms of wing B. Is this sufficient evidence that Brand A mattresses are inferior to Brand B mattresses? Why or why not?

2. A website that promotes a nutrient supplement claims that the supplement reduces attention deficit hyperactivity disorder. The claim is based on the fact that 87% of the users who responded to an online survey at the website, reported that their ability to concentrate and do work had substantially improved after 2 weeks of taking the supplement.
   (a) Is that sufficient evidence of the effectiveness of the supplement?
   (b) Suppose these testimonials reflect the experience of *all* persons who took the supplement. Is that sufficient evidence of its effectiveness? Explain why or why not?

3. Researchers (Stommel, Olomu, Holmes-Rovner, Corser, & Gardiner, 2006) have attributed historical improvements in the survival of postdischarge ambulatory-care-sensitive patients to *quality improvement in care* between 1994 and 2003. Read the article and make a list of all possible *alternative* hypotheses that may account for why survival rates have improved over this 10-year span.

4. List as many sources of measurement error as possible when it comes to measuring a patient's BP.

REFERENCES

Centers for Disease Control and Prevention (CDC). (2012). *Second national report on biochemical indicators of diet and nutrition in the U.S. population 2012.* Retrieved from http://www.cdc.gov/nutritionreport/pdf/ExeSummary_Web_032612.pdf

Friedman, L. M., Furberg, C. D., & DeMets, D. L. (2010). *Fundamentals of clinical trials* (4th ed.). St. Louis, MO: Springer.

Horodynski, M., & Stommel, M. (2005). Nutrition Aimed at Toddlers (NEAT): Results from an intervention study. *Pediatric Nursing, 31*(5), 364–372.

Polit, D. F., & Beck, C. T. (2003). *Nursing research: Principles and methods* (7th ed.). Philadelphia, PA: Lippincott Williams & Wilkins.

Shadish, W. R., Cook, T. D., & Campbell, D. T. (2002). *Experimental and quasi-experimental designs for generalized causal inference.* Boston, MA: Houghton Mifflin Comp.

Stommel, M., & Wills, C. (2004). *Clinical research.* Philadelphia, PA: Lippincott Williams & Wilkins.

Stommel, M., Olomu, A., Holmes-Rovner, M., Corser, W., & Gardiner, J. C. (2006). Changes in practice patterns affecting in-hospital and post-discharge survival among ACS patients. *BMC Health Services Research, 6*, 140.

PART II. MODELS FOR CONTINUOUS/ INTERVAL-LEVEL OUTCOME MEASURES

CHAPTER 8

t-Test

In this section of the book, we discuss statistical models for continuous outcome or dependent variables. A *continuous* variable is one that, in principle, can take on any value within some range. However, in practice, all *measured* variables are *discrete*, as the precision of measurement is always limited by the measurement tool at hand. Take, for instance, time or age. Theoretically, we could divide time into nanosecond intervals, but practically this would be a complete waste of effort: The precision of measurement should depend on the purposes of measurement. Thus, in many health-related studies we measure the age of individual adults in years, those of babies sometimes in months or even weeks, but never in minutes or seconds. In practice then, even variables that are theoretically continuous end up as discrete numbers in our data sets. Important for the models in this section of the book is only that the outcome or dependent variables take on sufficiently many distinct values, so that they can "mimic" continuous variables. As a rule of thumb, we should not apply the statistical models for continuous variables presented in this section of the book to outcome variables with less than 8 to 10 distinct values.[1] In Part III of this book, we introduce other models that can be used instead, if outcome variables have fewer values. The other common property required for the application of the statistical models discussed in Part II is that the outcome variables should be measured at the interval or ratio levels of measurement. This, too, is implied in the use of models that employ as their basic building blocks means and variances. In fact, as the discussion of the *t*-test shows, it is just one member of the "family" of linear statistical models, which all share the assumption that means and variances can be computed and be given a meaningful interpretation when applied to the test variables in question.

VARIETIES OF *t*-TESTS

The *t*-test is one of the most commonly used statistical tests in the nursing and medical literature. The *t*-test is employed to determine, if two mean scores should be considered equal or different from each other. It comes in three versions:

1. The **one-sample** *t*-test compares a study sample mean to some predetermined or hypothesized population mean value.

---

[1] Just for starters: It makes no sense to assume that the error terms in statistical models come close to a normal distribution, if they can take on only very few discrete values.

2. The **independent-sample** t-test compares mean scores in two different groups, such as male and female patients or subjects in the treatment and control group of a randomized trial.

3. The **paired-sample** (dependent-sample) t-test compares mean scores for the same group of subjects measured at two different occasions/times.

The t-test is an *inferential* statistical test. Thus, the comparison of means envisioned here involves more than the calculation and description of two particular sample means. That would just be a matter of simple algebra. As we have seen in Part I of this book, the value of a statistical test is that it gives us a *context* in which we can interpret a particular sample result. That context involves assumptions about how a particular data set was generated. Thus, when we interpret results from a t-test, it matters whether we are analyzing data from an *experimental* study with *prior random assignment* of subjects to treatment and control group,[2] or data from an *observational* study with *random sample selection*,[3] or data from a *nonexperimental* study using a *convenience sample*.[4]

THE ONE-SAMPLE t-TEST

This version of the t-test is not often employed in the research literature but it does have its uses, as when we compare a sample mean on a measure of interest to existing population norms. For instance, Humphreys, Lee, Neylan, and Marmar (2001) compared mean scores on the subscales of Derogatis's Brief Symptom Inventory to means from a normative population; or Horsted, Rasmussen, Meyhoff, and Nielsen (2007) compared mean scores on the SF-36 subscales, which measure physical and psychological functioning, to Danish population norms. In such situations, researchers start with a hypothesized population value of a mean score and test, if the observed study sample mean is consistent with the hypothesized population mean. In effect, researchers would be asking whether the study sample could have been a random sample drawn from this population.

In order to conduct the test, we need the following information:

1. Observed sample mean, $\bar{x}$

2. Observed sample standard deviation, s

3. Sample size, n

As we already saw in Chapter 6, with this information in hand we can estimate the standard error of the mean (SEM), $s/\sqrt{n}$. In turn, this would allow us to construct relevant confidence intervals (CIs) as well as hypothesis tests. However, for the t-test to be validly applied, the data must meet several assumptions (see Box 8.1). Most of these assumptions can actually be tested using the data at hand, as long as the sample size is reasonably large.

---

[2]The classic example would be the randomized clinical trial.

[3]The best examples in the health care field would be the surveys conducted by the National Center for Health Statistics, such as the National Health Interview Survey or National Health and Nutrition Examination Survey, whose purpose is to obtain health-related information from representative samples of the U.S. resident population.

[4]Many observational clinical studies rely on study samples from particular clinical settings, which may or may not be representative of larger patient target populations.

The first assumption concerning the interval level of measurement of the test variable derives from the simple fact that the *t*-test requires the calculation of sample means and sample standard deviations. The second assumption refers to the requirement that individual test scores are independent of each other, that is, that the score of some individual (*i*) does not influence or predict the score of another individual (*j*). In addition, the *t*-test presupposes that the test variable approximates a normal distribution in the *population* from which the sample is drawn. These assumptions for the valid application of the *t*-test are the same as those that underlie the *z*-test or normal-distribution test, which we already employed in Chapter 6.

BOX 8.1	ASSUMPTIONS OF THE ONE-SAMPLE *t*-TEST

1. Interval/ratio level of measurement for test variable
2. Independence of individual observations (uncorrelated error terms)
3. Normally distributed variable in population
4. Randomly drawn sample

What, then, is the difference between the *t*-test and the *z*-test? If the data meet all the assumptions listed in Box 8.1 and we have *prior knowledge of* the size of the *population* standard deviation σ, then we can indeed employ the *z*-test to test for mean differences, regardless of sample size. Recall, however, from Chapter 6 that, in most situations, we do not know the population standard deviation and have to *estimate* it from a single study sample. In that case, the use of the normal distribution is only legitimate for reasonably large study samples: We used $n > 120$ as a benchmark. When we estimate the SEM using information from a particular study sample, we introduce additional uncertainty into our estimates, as sample standard deviations are subject to sampling fluctuations as well. It is for this reason that we employ the *t*-distribution, rather than the normal distribution, to mimic the shape of the sampling distribution of the mean.

The *t*-distribution was so named by its inventor William Gosset, who published it under his pen name "Student" (1908). It actually comprises a family of distributions, shaped very similar to that of the normal distribution (see the graphs in Figure 8.1). Like the normal distribution, the *t*-distributions are completely symmetric, that is, the means of these distributions are also their medians and modes. The principle difference from the normal distribution is that *t*-distributions for small samples are somewhat flatter in the middle and have thicker tails. This is a reflection of the fact that the standard error estimates, $s/\sqrt{n}$, from small samples are subject to larger sampling fluctuations, resulting in the flatter shape of the distributions. However, for samples larger than $n = 120$, the *t*-distribution is barely distinguishable from the normal curve. As *n* grows in size, the *t*-distribution converges to the normal distribution.

Figure 8.1 shows two *t*-distributions, one with 2 "degrees of freedom" (df; in light gray), and the other with 6 "df" (in dotted line). Figure 8.1 also contains the standard normal distribution (in dark gray), $N(0, 1)$, for comparison. For all three of these probability distributions, the graphs show the 95% confidence limits. For instance, for the graph of the *t*-distribution with 6 df (dark curve), 95% of the area under the curve is encompassed within the limits of -2.45 and $+2.45$ standard errors. Thus, if we repeatedly drew random samples of size 7 (df $= 7 - 1 = 6$) from the same target population, the sampling distribution of the corresponding sample means would follow the shape of this *t*-distribution, with 95% of all

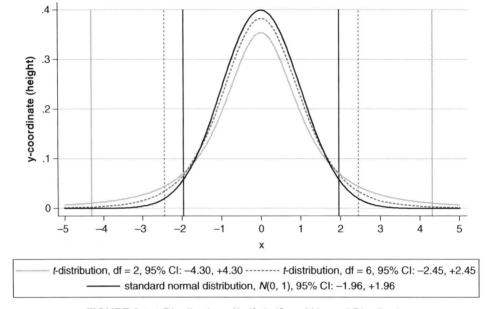

FIGURE 8.1 t-Distributions (2 df, 6 df) and Normal Distribution.

sample means falling within ±2.45 standard errors of the population mean. Similarly, for means of samples of size 3 (df = 3 − 1 = 2), we would expect the sampling distribution to follow the t-distribution with 2 df (light gray). This distribution has a much wider 95% CI with limits of ±4.30 standard errors.

In practice, we do not have to calculate the appropriate t-values and their associated probabilities from graphs like in Figure 8.1. We either use tables, like the one in Appendix C, or standard statistical software packages to obtain the appropriate values. As we already noted, with increasing sample sizes (and degrees of freedom), the t-distribution converges toward the normal distribution. Already at 120 df, the 95% confidence limits are very similar to those of the normal distribution: ±1.98 for the t-distribution (with 120 df) versus ±1.96 for the normal distribution; the 99% CI limits are ±2.62 for the t-distribution (with 120 df) versus ±2.58 for the normal distribution. Because of this convergence of the t-distribution and normal distribution for larger df, statistical software does not distinguish between t-tests and tests based on the normal distribution: with higher df, the normal distribution is automatically "built into" the t-distribution tests.

Conducting a One-Sample t-Test

If our data meet the assumptions for the one-sample t-test, all we need to do is construct the relevant test statistic. In the one-sample test, we compare a sample mean, $\bar{x}$, calculated from observed data, to the hypothesized population mean, μ, and divide the difference between the two numbers by the *estimated* SEM: $(\bar{x} - \mu) / (s/\sqrt{n})$. This expression is the t-value we need to calculate the associated probability or p-value. The ratio expresses the difference between the observed sample mean and the hypothesized population mean in terms of the number of standard errors by which they differ. As the t-distributions also show distances from their means in terms of standard errors (Figure 8.1), we can use them to figure out the probabilities that an observed t-value exceeds any particular number.

TABLE 8.1 One-Sample *t*-Test

```
One-sample t-test
-------------------------------------------------------------------
Variable  |    Obs    Mean    Std. Err.   Std. Dev.   [95% Conf.   Interval]
--------+----------------------------------------------------------
birthwgt  |    100   7.2952   .1284983    1.284983    7.040232    7.550168
-------------------------------------------------------------------
    mean = mean(birthwgt)                                 t =    -1.4382
Ho: mean = 7.48                          degrees of freedom =        99

    Ha: mean ≠ 7.48
Pr(|T| > |t|) = 0.1535
```

Here is how it is done: Suppose we have birth-weight data from a sample of 100 newly born babies. We want to know if this sample comes from a target population that is similar to the overall U.S. population, with a mean birth weight of 7.48 pounds (CDC, 2012). All we need now is information on the relevant sample data. Table 8.1 shows the results from a STATA run.

For the variable "birthwgt" (birth weight in lbs) we have $n = 100$ observations (Obs = size of sample) with a mean birth weight of 7.2952 pounds. The sample standard deviation equals 1.284983. With a sample size of exactly 100, the estimated SEM equals: $s/\sqrt{n} = 1.284983/\sqrt{100} = 0.1284983$. Now, we want to test if the observed sample mean of 7.2952 is consistent with our hypothesis that the sample comes from a population with a true mean of 7.48. Thus, our null hypothesis is $H_0: \bar{x} = \mu = 7.48$.[5] Our alternative hypothesis, H_A, is that our sample does not come from a population with mean 7.48. As we cannot know prior to having seen the data whether the sample mean will be smaller or larger than the hypothesized population mean, we state our alternative hypothesis as follows: $H_A: \bar{x} - \mu \neq 0$.

In short, we test the null hypothesis against the alternative hypothesis that the sample does not come from a population with mean 7.48, without specifying whether the difference will be positive or negative.

Before commencing with the calculations, we must also specify the significance level, that is, the risk that we commit a Type I error, if we reject the null hypothesis. Let us use the conventional significance level of $\alpha = 0.05$. From the *t*-distribution table in Appendix C, we learn that there is a 5% (two-sided) probability that *t*-values could be smaller than -1.984 or larger than $+1.984$ as a result of mere random sampling.[6]

Now, we are ready for the final test. Table 8.1 shows the observed sample mean to be equal to 7.295; thus, the difference between the sample mean and the hypothesized population mean is: $\bar{x} - \mu = 7.2952 - 7.48 = -0.1848$. Dividing this difference by the estimated SEM yields our test statistic: $t = (\bar{x} - \mu)/(s/\sqrt{n}) = (-0.1848)/0.1284983 = -1.4382$. The absolute value of this *t*-value is *smaller* than the *t*-value corresponding to the 0.05 significance level. That implies that the observed sample mean differs from the hypothesized population mean by less than the critical value; so we will *not* reject the null hypothesis. In fact, Table 8.1 shows that the probability that a random sample from a population with mean $\mu = 7.48$ produces a sample mean of $\bar{x} = 7.2952$, thus differing from the population mean by at least ± 1.4382 standard errors, is equal to .1535.

---

[5] Of course, this implies that $\bar{x} - \mu = 0$.

[6] As $n = 100$, df $= n - 1 = 99$. Appendix C only shows the *t*-values and probabilities for df $= 100$, instead of df $= 99$. However, the differences are so small that they can be neglected in practice. Using the STATA software, the actual *t*-values corresponding to a two-sided significance level of 0.05 for the *t*-distribution with 99 df are ± 1.984217.

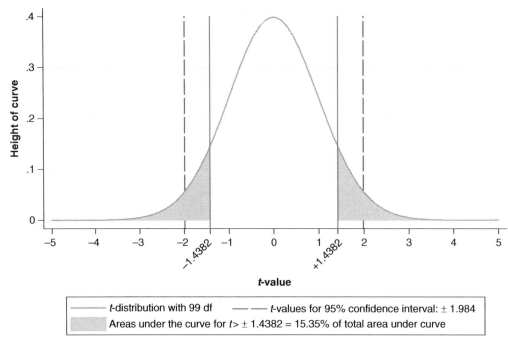

FIGURE 8.2 *t*-Distribution With 99 Degrees of Freedom (df).

Figure 8.2 provides a graphical illustration of this one-sample *t*-test. It shows the *t*-distribution with 99 df, which is centered on the null value of H_0: $\bar{x} - \mu = 0$. The solid vertical lines are located at the observed sample *t*-values of $t = \pm 1.4382$. The gray areas to the left and right of these *t*-values indicate the probability that a random sample might return a *t*-value exceeding the absolute magnitude of $|t| = |\pm 1.4382|$. That joint probability equals .1535, with separate probabilities of .07675 for the occurrence of *t*-values smaller than −1.4382 or larger than +1.4382. Figure 8.2 also shows the (dashed) vertical lines for the *t*-values corresponding to the significance level of 0.05 (or confidence level of 0.95). If the null hypothesis is true, then 95% of all random samples would return sample means that lie between ±1.984 standard errors of the null-hypothesis value. As we can see, the observed sample *t*-value lies inside the 95% confidence limits. Thus, we do not reject the null hypothesis because we want to limit the Type I error to 0.05.

Finally, Table 8.1 provides estimates for the limits of the 95% CI: the CI ranges from 7.040232 to 7.550168. As we have seen, 95% CIs for a *t*-distribution with 99 df are bounded by *t*-values of ±1.984. Thus, as long as sample means do not differ by more than 1.984 standard errors from the (hypothesized) population mean, they fall within the 95% CI. With our estimate for the SEM being 0.1284983 (Table 8.1), we can now construct the 95% CI:

$$\bar{x}_i - 1.984 \times \text{SEM} < \mu < \bar{x}_i + 1.984 \times \text{SEM}$$

$$7.2952 - 1.984 \times .1284983 > \mu < 7.2952 + 1.984 \times .1284983$$

$$7.2952 - 0.254968 < \mu < 7.2952 + 0.254968$$

$$7.040232 < \mu < 7.550168$$

Testing the Assumptions for the *t*-Test

Earlier in this book we emphasized that any statistical test is valid only if the data fit the assumptions of the test, at least in an approximate way. The *t*-test is actually a **robust test**, which means that some deviation from the normality assumption about the population distribution of the test variable is not a big problem. More specifically, a robust test will return *p*-values that are similar to the ones obtained, if all the assumptions of the test are fulfilled. Part of the reason for this robustness is due to the already-mentioned Central Limit Theorem (Chapter 5): Large samples produce sampling distributions that are close to normal in shape, even if the underlying population distributions are not normal. Nonetheless, with smaller samples in particular, outliers can have pronounced effects on the standard deviations computed from a study sample; likewise, substantial skew in distributions also leads to large increases in sample standard deviations. As a result, estimates of the SEM are also affected, making the *t*-test less powerful, as larger standard errors increase the chance of a Type II error. How then do we detect pronounced deviations from normality?

Essentially, there are two methods to discover deviations from normality in the population: graphical methods and statistical tests. In Chapter 3, we introduced the box-and-whisker plot (Figure 3.4), which offers an easy way to check for the existence of outliers and skew (or asymmetry) of a *sample* distribution. The histogram (Figure 3.6) also provides a way of checking for approximate normality of a *sample* distribution. Another common graphical device is the (cumulative) normal probability plot. It is constructed by first ordering the values of a particular variable from lowest to highest; then one computes the proportion of cases that fall below the lowest 1%, 2%, 3%, . . ., 100% of the empirical distribution; and, finally, one compares the cumulative proportions from the empirical distribution to the probability of occurrence expected in a normal distribution. The plot is constructed in such a way that under perfect congruence of the variable and the normal distribution, all data points should lie on a straight diagonal line, as the cumulative probability of the empirical and the ideal normal distribution would progress at the same rate. Figure 8.3 offers an example for the data with the birth weights of 100 babies. The figure shows that the empirical distribution mirrors that

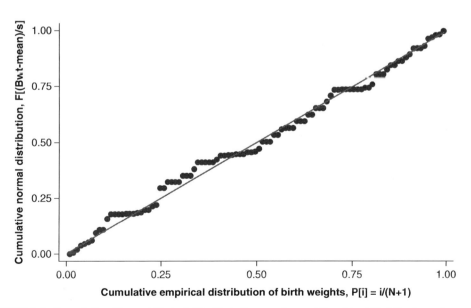

FIGURE 8.3 Cumulative Normal Probability Plot: Comparison of Empirical Distribution of 100 Birth Weights to Normal Distribution.

of the normal distribution quite closely: The increases in the cumulative proportions of cases in the empirical distribution are almost identical to those in the normal distribution; thus, no substantial skew or outliers can be observed.

Another way of testing the normality assumption would be to use a formal statistical test. Recall that the normality assumption refers to the distribution of a variable in the *population* from which the sample is drawn. As samples rarely reflect the population distributions exactly, some deviation from the normality assumption may well be within expected sampling chance. One test to use would be the Kolmogorov–Smirnov (K–S) test,[7] which compares the shape of an empirical sample distribution from a particular data set to an ideal distribution like the normal distribution. Its null hypothesis is that the sample data could have come from a normal distribution, with the alternative hypothesis that the sample data most likely come from a nonnormal distribution. Under this assumption, a p-value less than .05 would lead us to reject the null hypothesis, that is, it is unlikely that the sample comes from a cumulative normal distribution. For the baby weight data we find that $p > .682$, when testing the null hypothesis of the K–S test. Thus we accept that these data come from a normal population distribution.

There is, however, a caveat when using statistical tests to see whether sample data could have come from normal population data: If study samples are very small ($n < 30$), such tests lack the requisite power to detect deviations from normality; on the other hand, if study samples are quite large (say $n > 1000$), then even trivial deviations from normality are "statistically significant." Thus, there is no single foolproof test; however, the combination of graphical inspections and specific tests will alert us to major violations of the normality assumption.

THE INDEPENDENT-SAMPLE *t*-TEST

The independent-sample *t*-test is frequently encountered in the medical and nursing literature (Bentley, 2006; Dombrowski, Yoos, Neufeld, & Tarshish, 2012; Meydani et al., 2004). This version of the *t*-test compares *two* group means, with the null hypothesis being that the underlying population means are equal: $H_0: \mu_1 = \mu_2$ or $\mu_1 - \mu_2 = 0$. Here are the assumptions of this *t*-test:

BOX 8.2	ASSUMPTIONS OF THE INDEPENDENT-SAMPLE *t*-TEST

1. Interval/ratio level of measurement for test variable
2. Independence of individual observations (uncorrelated error terms)
3. Normally distributed variable within *both* populations compared
4. Equal variances (or standard deviations) within *both* populations
5. Randomly drawn sample

The independent-sample *t*-test is used with data from both randomized intervention studies (clinical trials) and observational studies. In the case of a randomized study, both groups come from the same population, with sample group differences due to the results of the randomization process. In the case of an observational group criterion, like sex, which cannot be randomly assigned, the groups come from separate populations in which the test variable may have differently shaped distributions. While it is advisable to test for the equality of variances (or standard deviations) prior to all group mean comparisons, this is particularly relevant in the comparison of two naturally occurring populations.

---

[7]Available in all common statistical software packages, for example, SPSS, STATA, and SAS.

Conducting an Independent-Sample *t*-Test

As with the one-sample *t*-test, we can test the normality assumption using the graphical and statistical testing methods outlined earlier. However, it is important to note that the normality assumption refers to the distribution of the test variable *within* each of the two groups being compared. Furthermore, when we estimate the SEM difference between the *two* comparison groups, we encounter an additional problem: With two groups, we could obtain two different estimates of population standard deviations. While we still use as our test statistic the mean difference between the two comparison groups divided by the standard error, $(\bar{x}_1 - \bar{x}_2)/\text{SE}$, the estimate of the SEM difference relies on a weighted sum of the two variances involved:

$$\text{SE} = \sqrt{\frac{s_1^2}{n_1} + \frac{s_2^2}{n_2}}$$

If the variances in the two groups are the same, then we estimate the SEM difference using a modified expression, which includes a single estimate of the sample standard deviation that is the square root of the weighted *average* of the two variances involved:

$$\text{SE} = \sqrt{\frac{(n_1 - 1)s_1^2 + (n_2 - 1)s_2^2}{n_1 + n_2 - 2}} \times \sqrt{\frac{1}{n_1} + \frac{1}{n_2}}$$

While it is not essential to remember the particular formulas for the estimation of the standard errors of the mean difference, it is important to check whether assumption 4 in Box 8.2 about equal variances in the comparison groups is violated. If yes, we need to modify the *t*-test accordingly. To see whether the assumption of equal variances holds for the two independent groups, we first conduct a test of the equality of *variances* between the two groups *before* applying the *t*-test for the equality of group *means*. This test of the equality of variances is also known as Levene's (variance-ratio) test.

Going back to the birth-weight data from a sample of 100 newly born babies, we find that 50 of these babies are female and 50 are male. We are interested in finding out whether the mean birth weights in these two groups differ in the populations from which they were drawn. *Prior* to applying the *t*-test, we conduct the Levene's variance-ratio *f*-test. The results are given in Table 8.2:

TABLE 8.2 Levene's *f*-Test of Equality of Variances Prior to *t*-Test of Equality of Means

Variance ratio test

Group	Obs	Mean	Std. Err.	Std. Dev.	[95% Conf.	Interval]
male	50	7.2892	.2029456	1.435042	6.881366	7.697034
female	50	7.3012	.1597898	1.129885	6.98009	7.62231
combined	100	7.2952	.1284983	1.284983	7.040232	7.550168

ratio = sd(male) / sd(female)   f =   1.6131
Ho: ratio = 1   degrees of freedom =   49, 49

Ha: ratio ≠ 1
2*Pr(F > f) = 0.0975

TABLE 8.3 Independent/Two-Sample *t*-Test of Equality of Means

```
Two-sample t-test with equal variances
------------------------------------------------------------------------
    Group |    Obs     Mean    Std. Err.   Std. Dev.   [95% Conf.   Interval]
----------+-------------------------------------------------------------
     male |     50   7.2892    .2029456    1.435042    6.881366    7.697034
   female |     50   7.3012    .1597898    1.129885    6.98009     7.62231
----------+-------------------------------------------------------------
 combined |    100   7.2952    .1284983    1.284983    7.040232    7.550168
----------+-------------------------------------------------------------
     diff |            -.012    .2583016               -.5245911   .5005911
------------------------------------------------------------------------
     diff = mean(male) – mean(female)                    t =    -0.0465
Ho:  diff = 0                             degrees of freedom =         98

Ha:  diff ≠ 0
Pr(|T| > |t|) = 0.9630
```

The only pieces of descriptive information in Table 8.2 that are relevant to the variance-ratio test are the two standard deviations of birth weight among male (1.435042) and female babies (1.129885). Squaring them gives us the respective variances: 2.059346 (male) and 1.276640 (female). If the variances are equal, as stipulated in the null hypothesis for this test, the ratio of the variances must be: $H_0 = 1$. The test statistic, which is a ratio of two variances, s_1^2/s_2^2, has a sampling distribution shaped like the F-distribution with 49 df in the numerator and 49 df in the denominator.[8] For the data in Table 8.2, we have $f = 2.059346/1.276640 = 1.6131$. Here we only ask: What is the probability of observing a sample *f*-ratio as large as 1.6131, if the null hypothesis is true, which would imply the *f*-ratio in the respective target *population* is equal to 1? Table 8.2 provides the answer: $p = .0975$. As our conventional significance-level criterion of $\alpha = 0.05$ would lead us to reject the null hypothesis only if $p \le .05$, we accept H_0. Thus, for the subsequent *t*-test, we assume that the variances for birth weight are approximately equal among male and female babies in the population.

After this preliminary variance-ratio test, we are now ready to conduct the *t*-test for equality of group means. Table 8.3 provides the results from the independent-sample *t*-test, with equal variances assumed in both population groups.

Table 8.3 offers information on combined as well as separate descriptive statistics for the male and female babies. We learn that each gender group contains 50 babies, with mean birth weights of 7.2892 pounds among male and 7.3012 pounds among female babies, resulting in a difference of $7.2892 - 7.3012 = -0.012$. To get the relevant test statistic or *t*-value, we express this mean difference in terms of standard error units: $t = (\bar{x}_1 - \bar{x}_2)/SE = -0.012/0.2583 = -0.0465$. Then we locate this *t*-value on the relevant *t*-distribution, which, in this case, has 98 df. Recall from the earlier discussion that the df are generally computed as: sample size minus the number of population parameters to be estimated. In a two-sample *t*-test, we estimate two population means; thus, the df of this test equal: $df = n - 2$. In the example data, we get: $df = 100 - 2 = 98$. Locating a *t*-value of -0.0466 on the *t*-distribution with 98 df yields a *p*-value of $\ge.936$ (the software provides the *p*-value at the bottom of Table 8.3). In other words, if we were to *reject*

---

[8]More discussion on the *f*-distribution follows in Chapter 9 on one-way ANOVA.

the null hypothesis that there is no difference in the mean birth weight of the male and female babies, we would be almost certainly wrong, as the Type I error for a rejection of H_0 is >0.96. Thus, we accept the null hypothesis of no mean difference.

Table 8.3 also provides estimates for the 95% CI of the mean difference. The 95% CIs for a *t*-distribution with 98 df are bounded by *t*-values of ±1.9844675.[9] This yields the 95% CI for the mean difference in birth weight between male and female babies:

$$-0.12 - 1.9844675 \times 0.2583016 < \mu_m - \mu_f < -0.12 + 1.9844675 \times 0.2583016$$

$$-0.5245911 < \mu_m - \mu_f < 0.5005911$$

Notice, that the 95% CI contains the null value of 0. As the observed sample mean difference of −.012 differs very little from the null value, the null value lies inside the 95% CI, confirming that there is no "statistically significant" difference.[10]

Finally, if the Levene's variance-ratio test had led to the *rejection* of the null hypothesis that the *variances* in the comparison groups can be considered equal in magnitude, then we would still have proceeded with the *t*-test for the equality of means, but that test would use a *t*-distribution with *modified* df, known as Welch's test (Welch, 1947). Some software packages print out the *p*-values for the Levene's test and Welch's correction to the *t*-test automatically (SPSS), in others, it must be requested (STATA, SAS).

THE PAIRED-SAMPLE *t*-TEST

In the previous discussion of the independent-sample *t*-test, we introduced a statistical model that rests on the assumptions listed in Box 8.2. For paired (or dependent) sample data, the assumption of independence of individual observations (or uncorrelated error terms) cannot be maintained. Such data often consist of repeated measures on the same individuals, as would be the case with a pretest–posttest design, where a sample of patients is first tested for their blood pressure, then asked to exercise 15 minutes on a treadmill, followed by a second reading of their blood pressure. Paired data may also involve purely observational data, as when measuring the height and weight of a sample of adolescents at two different times spaced 1 year apart. In either case, we would expect that the earlier and later measures taken from the same individual would be correlated. Paired or correlated data also arise with samples consisting of *matched pairs*, sharing an important characteristic with respect to the test variable. For instance, in a randomized block design for a hypertension intervention trial, researchers may want to make sure that, for each hypertensive female smoker aged 45 in the treatment group, there will be another individual with the same characteristics in the control group. Alternatively, in an observational study of nutrition, two children living in the same household would be expected to have similar ("correlated") diets. Given the lack of independence among paired observations, a modified version of the *t*-test is used to test for *changes* in mean scores over time or differences

---

[9]While df = $n - 2$ = 98, Appendix C shows the *t*-values and probabilities for df = 100, which are still "close enough." Using the STATA software, the actual *t*-values corresponding to a two-sided significance level of 0.05 for the *t*-distribution with 98 df are ±1.9844675.

[10]*Note*: The sample mean difference always lies within the 95% CI, as CIs are constructed around the sample estimates; however, the hypothesized null value of no mean difference may or may not lie within the CI, depending on how the sample data fall out.

TABLE 8.4 Sample Data for Paired t-Test: Two Diastolic Blood Pressure Readings Taken 2 Months Apart

ID	x_{i1} (TIME 1)	x_{i2} (TIME 2)	$D_i = x_{i2} - x_{i1}$	$D_i - \bar{D}$	$\sum(D_i - \bar{D})^2$
1	92	86	−6	0	$(0)^2 = 0$
2	94	90	−4	2	$(2)^2 = 4$
3	96	92	−4	2	$(2)^2 = 4$
4	98	92	−6	0	$(0)^2 = 0$
5	100	95	−5	1	$(1)^2 = 1$
6	102	91	−11	−5	$(-5)^2 = 25$
$n = 6$	$\bar{x}_{.1} = 97$	$\bar{x}_{.2} = 97$	$\bar{D} = -6$	$\sum(D_i - \bar{D}) = 0$	$\sum(D_i - \bar{D})^2 = 34$

in mean scores among *matched* pairs. This version of the t-test is also quite common in the clinical literature (Mallory, 2003).

The paired-sample t-test compares two mean scores for *related* or *paired* groups. In order to demonstrate the inferential logic of the paired t-test, we use a hypothetical example. Table 8.4 shows data from a small study of six hypertensive primary care patients, who are assumed to have taken a hypertension-reducing drug every day for a period of 2 months.

The table shows individual diastolic blood pressure (DBP) readings taken at time 1, before the drug therapy commenced (x_{i1}), and a second reading at time 2, 2 months into the therapy (x_{i2}). At the bottom of the table several descriptive statistics are listed, including the mean DBP before the start of the drug therapy $(\bar{x}_{.1} = 97)$, the mean DBP 2 months later, $(\bar{x}_{.1} = 91)$, and the mean change score, representing the average change or decline in *paired* DBP scores over 2 months $(\bar{D} = -6)$. The data in the fourth column indicate that the decline in DBP scores varies among individuals, from (-4) to (-11). In short, the decline is not uniform, but shows individual change D_i *deviates* from the mean change score of $\bar{D} = -6$. By definition, the sum of all these deviations must always be 0: $\Sigma(D_i - \bar{D}) = 0$. The column on the right adds the sum of *squared* deviations of individual change scores from their mean; this measure is the basic building block for the variance and standard deviation (see Chapter 3). While these descriptive results tell us the story about the individuals *in this particular sample*, we need again the inferential t-test to provide a context for judging if the observed mean decline in DBP scores is "statistically significant" and not just a sampling fluke.[11]

Given the available data, it is not difficult to construct the new test statistic. We start with the six pairs of difference or change scores constructed from the 12 DBP readings. We have seen that, in this particular sample, the mean change score is $\bar{D} = -6$. We now need to express the difference between the sample mean change score, $\bar{D}$, and the hypothesized population mean change score, μ_δ, in terms of the appropriate standard error. Recall that we estimate the SEM scores using the formula: $\text{SEM} = s/\sqrt{n}$. The only modification for the paired

---

[11] Again, the presence of measurement error and sample selection would likely produce different change scores in different samples.

TABLE 8.5 Paired-Sample *t*-Test of Equality of Means

Paired t-test						
Variable	Obs	Mean	Std. Err.	Std. Dev.	[95% Conf.	Interval]
time2	6	91	1.21106	2.966479	87.88687	94.11313
time1	6	97	1.527525	3.741657	93.07337	100.9266
diff	6	−6	1.064581	2.607681	−8.736593	−3.263407

$$\text{mean(diff)} = \text{mean(var2 - var1)} \qquad\qquad t = -5.6360$$

$$\text{Ho: mean(diff)} = 0 \qquad\qquad \text{degrees of freedom} = 5$$

$$\text{Ha: mean(diff)} \neq 0$$
$$\Pr(|T| > |t|) = 0.0024$$

t-test is that, instead of the sample standard deviation *s* of the original scores x_i, we use the sample standard deviation of the individual *difference* scores, D_i:

$$s_{D_i} = \sqrt{\frac{\sum(D_i - \bar{D})^2}{n-1}} = \sqrt{\frac{34}{5}} = 2.6077$$

The SEM *change scores*, SE_{Di}, then becomes: $\text{SE}_{D_i} = s_{D_i}/\sqrt{n}$. For the data in Table 8.3, we get $\text{SE}_{D_i} = s_{D_i}/\sqrt{n} = 2.6077/\sqrt{6} = 1.0646$. As the *t*-value for the paired *t*-test is defined as $t = (\bar{D} - \mu_\delta)/\text{SE}_{Di}$, our test statistic becomes:

$$t = (\bar{D} - \mu_\delta)/\text{SE}_{Di} = (-6 - 0)/1.0646 = -5.636$$

The null hypothesis, as usual, states that there is no real difference in mean diastolic blood pressure before and after the drug treatment. In other words, we assume that the true mean *change*, which we denote by the Greek symbols μ_δ ("mu of delta" or the population mean change), equals 0. However, in our data, the observed sample mean change of $\bar{D} = -6$ differs quite a bit from the hypothesized population mean change of $\mu_\delta = 0$: We now know that $\bar{D}$ is 5.636 standard errors below the hypothesized population mean of 0.

All that is now left to find is the probability that a sample *t*-value would exceed ±5.636. The appropriate *t*-distribution to answer this question has 5 df (df = 6 − 1 = 5), as we only estimate *one* population parameter, that is, the mean of the paired change scores, of which there are *n* = 6. The probability of exceeding $|t \pm 5.636|$ is very low, namely $p \leq .00244$. That is, less than two in a thousand random samples of size 6 would produce this result by chance alone. Our conclusion would be that the two DBP means do differ: There is a "statistically significant" decline in diastolic BP, with an average decline of −6. Table 8.4 summarizes the results.

A note of caution: The paired-sample *t*-test (Table 8.5) allows us to evaluate *average* change in a *group* between two time occasions. It is less well adapted to estimating *individual* change. For instance, assume somewhat different data in Table 8.4: A mean change score of $\bar{D} = -6$ could also have occurred, if individuals 2 and 3 had shown no change at all (0), while individuals 1 and 4 had change scores of (−10). Thus, from the mean change score, we will not know, if *all* or *most* individuals in the patient sample showed a decline in DBP. In Chapter 10, we discuss the Pearson correlation and apply it to this problem. As we will see then, a high correlation would indicate that most, if not all individuals in the sample experience a change in the same direction.

Assumptions of the Paired-Sample *t*-Test

Box 8.3 provides a short list of the main assumptions underlying the application of the paired *t*-test. The test statistic for the paired *t*-test involves individual change scores between two variables, for which we compute means and standard deviations. This requires at least an interval-level measurement of the original variables. The paired *t*-test also assumes that the individual change scores in the underlying population are normally distributed; otherwise, we cannot assume that the sampling distribution of the test statistic has the shape of a *t*-distribution. Even though the paired original variables are likely to be correlated, the paired *t*-test elegantly circumvents this problem, in that the two original variables are converted into a single individual change score variable. There is every reason to assume that the *change* scores of *different* individuals are independent of each other, meaning that the change in individual *i* does not influence the change in individual *j*. As always, generalization beyond a particular study sample requires that the study sample is a probability sample from a specified target population.

BOX 8.3	**ASSUMPTIONS OF THE PAIRED-SAMPLE *t*-TEST**

1. Interval/ratio level of measurement for test variable
2. Independence of individual change scores
3. Normally distributed change scores within population
4. Randomly drawn sample

SUMMARY

The *t*-test is a useful, and frequently used, inferential statistical test that allows us to determine whether *two* sample means (paired or unpaired) come from populations with the same or different means. The *t*-test can also be used to determine whether a sample mean differs from a predetermined population mean. *t*-tests may be applied to observational data as well as randomized clinical trial data. In the latter case, the *t*-tests are often used to gauge the success of the randomization at baseline, or they may be used to determine whether the mean outcome scores in an intervention group differ from those in the control group. For all applications of the *t*-test, we assume an interval level of measurement of the test variable as well as approximately normally distributed test variables in the underlying populations. While the *t*-tests are robust, extreme skew or substantial outlier problems may invalidate the use of the *t*-distribution to obtain correct *p*-values. In those cases, researchers may sometimes be able to "normalize" skewed distributions (see Appendix D) or may choose alternative "distribution-free" or "nonparametric" tests, which do not make these assumptions. Chapter 16 introduces some of these alternative tests.

As the *t*-test can only be used in the comparison of two means, it remains limited in its applications. In the following chapter(s), we introduce several analysis-of-variance (ANOVA) and regression models, which can be considered generalizations of the *t*-test, allowing for the comparison and modeling of multiple mean outcomes.

LITERATURE APPLICATION

Read: Kim, I. S., Chung, S. H., Park, Y. J., & Kang, H. Y. (2012). The effectiveness of an aquarobic exercise program for patients with osteoarthritis. *Applied Nursing Research, 25*(1), 181–189.

(a) Provide a very brief (three to four sentences) summary of what this study is about.

(b) Define precisely the target population to which the statistical analysis can be generalized (be sure to mention ALL exclusion criteria applied).

(c) List all dependent/outcome variables, provide a clear definition of them, and determine their level of measurement.

(d) List the main independent/explanatory variable in the study.

(e) List all instances of *t*-tests in this article; formulate the null hypothesis for each test and state in a sentence what the associated probability value indicates.

(f) In Table 5, the authors show "changes in dependent variables between the experimental and control groups"; however, the authors did not conduct paired *t*-tests, but independent-sample *t*-tests. What outcome measures were compared across the two groups?

(g) Given the information in the column titled "diff" in Table 5, perform separate paired *t*-tests within the experimental and control groups. Are all paired *t*-tests "statistically significant" at the $\alpha = 0.05$ level?

EXERCISES

1. In a preliminary study of a new antihypertensive drug, researchers obtained a baseline mean diastolic BP of 94 mmHg. After 4 weeks of taking the new drug, these same patients had a mean diastolic BP of 86. The standard deviation of this mean difference was SD = 26 and the total study sample had a size of $n = 169$ patients. Which of the following conclusions is correct?
   (a) The findings are statistically significant: We can reject the null hypothesis that the mean diastolic BP did not decline over time.
   (b) Given the information provided, we cannot compute the relevant *t*-value.
   (c) The standard error of the test statistic (mean difference) is 26; thus, the *t*-value is $-0.31 (= -8/26)$.
   (d) As the *t*-value equals -4.0 and the probability of such a *t*-value occurring by chance is less than 1 in 1,000, we conclude that the decline in diastolic BP measures is just a random occurrence, and not "for real."
   (e) The 95% CI for the test statistic includes the null value of 0. Thus we conclude that the antihypertensive drug treatment is effective.

2. You have the following information about a random sample of adult Michigan Medicaid recipients: The mean sample weight of 900 randomly chosen subjects is 145 pounds, and the sample variance of the weight variable is 441. Which of the following values show the 95% CI for the mean weight of the target population (adult Michigan Medicaid recipients)?
   (a) 145 ± 1.121
   (b) 145 ± 1.8

    (c) 145 ± 1.372
    (d) 145 ± 1.764
    (e) 145 ± 2.178

3. The Central Limit Theorem asserts:
    (a) That the distribution of variables in the population follows the normal distribution, if populations are large
    (b) That the distribution of sample means follows the distribution of sample values
    (c) That the distribution of variables in the study sample follows the normal distribution if samples are large
    (d) That the sampling distribution of the mean of large samples is normally distributed, even if the population distribution of the variable in question is not normally distributed
    (e) Normality of variables can be assumed, when we have a large number of samples

4. The following table shows the weights of 10 individuals, who enrolled in a physical exercise class scheduled three times a week for 2 months, at the time of enrollment.

SEX	WEIGHT AT TIME 1	WEIGHT AT TIME 2
1	78	74
1	59	56
1	62	57
1	64	62
1	71	65
2	93	90
2	78	79
2	69	65
2	82	79
2	86	81

    (a) Using a hand calculator, compute the t-value to test the null hypothesis that there is no statistically significant difference between the average weight of women (sex = 1) and men (sex = 2) at time 1.
    (b) Using a hand calculator, compute the t-value to test the null hypothesis that there is no statistically significant difference between the average weight of women (sex = 1) and men (sex = 2) at time 2.
    (c) Using a hand calculator, compute the t-value to test the null hypothesis that there is no statistically significant difference between the average weight of women (sex = 1) at time 1 and time 2.
    (d) Using a hand calculator, compute the t-value to test the null hypothesis that there is no statistically significant difference between the average weight of men (sex = 2) at time 1 and time 2.
    (e) Using a hand calculator, compute the t-value to test the null hypothesis that there is no statistically significant difference between the average weight of all individuals (men and women) at time 1 and time 2.

Notes:
1. For all tests, the statistical significance criterion is $\alpha = 0.05$.
2. The *t*-distribution table in Appendix C shows the appropriate cut-off points. (*Tip*: Make sure to choose the *t*-distribution with the appropriate df.)
3. Check your results using a statistical software of your choice (SPSS, Minitab, STATA, SAS, etc.) or Microsoft Excel.

REFERENCES

Bentley, R. (2006). Comparison of traditional and accelerated baccalaureate nursing graduates. *Nurse Educator*, *31*(2), 79–83.

Centers for Disease Control and Prevention (CDC). (2012). Births: Final data for 2012. *National Vital Statistics Reports*, *61*(1), 1–72.

Dombrowski, W., Yoos, J. L., Neufeld, R., & Tarshish, C. Y. (2012). Factors predicting rehospitalization of elderly patients in a postacute skilled nursing facility rehabilitation program. *Rehabilitation*, *93*(10), 1808–1813.

Gosset, W. S. (Student). (1908). The probable error of a mean. *Biometrika*, *6*(1), 1–25.

Horsted, T. I., Rasmussen, L. S., Meyhoff, C. S., & Nielsen, S. L. (2007). Long-term prognosis after out-of-hospital cardiac arrest. *Resuscitation*, *72*(2), 214–218.

Humphreys, J., Lee, K., Neylan, T., & Marmar, C. (2001). Psychological and physical distress of sheltered battered women. *Health Care for Women International*, *22*(4), 401–414.

Mallory, J. L. (2003). The impact of a palliative care educational component on attitudes toward care of the dying in undergraduate nursing students. *Journal of Professional Nursing*, *19*(5), 305–312.

Meydani, S. N., Leka, L. S., Fine, B. C., Dallal, G. E., Keusch, G. T., Singh, M. F., & Hamer, D. H. (2004). Vitamin E and respiratory tract infections in elderly nursing home residents. *The Journal of the American Medical Association*, *292*(7), 828–836.

Welch, B. L. (1947). The generalization of "Student's" problem when several different population variances are involved. *Biometrika*, *34*(1/2), 28–35.

CHAPTER 9

One-Way Analysis of Variance

In the last chapter, we introduced the *t*-test, a statistical model for comparing the magnitudes of two mean scores. While often useful, it is a model of limited applicability. For many health-related studies, we need models to examine more complex data patterns. For example, in the classic pretest/posttest randomized control group design, we end up with two baseline mean scores (intervention and control group) and two posttest mean scores (again for the intervention and control group) after the experimental stimulus has been administered (Oenema, Burg, & Lechner, 2001). Thus, to take full advantage of the data generated by such a study, we would need to be able to evaluate simultaneously all the patterns arising among four mean scores. Other common study designs in the nursing and medical literature involve even more measurements: many intervention studies have repeated follow-up measures (within-subjects variation), commonly between two and six such measures (Manchikanti, Cash, McManus, Pampati, & Fellows, 2012). Randomized controlled trials involve often more than just two comparison groups (between-subjects variation), for example, when the intervention arm is split into multiple groups distinguished by different treatment combinations or different dosages of a drug they receive (Suh, 2012), or the intervention consists of a combination of different treatments or drugs all of which are tested simultaneously in a single study (Epstein, Sidani, Bootzin, & Belyea, 2012). Such studies may also have several outcome variables to keep track of. Many observational studies also have more complex designs. For instance, panel studies are a major source of information about the health states of individuals, as they involve following individuals over lengthy time periods, allowing us to observe patterns of growth and decline (Soto-Campos, 2007). In short, we need a generalized method of comparing means scores in multiple groups and over multiple occasions within groups.

One important class of statistical models for continuous outcome/dependent variables that can accommodate all the mentioned complications is the **analysis of variance (ANOVA)** model. All of the ANOVA models are based on the principle of *decomposition of variance*, hence the name ANOVA. In this chapter, we demonstrate the basic idea of how variance is decomposed, starting with the simplest between-subjects model: the one-way ANOVA. This statistical model makes the same assumptions about the nature of the data as the independent-sample *t*-test (see Box 9.1).

To fix the idea of decomposition of variance, we present some made-up sample data, with numbers selected for computational convenience. Suppose that a randomized clinical trial of the effectiveness of a physical therapy intervention is being conducted among

BOX 9.1	ASSUMPTIONS OF THE ONE-WAY ANOVA

- Interval/ratio level of measurement for test variable
- Independence of individual observations (uncorrelated error terms)
- Normally distributed variable in population groups compared
- Equal variances (or standard deviations) within *all* comparison populations
- Randomly drawn/assigned study sample

10 elderly residents of an assisted-living facility. The goal of the study is to see whether the intervention has an effect on alleviating physical impairments, measured as the number of functional limitations in activities of daily living (ADL). (In this case, 11 activities such as dressing oneself, eating, or walking are considered. That means a person's impairment score can vary from 0 [no limitation in ADL] to 11 [need for assistance in all ADL].) Five nursing home residents are exposed to a daily hour of tailor-made exercises with a physical therapist for 3 months (intervention group). Five other nursing home residents participate daily in a card game club (control group). Assignment to either group is based strictly on the luck of the coin.[1] In the following, we consider only two variables:

- The independent variable or factor[2] is symbolized as X_g, which indicates the treatment exposure: g takes on two values—1 = intervention (physical therapy) group, 2 = control (card game) group.

- The dependent variable Y_{ig} is a score that represents a count of the functional impairments in ADL for each study participant at the end of the study period: i is a subscript for the individual study participant (in this example, case numbers vary from 1 through 10) and g represents again the exposure group an individual belongs to.

Table 9.1 contains the data and a few calculations necessary for the analysis. Our main goal is to show that the *mean* number of ADL impairments among residents who received the physical therapy intervention is *lower* than the *mean* impairment score among residents who participated in the card-playing club. We accomplish this goal by the establishing to what extent ADL impairment scores vary systematically according to treatment exposure. As the *Y*-values in Table 9.1A show, there are substantial differences in impairment scores among the 10 individuals. This between-subjects variation is to be expected, as each resident brings unique physical attributes and health histories to the situation. In addition, it is unlikely that all individuals, exposed to the same therapy, would show exactly the same reaction. Then there is the problem of measurement: Establishing whether or not a nursing home resident should be considered "dependent" in an activity like eating or walking is, to some extent, a judgment call. Thus, even trained observers might disagree in a particular case.[3] For all these reasons, it is not surprising to find lots of between-subjects variation in ADL impairment scores. If we want to make sense out of these data, we need to find a way of distinguishing "systematic"

---

[1]Particularly with a small sample, researchers would normally use blocked randomization to reduce across-group variability of other important predictor variables such as age.

[2]In experimental studies, the independent variable is often called the independent "factor."

[3]However, the use of multiple observers/judges allows us to estimate the consistency and thus the *reliability* of such judgments; see Chapter 21 for more on measurement reliability.

TABLE 9.1 Data for Study on the Impact of a Physical Therapy Intervention on Physical Functioning Among Residents of an Assisted-Living Facility

(A) TOTAL SAMPLE (INTERVENTION + CONTROL GROUPS)				
ID	X_g	Y_{ig}	$(Y_{ig} - \bar{\bar{Y}}_{..})$	$(Y_{ig} - \bar{\bar{Y}}_{..})^2$
1	1	1	$1 - 6 = -5$	$(-5)^2 = 25$
2	1	3	$3 - 6 = -3$	$(-3)^2 = 9$
3	1	5	$5 - 6 = -1$	$(-1)^2 = 1$
4	1	7	$7 - 6 = 1$	$(1)^2 = 1$
5	1	9	$9 - 6 = 3$	$(3)^2 = 9$
6	2	3	$3 - 6 = -3$	$(-3)^2 = 9$
7	2	5	$5 - 6 = -1$	$(-1)^2 = 1$
8	2	7	$7 - 6 = 1$	$(1)^2 = 1$
9	2	9	$9 - 6 = 3$	$(3)^2 = 9$
10	2	11	$11 - 6 = 5$	$(5)^2 = 25$
		$\sum Y_{ig} = 60$	$\sum (Y_{ig} - \bar{\bar{Y}}_{..}) = 0$	$\sum (Y_{ig} - \bar{\bar{Y}}_{..})^2 = 90$

Total sample (grand) mean: $\bar{\bar{Y}}_{..} = \frac{1}{n}\sum Y_{ig} = 60/10 = 6$

(B) SUBJECTS EXPOSED TO PHYSICAL THERAPY (INTERVENTION GROUP 1)				
ID	X_1	Y_{i1}	$Y_{i1} - \bar{Y}_{.1}$	$(Y_{i1} - \bar{Y}_{.1})^2$
1	1	1	$1 - 5 = -4$	$(-4)^2 = 16$
2	1	3	$3 - 5 = -2$	$(-2)^2 = 4$
3	1	5	$5 - 5 = 0$	$(0)^2 = 0$
4	1	7	$7 - 5 = 2$	$(2)^2 = 4$
5	1	9	$9 - 5 = 4$	$(4)^2 = 16$
		$\sum Y_{i1} = 25$	$\sum (Y_{i1} - \bar{Y}_{.1}) = 0$	$\sum (Y_{i1} - \bar{Y}_{.1})^2 = 40$

Intervention group 1 mean: $\bar{\bar{Y}}_{..} = \frac{1}{n}\sum Y_{ig} = 25/8 = 5$

(C) SUBJECTS EXPOSED TO CARD CLUB (CONTROL GROUP 2)				
ID	X_2	Y_i	$(Y_{i2} - \bar{Y}_{.2})$	$(Y_{i2} - \bar{Y}_{.2})^2$
6	2	3	$3 - 7 = -4$	$(-4)^2 = 16$
7	2	5	$5 - 7 = -2$	$(-2)^2 = 4$
8	2	7	$7 - 7 = 0$	$(0)^2 = 0$
9	2	9	$9 - 7 = 2$	$(2)^2 = 4$
10	2	11	$11 - 7 = 4$	$(4)^2 = 16$
		$\sum Y_{i2} = 35$	$\sum (Y_{i2} - \bar{Y}_{.2}) = 0$	$\sum (Y_{i2} - \bar{Y}_{.2})^2 = 40$

Control group 2 mean: $\bar{Y}_2 = \frac{1}{n_2}\sum Y_{i2} = 35/5 = 7$

variation in impairment scores, attributable to the treatment levels, from other, "unexplained" sources of variation in impairment scores.

A useful way to start is with a measure of the overall variation in the scores of the dependent variable. This is called the **total sum of squares** (**TSS**; see the last column of Table 9.1A: $\sum(Y_{ig} - Y..)^2 = 90$. In words, we subtract from each observed ADL impairment score Y_{ig} of individual i in group g the grand or overall sample mean, $\bar{\bar{Y}}$, square the difference, and sum over all individuals. This TSS is always a positive number, as all individual deviations from the sample mean are squared. In the limiting case, when all individuals have exactly the same score, the TSS is zero; but then, there is no variation to explain!

Next, we construct a measure that represents individual variation in Y_{ig} scores that is *not* accounted for by the treatment variable or factor. As individuals *within* each group or factor level are exposed to the *same* treatment (physical therapy *or* card-playing club), individual variation *within* each group *cannot* have been caused by the variation *of* the factor levels. We thus choose the **within-group sum of squares (WGSS)** as our measure of individual variation *unaccounted for by the factor* in question. The WGSS represents the sum of all squared deviations of individual scores of Y_{i1} and Y_{i2} from their respective factor level group means: $\bar{Y}_1$ and $\bar{Y}_2$ (see the last columns of Table 9.1B and C: $\sum(Y_{i1} - Y_{.1})^2 + \sum(Y_{i2} - Y_{.2})^2 = 40 + 40 = 80 = WGSS$).

Finally, we compute the amount of variation in Y_{ig} that *can* be attributed to X_g, also known as the **between-group sum of squares (BGSS)**. This measure can be obtained in *two* ways:

1. *Directly*, by summing the squared deviations of the group means from the grand mean for all cases in a group: $\sum(\bar{Y}_{.1} - Y_{..})^2 + \sum(\bar{Y}_{.1} - \bar{\bar{Y}}_{..})^2 = 5 \times (5 - 6)^2 + 5 \times (7 - 6)^2 = 5 + 5 = 10$.

2. *Indirectly*, by subtracting the WGSS (also called the "error sum of squares" or "unexplained sum of squares") from the TSS: TSS $-$ WGSS $=$ BGSS $\rightarrow 90 - 80 = 10$.

Look at what we have accomplished! We have divided the total variation in the scores of an outcome variable into two groups: explained and unexplained variation. The unexplained or "error" variation reflects individual differences among study participants regardless of which study arm they were assigned to. Because of the random assignment, we should expect that within-group variances of individual scores are quite similar in the two comparison groups. In fact, the ANOVA model makes the stronger assumption that scores *within factor levels* (i.e., within the groups defined by the factor) are normally distributed.

The explained variation captures the systematic differences in mean scores across treatment levels. The more the means differ, the larger the BGSS. If participants in a clinical trial are randomly assigned to their respective treatment levels *and* efforts are made to control the environment, *we are able to interpret the mean differences in causal terms*, as in a well-designed experiment the exposure to different treatment levels is the *only* systematic difference between subjects in the treatment and the control group.

There is one question that we have not yet addressed. Should we consider *any* difference in mean outcome scores as evidence of the causal effectiveness of the treatment? From our discussion of the *t*-test in the last chapter, we know that the answer is "no." Recall that after random assignment, some observed differences between the group *means* should be expected, as is reflected in the sampling distribution of such mean differences. Thus, what we need now is a variance-based test statistic, on the basis of which we can decide to what extent the observed differences between the comparison groups are likely to be the result of mere chance events.

In ANOVA, this test statistic is the ratio of two variances: the between-group variance divided by the within-group variance. This test statistic is also known as the *f*-ratio in honor of the statistician R. A. Fisher, who worked it out for the first time. How do we obtain estimates of the two variance measures? In general, variances are defined as *average squared deviations from a mean*, or in short *mean squares*. We already obtained measures of the *sums of squared deviations* (refer to the computations for BGSS and WGSS); the only remaining issue now is to divide these sums of squares by the appropriate numbers to get the mean squares.

When we estimate variances or mean squares from sample data, we divide the sum of squares not by *n*, the number of cases or observations in the sample, but instead, we divide by the **degrees of freedom**. The degrees of freedom are calculated by subtracting from the number of *independent* observations involved the number of population parameters to be estimated, which is the same as the number of *linear restraints* imposed on the independent observations. The concept of degrees of freedom is a frequent source of confusion, but its meaning can be illustrated in a straightforward manner (see Box 9.2).

BOX 9.2	THE CONCEPT OF DEGREES OF FREEDOM

In order to compute a *sum of squared deviations from a mean*, we must already know the mean. However, if the mean is given, it is easy to see that *only n − 1 deviations from the mean are free to vary, while the last deviation is fixed*. That is the linear constraint.

Example: Suppose you start with a sample of three numbers: 5, 7, and 9. The mean of these three numbers is 7. If we know that two of the numbers are 7 and 9 and all three numbers are subject to the constraint that their mean equals 7, then the third number must have the value of 5. In this sense, it is "fixed" and no longer free to vary.

Now we are ready to construct the test statistic, which helps us decide whether or not the observed differences in sample group means are "statistically significant" (see Table 9.2).

With the ANOVA model, the test for the mean differences between comparison groups is *indirect*. The test statistic consists of the ratio of the *systematic* or **between-group variance** in the numerator and the *error* or **within-group variance** in the denominator. Both variances are themselves ratios of the familiar sums of squares, BGSS and WGSS, and their requisite degrees of freedom (see the column titled "Mean Squares" in Table 9.2).

Let us take a closer look at the between-group variance. There are *k* group means; in this example *k* = 2, as we have only one treatment and one control group. These two group means are subject to one constraint: Together they must average out to the total sample mean. Thus, the associated degrees of freedom are *k* − 1, or 1 in the two-group case.

Now we look at the within-group variance. Its numerator (WGSS) actually combines two sums of squares calculated from data within the treatment and control groups. The computation of the WGSS for the five cases in the treatment group is subject to the constraint that their scores average out to the treatment group mean. The same constraint occurs within the control group. Consequently, the overall WGSS is subject to two constraints or, in general, to as many constraints as there are comparison groups. This leaves us with *n* − *k* degrees of freedom for the WGSS.

TABLE 9.2 ANOVA Table for a Single-Factor (Two-Groups) Between-Subjects Design

SUM OF SQUARES	DEGREES OF FREEDOM	MEAN SQUARES (VARIANCES)
BGSS = $\sum(\bar{Y}_{.1} - \bar{\bar{Y}}_{..})^2 + \sum(\bar{Y}_{.2} - \bar{\bar{Y}}_{..})^2 = 10$	$k - 1 = 2 - 1 = 1$	BGSS/$k - 1 = 10/1 = 10$
WGSS = $\sum(Y_{i1} - \bar{Y}_{.1})^2 + \sum(Y_{i2} - \bar{Y}_{.2})^2 = 80$	$n - k = 10 - 2 = 8$	WGSS/$n - k = 80/8 = 10$
TSS = $\sum(Y_{ig} - \bar{\bar{Y}}_{..})^2 = 90$	$n - 1 = 10 - 1 = 9$	TSS/$n - 1 = 90/9 = 10$
f-ratio = (BGSS/$k - 1$)/(WGSS/$n - k$) = 10/10 = 1; f-probability = .3466		

k, number of factor levels or group categories defined by the independent variable; n, number of cases in the sample.

The TSS is also subject to one constraint, as its computation already assumes a known sample mean. Its degrees of freedom are $n - 1$. Note how all the degrees of freedom for the variance components add up: Just like TSS = BGSS + WGSS, so does $n - 1 = k - 1 + n - k$.

We already emphasized the indirect nature of the ANOVA test statistic. The *f-ratio* is the ratio of the systematic or between-group variance (BGSS/$k - 1$) to the error or within-group variance (WGSS/$n - k$). It is now clear *that the greater the differences between the group means, the larger the between-group variance relative to the within-group variance.* If all group means in the sample are exactly equal, the between-group variance equals zero, and the *f*-ratio also equals zero. Of course, under conditions of random assignment, we do *not* expect all the group means to be *exactly* equal, *even if the null hypothesis is true and the intervention or treatment has no effect.* The reason for this is, of course, that mere random distribution of cases across the comparison groups is likely to make for some observable group differences. However, if the *f*-ratio grows larger and larger, it becomes less and less plausible to argue that mere random assignment produced it.

All we need to know now is the shape of the sampling distribution of *f*-ratios, computed from a large number of samples generated either through random assignment in an experiment or through random sampling from the same target population. If we know the shape of the sampling distribution, we can determine the probabilities that are attached to *f*-ratios of a given magnitude or larger. As Fisher and Yates (1938) have shown, the *f*-ratio follows the eponymous *f*-distribution, which is again a family of distributions whose exact shapes depend on the degrees of freedom in the numerator and denominator of the *f*-ratio. As with the *t*-distribution, the requisite probabilities can be obtained from tables (see Appendix E) or directly from statistical software. Figure 9.1 shows the *f*-distribution with one degree of freedom in the numerator and eight degrees of freedom in the denominator and the associated cut-off point for the 0.05 significance level.

With this information, we can now decide whether an observed *f*-ratio in a particular sample is likely or unlikely to occur, should the null hypothesis be true, that is, under the assumption that the intervention is not effective. If the observed *f*-ratio is associated with a probability of <.05, we would reject the null hypothesis using the customary significance level of $\alpha = 0.05$.

In our example (Table 9.2), the observed *f*-ratio is equal to 1. As can be seen from Figure 9.1, the critical *f*-value = 5.3177, meaning, for this *f*-distribution (df1 = 1, df2 = 8) only *f*-values equal to or larger than 5.3177 occur by chance in less than 5% of all random samples. With the observed *f*-ratio being smaller than the critical value, we would *not* reject the null hypothesis. In fact, as is shown in Table 9.2, the probability that a random sample

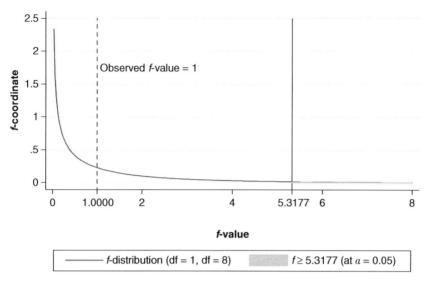

FIGURE 9.1 f-Distribution With Cut-Off for f-Value at $\alpha = 0.05$.

returns an f-ratio of 1 or larger is equal to .347. Thus, we conclude that the observed sample difference in group means of 2 (= 7 − 5) *is well within sampling chance*: Almost 35% of all random assignments alone would result in f-ratios of this magnitude or larger. It follows that we do *not* have strong evidence that the physical therapy intervention makes any difference. We would say that the observed differences between the groups fail to reach "statistical significance."

The reader might now wonder why we went through all the trouble of calculating a new, complicated test statistic, when in fact the t-test introduced in the last chapter could have done the job. In fact, it can be shown that for a *two*-group comparison, there is a simple relationship between the t- and the f-statistic: $f = t^2$.[4] Every other statistic associated with the t-test or the one-way ANOVA, from p-values to confidence intervals, is identical. However, as we already mentioned, the great virtue of the ANOVA approach is that *it is perfectly general* and applies to all kinds of complicated study designs. Just imagine a four-group comparison, as in a drug trial with one control group and three groups who get different dosages of the drug. The fundamental test of the effectiveness of the interventions would still be the f-statistic. Only this time, the WGSS and BGSS are calculated from four comparison groups. Otherwise, the logic is the same: Larger treatment effects translate into larger observed mean *differences* among the comparison groups, thus increasing the between-group variance relative to the within-group variance. When f-ratios become larger, the probability of a mere chance effect declines, and we become more confident in our conclusion that the treatment(s) must have produced real differences. This is the principle; everything else is just elaboration.

---

[4]This relationship between the t- and the f-statistic does *not* hold for models with more than 1 df in the numerator of the f-ratio.

ONE-WAY ANOVA WITH MULTIPLE GROUPS

We already mentioned that many clinical trials involve the comparisons of more than two groups. In addition, in both randomized trials and observational studies, it is common practice to compare mean scores for multiple groups defined by the categories of a nominal variable. Study participants' characteristics, such as race/ethnicity or marital status, are cases in point. For instance, we may be interested in knowing whether babies have different mean birth weights depending on whether they are non-Hispanic Caucasians, Latinos/Hispanics, African Americans, or part of some other ethnic group. Table 9.3 provides an example from a study of birth weights of 100 babies in low-income families.

The descriptive information in Table 9.3 tells us that the 41 non-Hispanic Caucasian babies in the study sample had the highest mean birth weight (7.56 lbs), followed by the 42 Hispanic babies (7.33 lbs), 3 babies from other ethnic groups (6.27 lbs), and 14 African American babies (6.26 lbs). Of course, a different sample drawn from the same target population would have given us somewhat different sample means. So the question arises: Do these data provide strong enough evidence for us to conclude that mean birth weights in the target population differ for babies from these four groups?

Just as with the t-test, before we apply the f-test, we must first establish whether the variances of the test variable can be considered equal across the four comparison groups. For the t-test, we used Levene's variance-ratio test; here we use Bartlett's equality of variance test, which is a chi-square test with three degrees of freedom. The null hypothesis for this test states that all within-group variances (or standard deviations) are equal. The observed p-value for this test is $p \geq .815$ (see Table 9.3). Thus, the probability that the null hypothesis is true is very high and we accept it and proceed to the f-test concerning the equality of group means.

The null hypothesis concerning the group means is H_0: $\mu_1 = \mu_2 = \mu_3 = \mu_4$, that is, the mean birth weights are the same among all four population groups. We would accept this null hypothesis, if the observed f-ratio is smaller than the critical value of $f = 2.699$, as only f-values *larger* than 2.699 occur by chance *less* than 5% of the time (see the f-distribution table in Appendix E).[5] Table 9.3 shows the observed f-value to be 4.44. The corresponding p-value is $p \leq .0058$ for the f-distribution with df1 = 3 and df2 = 96. Thus, we can reject the null hypothesis and conclude that *at least some of the group means* differ from each other significantly.

Having established that there are some group mean differences, we may want to know which group means differ from which other group means. As there are four groups, there are six independent pairwise comparisons possible,[6] which can be tested employing the standard independent-sample t-test. Table 9.3 shows all possible sample group mean *differences* and, underneath, a p-value associated with the null hypothesis that the mean difference in question is equal to zero. For example, the mean sample birth weight among African American babies

---

[5]Appendix E does not show f-values for the required f-distribution with df1 = 3 and df2 = 96; instead, it shows only the f-values for f-distributions with df1 = 3, df2 = 60 and df1 = 3, df2 = 120. The corresponding f-values are 2.758 and 2.680. A rough approximation can be obtained through linear extrapolation: $2.68 + (2.758 - 2.68) \times [(120 - 96)/(120 - 60)] = 2.711$. In practice, computer software will print out the exact f-value.

[6]$(4 \times 3)/2 = 6$; the pairs of group means are: 1–2, 1–3, 1–4, 2–3, 2–4, 3–4, where 1 = non-Hispanic Caucasian, 2 = Latinos/Hispanics, 3 = African American, 4 = Other ethnic group(s).

TABLE 9.3 One-Way Analysis of Variance

| Race/ Ethnicity | Summary of Child's birth weight (lbs) | | |
	Mean	Std. Dev.	Freq.
NH Cauc	7.557	1.2496	41
Lat/Hisp	7.334	1.2302	42
AfrAmer	6.259	1.1862	14
Other	6.273	1.8894	3
Total	7.243	1.3132	100

Analysis of Variance

Source		SS	df	MS	F	Prob > F
Between groups	(BGSS)	20.7825	3	6.9275	4.44	0.0058
Within groups	(WGSS)	149.9361	96	1.5618		
Total	(TSS)	170.7186	99	1.7244		

Bartlett's test for equal variances: chi2(3) = 0.9423   Prob>chi2 = 0.815

Comparison of Child's birthweight (lbsoz) by Race/Ethnicity
(Bonferroni)

Row Mean– Col Mean	NH/Cauc	Lat/Hisp	AfrAmer
Lat/Hisp	−.223 1.000		
AfrAmer	−1.298 0.007	−1.076 0.038	
Other	−1.284 0.535	−1.061 0.952	.015 1.000

is 1.298 lbs lower than among non-Hispanic Caucasian babies (7.557 − 6.259 = 1.298). The associated p-value is .007; thus, we reject the null hypothesis, as there is less than a 1% chance that this sample mean difference is a random occurrence. By contrast, all the mean differences involving the Other group are nonsignificant. This should not be surprising, as statistical tests involving samples of $n = 3$ lack the requisite power, even if the (descriptive) sample differences are large.

The results in Table 9.3 also show that differences among racial and ethnic groups account for 12.2% of the variation in babies' birth weight (BGSS/TSS = 20.7825/170.7186 = 0.1217). In ANOVA, this statistic (variance accounted for by an independent variable or variables) is known as **eta-squared (η^2)**. Thus, rejecting the null hypothesis for the f-test is equivalent to rejecting the null hypothesis that $\eta^2 = 0$.

MULTIPLE COMPARISONS AND THE APPROPRIATE
SIGNIFICANCE-LEVEL CRITERION

When we compare more than two groups, a new issue arises in statistical analysis: the effect that **multiple comparisons** have on the choice of appropriate significance levels. For the most part, we have employed the conventional significance level of $\alpha = 0.05$, meaning we were willing to accept a Type I error of 5% for our tests.[7] But when three or more comparison groups are involved, there are also additional **contrasts** that can be tested. For instance, in a study with four groups, there are six pairwise comparisons or contrasts. Let us assume for each of the six t-tests we set an α-level of 0.05. That is, on each individual test we run a 5% risk of concluding there is a difference when there is none. As the probabilities associated with independent comparisons are independent of each other, we can multiply them. Furthermore, with a Type I error of 0.05, the probability of *not making a Type I error* is .95. Again, with independent t-tests, the probability of not making a Type I error in *two* t-tests is $.95 \times .95 = .9025$. For six independent comparisons we get: $.95^6 = .735$. Thus, .735 is the probability of not committing *any* Type I error in the six tests. It follows that there is a 26.5% probability that we commit *at least one* Type I error ($1 - .735 = .265$) in six independent tests! It is apparent from this that the more tests we undertake, the more likely it becomes that we commit a Type I error: In short, we would conclude there is some effect, when in fact there is only random noise. This is the problem with multiple comparisons.[8]

One way to guard against the deteriorating α-values is: (a) to refrain from interpreting pairwise comparisons, as long as the overall f-test is not significant ($p > .05$), and (b) to adjust the significance level (α) to account for multiple comparisons.

A simple way to adjust α is to use the Bonferroni criterion for multiple tests (Dunn, 1961): If there are m tests to be performed, set the significance level for each individual test at $\alpha_{new} = \alpha/m$. For the example in Table 9.3, we get $\alpha = 0.05/6 = 0.0083$. Using this new criterion, we would reject the null hypothesis (and accept that there is a mean difference in birth weights) *only* for the comparison of African American babies and non-Hispanic Caucasian babies. As we will have more occasions to see, multiple comparisons arise in many analysis situations.

SUMMARY

In this chapter we introduced the one-way ANOVA model and, with it, the fundamental idea underlying all linear models with continuous/interval-level dependent variables: the decomposition of variance into explained variance, or joint covariance between the dependent and independent variable(s), and unexplained or error variance. This distinction is the basis for the overall **goodness-of-fit test** of linear models: the f-test.

As we will see in the following chapters, more complex ANOVA models and linear regression models are all based on the same principle of decomposition of variance. It is for this reason that this principle is fundamental in understanding linear models and interpreting them correctly.

---

[7]Recall that in drug trials, depending on the prior state of development, adjustments to Type I and Type II errors are sometimes made (see discussion in Chapter 6).

[8]It is a common problem in clinical research reports, as when researchers only offer information on their "statistically significant" results without telling the reader how many tests were run in the first place.

Read: den Uil-Westerlaken, J., & Cusveller, B. (2013). Competencies in nursing students for organized forms of clinical moral deliberation and decision-making. *Journal of Nursing Education and Practice*, 3(11), 93–100.

(a) Provide a very brief (three to four sentences) summary of what this study is about.

(b) Define precisely the target population to which the statistical analysis can be generalized.

(c) List all dependent/outcome variables, provide a clear definition of them, and determine their level of measurement.

(d) List the main independent/explanatory variable in the study.

(e) State the null hypothesis for each one-way ANOVA test performed.

(f) Do the authors offer evidence that the assumptions of the one-way ANOVA tests are met?

(g) Do the authors provide a statistical test that moral deliberation and decision making (MDD) knowledge scores "increase faster" during the nursing education than MDD attitude scores?

(h) Does the comparison of MDD scores for the three groups of nursing students offer a test of how nursing students "gain" competencies over the course of their education?

EXERCISES

1. The results from a one-way ANOVA show the following output: BGSS = 15,000; WGSS = 45,000; $k = 4$ (k = number of group means compared); $n = 304$ (n = sample size).
   (a) Compute the f-value/ratio (with a calculator).
   (b) What percentage of variance is accounted for by the independent factor?
   (c) How large is the error variance?
   (d) Does the f-value indicate a significant association between the dependent and independent variables? (*Tip*: Use the f-distribution table in Appendix E.)

2. In a one-way ANOVA table, the BGSS = 120, the TSS = 520; the study sample comprises 204 study participants, and the one-way ANOVA compares mean scores among four comparison groups (three intervention groups with different dosages and one control group). What is the value of the f-ratio?

3. In a study comparing depression symptoms among randomly selected autoworkers in a large factory, a researcher finds the following sample mean scores on the Center of Epidemiologic Studies-Depression scale (CES-D): 12.7 (among 400 nonsmokers), 13.8 (among 169 former smokers), 15.6 (among 144 current smokers). The f-test for the one-way ANOVA results in a p-value under the null hypothesis of >.14. The t-test comparing nonsmokers and former smokers yields a p-value of >.23, the t-test comparing nonsmokers and current smokers yields a p-value of <.03, and the t-test comparing former smokers and current smokers yields a p-value of <.06.
   (a) Can we say anything about the association of smoking status and depression symptoms among the autoworkers?
   (b) The TSS for the one-way ANOVA = 17,750 and $\eta^2 = 20\%$. What is the value of the *error variance*?

(c) Can we draw any causal conclusion from a study such as this about the effects of smoking on depression? Why or why not?

(d) What should the level of significance be for the *t*-tests in this study?

4. A randomized sleep deprivation study involving three groups of 12 subjects each is designed to test the effects of sleep deprivation on reaction times. The overall *f*-test associated with the one-way ANOVA is 7.65.

(a) Provide the degrees of freedom associated with the *f*-test.

(b) Can we conclude that different levels of sleep deprivation have an effect on reaction time?

REFERENCES

Dunn, O. J. (1961). Multiple comparisons among means. *Journal of the American Statistical Association, 56*(293), 52–64.

Epstein, D. R., Sidani, S., Bootzin, R. R., & Belyea, M. J. (2012). Dismantling multicomponent behavioral treatment for insomnia in older adults: A randomized controlled trial. *Sleep, 35*(6), 797–805.

Fisher, R. A., & Yates, F. (1938). *Statistical tables*. Edinburgh, UK: Oliver & Boyd.

Manchikanti, L., Cash, K. A., McManus, C. D., Pampati, V., & Fellows, B. (2012). Results of 2-year follow-up of a randomized, double-blind, controlled trial of fluoroscopic caudal epidural injections in central spinal stenosis. *Pain Physician, 15*(5), 371–384.

Oenema, A., Brug, J., & Lechner, L. (2001). Web-based tailored nutrition education: Results of a randomized controlled trial. *Health Education Research, 16*(6), 647–660.

Soto-Campos, G. (2007). A model of cognitive decline using data from a longitudinal study of aging: The variable of difficulty in managing money as a function of typical Alzheimer's disease risk factors. *The International Journal of Aging and Society, 1*(1), 65–74.

Suh, E. E. (2012). The effects of P6 acupressure and nurse-provided counseling on chemotherapy-induced nausea and vomiting in patients with breast cancer. *Oncology Nursing Forum, 39*(1), E1–E9.

CHAPTER 10

Linear Regression and Pearson's *r* Correlation

In Chapter 9, we introduced one-way analysis of variance (ANOVA) to model the relationship between one interval- or ratio-level dependent variable and one nominal or categorical independent variable. If the data meet the assumptions listed in Box 9.1, we can use the ANOVA model to examine whether mean scores of the dependent variable are equal to or different from each other for all the categories of the independent variable. In the example in Chapter 9, we showed that at least some of the mean birth weights of babies from four different racial or ethnic groups differed from each other, with sample estimates of 7.56 lbs for non-Hispanic Caucasian babies, 7.33 lbs for Latino/Hispanic babies, 6.26 lbs for African American babies, and 6.27 lbs for babies from other ethnic groups. As membership in a racial or ethnic group constitutes a categorical variable without any inherent ordering, we could recode the categories of the independent variable yielding a different ordering, as demonstrated in Figure 10.1. With categorical independent variables, all we can do is test whether group means differ from each other more than what is expected due to random fluctuations. However, suppose in the birth-weight example the independent variable is gestational age (measured in weeks of pregnancy). Gestational age is itself a ratio-level variable; accordingly, we may now ask whether there is a systematic relationship between *mean* birth weights and weeks of gestation. Using data from 400 babies, the graph in Figure 10.2 appears to indicate that there is indeed a tendency for mean birth weights to grow with the length of the pregnancy. In fact, when we draw a (solid) line of "best fit" through the scatter of data, it seems that the increase in mean birth weights follows almost a *linear* pattern; that is, for each additional week of gestation, the mean birth weights seem to increase by a fixed amount. If that is the case, then we can describe this relationship in a much more succinct fashion, instead of comparing multiple mean scores using the one-way ANOVA model. For the birth-weight example with data on 22 weeks of gestation, instead of estimating 22 separate mean birth-weight scores, we could use a much more parsimonious way of describing the relationship: a single linear equation that depicts the relationship between birth weights and weeks of gestation, $Y_i = \beta_0 + \beta_1 X_i + \varepsilon_i$, where Y_i represents the birth weight of individual babies in the population, X_i represents gestational age, measured in weeks, β_0 and β_1 are the intercept and the slope coefficients of the linear equation, and ε_i stands for the error term[1] or the deviation of an individual's birth weight from the birth weight predicted by the equation for a particular gestational age (X_i).

---

[1] Error terms in linear regression models are often called "residuals."

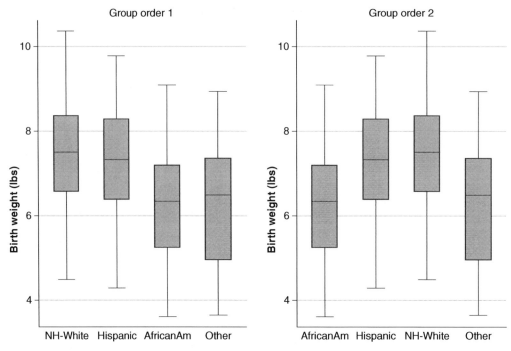

FIGURE 10.1 Mean Birth Weight by Race/Ethnicity.

As always, the population parameters (the intercept and the slope) are unknown; consequently, we have to *estimate* their values using sample data: $Y_i = b_0 + b_1 X_i + e_i$. That is, we need to find values for b_0 and b_1 that draw the line in such a way that it provides a "best fit" to the scatter of data. The criterion for best fit in linear regression models is known as the **least squares criterion**. In Figure 10.2, we added two (dashed) vertical lines at $X = 29$ and

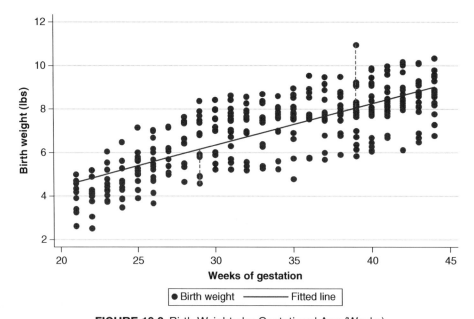

FIGURE 10.2 Birth Weights by Gestational Age (Weeks).

TABLE 10.1 Simple Linear Regression: Birth Weights on Gestational Age

```
regress birthweight (bwt) gestation

   Source |      SS        df        MS              Number of obs  =     400
  --------+---------------------------------         F(1, 398)      =  688.02
    Model |   671.2265      1      671.22640         Prob > F       =  0.0000
 Residual |   388.2844    398        .97559          R-squared      =  0.6335
  --------+---------------------------------         Adj R-squared  =  0.6326
    Total |  1059.5109    399       2.65542          Root MSE       =  .98772


      bwt |    Coef.    Std. Err.     t      P>|t|    [95% Conf.   Interval]
  --------+----------------------------------------------------------------
gestation |   .19030     .00726     26.23    0.000     .17604      .20456
    _cons |   .63135     .25141      2.51     0.012     .13710     1.12562
  ------------------------------------------------------------------------
```

$X = 39$ weeks of gestation. These lines show the distance between the birth weights of two particular babies and the predicted birth weight for all babies born after 29 or 39 weeks, which is represented by the height of the straight (regression) line. These distances are the "errors" or "residuals" resulting from the imposition of the straight line on the data points. According to the least squares criterion, the values for the regression coefficients, b_0 and b_1, are chosen in such a way that the sum of the squared deviations of all data points from the regression line is minimized: $\min(\sum(e_i)^2 = \sum(Y_i - \hat{Y})^2 = \sum(Y_i - b_0 - b_1 X_i)^2)$. As it turns out, if we set b_0 and b_1 equal to the following expressions:

$$b_1 = \frac{\sum(X_i - \bar{X})(Y_i - \bar{Y})}{\sum(X_i - \bar{X})^2}$$

$$b_0 = \bar{Y} - b_1\bar{X},$$

we obtain the equation for the regression line that minimizes the squared residuals from the regression line.[2]

Now, let us look at the output from the linear regression model, run on the birth-weight data (Table 10.1). In the lower half of the table, you see a column labeled "Coef." The numbers in that column are the estimates for the linear regression coefficients, with the intercept b_0 labeled the "constant" and the slope coefficient associated with the predictor variable b_1 labeled after the independent variable, with which it is associated ("gestation"). With this information, we can now write the estimated regression equation:

$$\hat{Y} = 0.631 + 0.190X$$
$$(0.251)\ (0.007),$$

where $\hat{Y}$ refers to the predicted birth weight, and X to the gestational week(s). The equation shows a regression intercept of $b_0 = 0.631$ and a regression slope coefficient of $b_1 = 0.190$, with their respective standard errors in parenthesis below them.

---

[2]For the reader familiar with some calculus, we obtain the derivatives of the equation $\sum(Y_i - b_0 - b_1 X_i)^2$ with respect to b_0 and b_1 and set them to zero: $\partial\sum(Y_i - b_0 - b_1 X_i)^2/\partial b_0 = 0$, $\partial\sum(Y_i - b_0 - b_1 X_i)^2/\partial b_1 = 0$. Solving these equations will yield the "normal equations," which in turn will yield the expressions for b_0 and b_1.

What does this equation tell us? For the moment, we ignore the standard errors and focus right away on the regression equation itself. It predicts that, for every increase in the X variable by *one* unit, the dependent Y variable increases by 0.19 units. Thus, for each additional week of gestation, the *average* birth weight increases by 0.19 pounds. If we substitute certain values for X, we can calculate the predicted $\hat{Y}$ value. Assume we have two babies, one born after 30, the other after 36 weeks of gestation. According to our regression equation, we predict the following birth weights:

$$\hat{Y}_{30} = 0.631 + 0.190(30) = 6.33; \quad \hat{Y}_{36} = 0.631 + 0.190(36) = 7.47$$

These predictions tell us that we expect the average birth weight of a baby born after 30 weeks of gestation to be 6.33 pounds and, after 36 weeks of gestation, that average is estimated to be 7.47 pounds.

Now let us go back and focus on the standard errors associated with these regression coefficients. As with estimates of means and mean differences in ANOVA, estimates of regression coefficients will vary depending on the particular study sample drawn. In fact, it can be shown that, if the data meet the assumptions of the linear regression model (see Box 10.1), the regression coefficients (both intercept and slope coefficients) each are distributed like the t-distribution with $n - 1$ degrees of freedom (df). Just like we obtained the relevant t-value in a one-sample t-test by dividing the difference between the observed sample mean and the hypothesized population value by its standard error, we do the same here: We divide the difference between the sample estimate of a regression coefficient and zero by its standard error and we obtain the requisite t-value. In Table 10.1, we get an intercept estimate of 0.63135 with a standard error of 0.25141; thus, we obtain a t-value of $t = 0.63135/0.25141 = 2.51$; similarly, the t-value for the slope coefficient equals $t = 0.1903/0.00726 = 26.21$.

The value of this information is that we can now test our statistical hypotheses. First, we must establish the relevant null hypotheses. As in most situations, the null hypothesis posits the absence of a relationship or the absence of an effect. In the current example, this means that we hypothesize that gestational age is *not* related to variations in average birth weight. This implies that the regression coefficients would equal zero: H_0: $b_0 = 0$ and $b_1 = 0$. However, we know from our t-values that the intercept differs by 2.51 standard errors from 0 and the slope coefficient differs by 26.23 standard errors from 0. Consequently, it is highly unlikely that this data set comes from a population, in which gestational age and birth weight are *not* related. In fact, the output in Table 10.1 provides us with the relevant p-values: There is only a 1.2% chance ($p \leq .012$) that we commit a Type I error, if we reject the null hypothesis about the intercept, and there is a chance of less than 0.0005 that we commit a Type I error[3] if we reject the null hypothesis about the slope coefficient. In other words, we are very confident that there is a relationship between these two variables. That the regression coefficients differ from zero is also indicated by their respective 95% confidence intervals (CIs). Neither the CI for the intercept nor the CI for the slope coefficient include zero, that is, the null value.

When we interpreted the regression equation, $\hat{Y} = 0.631 + 0.190X$, we did not dwell on the value of the intercept, $b_0 = 0.631$. The reason is that, in this example, the intercept term has little meaning in itself. Technically, this value is the predicted mean birth weight, if $X = 0$; in other words, it answers the (nonsensical) question of what the expected mean birth weight would be after 0 week of gestation. This situation points to a general principle of caution that should be observed when interpreting the results from regression analysis: Predictions are

---

[3]Statistical software usually cuts off p-values after three digits. p-values $< .0005$ would be rounded to .000 and $p = .0005$ would be rounded to .001.

only valid within the range of available sample observations for the predictor variable(s). In the example used here, we had data for babies born between 22 and 44 weeks of gestation. Thus all predictions made on the basis of this model should be limited to this range and cannot be extrapolated beyond it.

THE ANOVA APPROACH TO LINEAR REGRESSION

Table 10.1 provides additional information about the regression model in the upper panel, which presents the results from an ANOVA. As with all ANOVA models, we start with the total sum of squares (TSS), which is our measure of the overall variation in the dependent scores; that is, in the current example, we compute the mean birth weight of *all* study sample babies, subtract it from each individual birth weight, square that difference, and sum it over all cases to obtain the TSS. Then we divide the TSS into two subsets: the **model sum of squares (MSS)**, also called the "**regression sum of squares**" **(RegSS)**, which represents variation in *mean* birth weights *associated with* the independent variable (gestation), and the **residual sum of squares (RSS)**, a measure of the *unexplained* variation in individual birth weights at each *given* level of gestational age. Of course, MSS + RSS = TSS and MSS/TSS = the percentage of variance accounted for by the regression model.

ANOVA AND REGRESSION TERMINOLOGY

In ANOVA, we used the term "between-group sum of squares" (BGSS) for systematic variation in test scores among group means, which is analogous to "regression sum of squares" (RegSS) in regression. "Model sum of squares" (MSS) is a term used with both ANOVA and linear regression models.

In ANOVA, the most common term for the measure of *unexplained* individual variation around group means is "within-group sum of squares" (WGSS); in regression analysis, the usual term for unexplained variation in individual scores is "residual sum of squares" (RSS). "Error sum of squares" (ESS) is also a term in common usage, referring to unexplained residuals in both regression and ANOVA.

The ANOVA results in Table 10.1 show that MSS/TSS = 671.23/1,059.51 = 0.6335. From this it follows that the linear regression model with gestational age as the predictor variable accounts for 63.35% of the variance in birth weight. In regression analysis, this ratio of model over total sum of squares is usually referred to as R-squared (R^2). The output in Table 10.1 does show that R-squared equals 0.6335.

In addition to the familiar decomposition of the sums of squares into MSS and RSS, in Table 10.1 we also are given the requisite df and the associated mean squares or variances. Finally, we have the, by now familiar,[4] f-ratio, comparing the magnitude of the model variance to the residual variance. In this example, $f = 671.2264/0.97559 = 688.02$. We do not need to look up the probability that an f-ratio equals or exceeds the value 688.02 on the f-distribution with numerator df = 1 and denominator df = 398, as the software already provides it: $p < .0005$. As in ANOVA, the null hypothesis for the f-test is that none of the independent variables of the regression equation have an effect on/are correlated with the outcome variable. With a p-value smaller than .0005, we reject this null hypothesis and accept the alternative hypothesis

---

[4]See Chapter 9.

that there is a relationship. Of course, in the current situation, we did not learn anything new beyond the t-test: This simple linear regression model[5] has only one independent variable: gestational age. Thus rejecting the null hypothesis for the t-test associated with the slope coefficient and for the overall f-test is the same thing. In fact, in the special case of a single independent variable, $f = t^2$. The output in Table 10.1 confirms this: $688.02 = 26.23^2$.

ASSUMPTIONS OF THE LINEAR REGRESSION MODEL

The use of the linear regression model requires that the data meet assumptions that are essentially identical to those for the ANOVA model. As with ANOVA, the dependent variable must be measured at the interval or ratio level of measurement; observations must vary independently from each other (in the example, one baby's birth weight has no effect on another baby's birth weight—assuming they are babies from different mothers); *within* each category formed by the independent variable (in the example, babies born during the same gestational week), birth weights are normally distributed in the relevant population ("error" terms are normally distributed) and have equal variances across the categories/levels of the independent variable. The only *additional* assumption, compared to one-way ANOVA, concerns the *linearity* of the relationship between the dependent and (interval/ratio-level) independent variable.

BOX 10.1	**ASSUMPTIONS OF LINEAR REGRESSION MODEL**

1. Interval/ratio level of measurement for outcome variable
2. Linearity of relation between dependent and independent (interval/ratio-level) variable(s)
3. Independence of individual observations (uncorrelated error terms)
4. Normally distributed error terms, that is, normally distributed variables within the categories defined by the independent variable
5. Equal variances (or standard deviations) within all comparison populations defined by the independent variable(s)
6. Randomly drawn study sample for population inferences

As in the case of ANOVA models, we need to examine whether the data conform to the assumptions of the model. Again, we use a mixture of graphical inspections and a few statistical tests. Figure 10.3 shows the residuals or error terms plotted against all the levels of the independent variable (ranging from 22 to 44 weeks of gestation). The assumption of equal variances seems to be borne out. In fact, a test for heteroskedasticity[6] (Cook–Weisberg) confirms no significant differences among the variances at different levels of gestation ($p \geq .67$ for H_0 that all variances are equal); this test is similar to Bartlett's test in one-way ANOVA. Likewise, the Kolmogorov–Smirnov test does not show any significant deviations from normality ($p \geq .239$). However, as the pattern of the residuals suggests, there seems to be some (slight) nonlinearity in the relationship between the dependent and independent variable. This issue is explored further in the following.

---

[5]A "simple," as opposed to a "multiple," regression model has only a *single* independent/predictor variable.

[6]This forbidding word is of Greek origin and means "unequal spread" or variance.

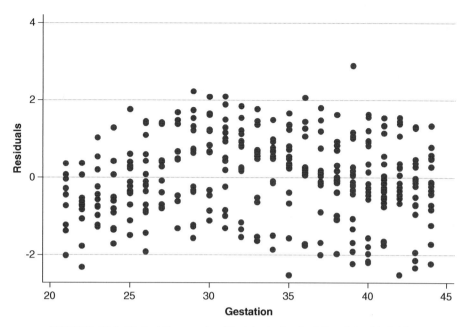

FIGURE 10.3 Plot of Regression Residuals Against Predictor Variable.

LINEAR REGRESSION WITH CATEGORICAL PREDICTOR VARIABLES

The similarity of ANOVA and linear regression models is no accident: Mathematically, they are actually the *same* model. That is, every *t*-test and ANOVA model can also be expressed as a linear regression model producing identical results. To see this, we compare output from the different procedures directly.

First, we use the independent-sample *t*-test to compare the mean birth weights of prematurely born babies to those of term babies. Of course, we would expect to reject the null hypothesis of no difference in this case. Table 10.2 shows the results, comparing the mean

TABLE 10.2 Independent-Sample *t*-Test: Birth Weight by Prematurity

```
. ttest bwt, by(premature)

Two-sample t-test with equal variances

---------------------------------------------------------------------
   Group |    Obs     Mean    Std. Err.   Std. Dev.   [95% Conf.   Interval]
---------+-----------------------------------------------------------
       0 |    281    7.8548    .06567     1.10076      7.7255      7.9841
       1 |    119    5.3086    .11267     1.22908      5.0854      5.5317
---------+-----------------------------------------------------------
combined |    400    7.0973    .08148     1.62955      6.9372      7.2575
---------+-----------------------------------------------------------
    diff |           2.5462    .12472                  2.3011      2.7914
---------+-----------------------------------------------------------
    diff = mean(0) - mean(1)                                t =    20.42
Ho: diff = 0                             degrees of freedom =      398

Ha:  diff ≠ 0
Pr(|T| > |t|) = 0.0000
```

birth weights from 119 premature babies (7.85 lbs) to the mean birth weight of 281 term babies (5.31 lbs). As expected, the *t*-value associated with this test is large ($p < .00005$) and we are confident that birth weights are generally lower for premature babies.

Now we run the same analysis as a linear regression model, with birth weight as the dependent variable, and the independent variable sex coded $X = 1$, if the baby is female, and $X = 0$, if the baby is male. Here is the regression analysis output:

TABLE 10.3 Linear Regression of Birth Weight on Prematurity (1 = yes, 0 = no)

```
. regress bwt premature

      Source |       SS          df       MS              Number of obs  =      400
-------------+------------------------------             F(1,  398)     =   416.82
       Model |    541.9898        1     541.9898          Prob > F       =   0.0000
    Residual |    517.5210      398       1.3003          R-squared      =   0.5115
-------------+------------------------------             Adj R-squared  =   0.5103
       Total |   1059.5108      399       2.6554          Root MSE       =   1.1403


         bwt |     Coef.    Std. Err.      t      P>|t|     [95% Conf.   Interval]
-------------+----------------------------------------------------------------------
   premature |   -2.5462     .12472     -20.42    0.000     -2.7914     -2.3011
       _cons |    7.8548     .06803     115.47    0.000      7.7211      7.9885
```

As we already discussed, an estimated linear regression equation with one independent variable takes on the general form of $\hat{Y} = b_0 + b_1 X_i$. Given the coefficients in Table 10.3, this translates into the following specific estimate of the equation:

$$\hat{Y} = 7.8548 - 2.5462 X_i$$

As X_i in this example is a dichotomous/binary variable, taking on the value 1 for babies born prematurely and 0 for term babies, we get the following mean birth-weight estimates for the two groups:

$$\hat{Y}_{prem} = 7.8548 - 2.5462(0) = 7.8548$$

$$\hat{Y}_{not\ prem} = 7.8548 - 2.5462(1) = 5.3086$$

The mean estimates from the independent-sample *t*-test and the linear regression are identical. So is the *t*-test itself. The slope coefficient in the regression model represents the *difference* in mean birth-weight scores between the term babies and the premature babies. The null hypothesis asserts that this coefficient does not differ from 0, which is the same null hypothesis as in the independent-sample *t*-test: The mean difference does not differ from 0. The resulting *t*-value is also identical (20.42).

The linear regression model can also be used to estimate one-way ANOVA models, but that requires the recoding of categorical independent variables with more than two categories. There are several ways of recoding categorical variables; here we focus on one popular method: **dummy coding** (Hardy, 1993). In the data set containing the birth weights of 400 babies, there is also information on the marital status of the mother. Among the 400 mothers, 232 were married at the time of the birth, 137 were single, and 31 were either divorced

TABLE 10. 4 Coding Schemes to Convert a Nominal Variable With *j* Categories to *j* – 1 Binary Dummies

Original Codes:	Coding Scheme 1:		Coding Scheme 2:		Coding Scheme 3:	
	single	div/sep	single	married	married	div/sep
Married (1)	0	0	0	1	1	0
Single (2)	1	0	1	0	0	0
Divorced/Sep. (3)	0	1	0	0	0	1
Reference group:	married		div/sep		single	

or separated. The original codes for the marital status variable were 1 = married, 2 = single, and 3 = divorced/separated (a combined category). In this form, we cannot use this variable in a regression model, because the category numbers 1, 2, 3 are *arbitrary* labels representing nominal categories. Consequently, it makes no sense of speaking of a "one-unit increase" in the independent variable, if we look at the difference between categories 1 and 2, or 2 and 3. Table 10.4 shows how the marital status variable with three categories can be represented by two binary variables, each coded (0, 1).

In general, a variable with *j* categories can be represented by *j* − 1 dummy-coded (0, 1) variables, as the mean of the default or "reference" category is represented by the intercept or constant coefficient in the regression equation. Here is how it works: Let us adopt Coding Scheme 1 from Table 10.4, for which we created two binary variables (0, 1): X_1 = single (coded 1, if the mother is single, coded 0 if she is not single) and X_2 = divorced/separated (coded 1, if the mother is divorced or separated, coded 0 if she is not divorced or separated). Thus we get the following regression equation with two independent dummy variables: $\hat{Y} = b_0 + b_1 X_1 + b_2 X_2$. It is apparent from this equation that $\hat{Y} = b_0 + b_1(0) + b_2(0) = b_0$, if X_1 and X_2 are both coded 0. In short, the default or reference category for this coding scheme, which is "married," is represented by the intercept/constant coefficient. Table 10.5 shows both the output from the one-way ANOVA and the linear regression model using the first dummy coding scheme from Table 10.4. It is easy to see that the linear regression model provides identical results to those from the ANOVA. As with the *t*-test, to recover the estimated group means, we substitute the estimates for the regression slope coefficients one at a time into the equation:

$$\hat{Y}_{married} = 7.35473 - 0.67539(0) - 0.33692(0) = 7.35373$$

$$\hat{Y}_{single} = 7.35473 - 0.67539(1) - 0.33692(0) = 6.67934$$

$$\hat{Y}_{divsep} = 7.35473 - 0.67539(0) - 0.33692(1) = 7.01781$$

Again, we see that the linear regression model is just an alternative representation of ANOVA with the underlying assumptions and mathematics being identical. This is apparent from the decomposition of the sums of squares, the variances (or mean squares) as well as the *f*-test. However, the regression output provides some additional information, most important of which is the result that the coefficient comparing the reference group of married women to the divorced or separated women (−0.33692) is *not* statistically significant ($p \geq .272$). In short, while the overall *f*-test is significant ($p \leq .0005$), meaning that *some* mean comparisons are statistically significant, the *t*-test comparing the birth-weight means for married and divorced/separated women is not. This test is identical to the independent-sample *t*-test comparing these two groups.

TABLE 10.5 Comparison of Output From One-Way ANOVA and Regression With Dummies

```
. oneway bwt marital, tab

                |            Summary of bwt
      marital   |     Mean       Std. Dev.      Freq.
----------------+-----------------------------------------
   1. married   |   7.3547285    1.5098641       232
   2.  single   |   6.6793358    1.7431223       137
   3. div/sep   |   7.0178065    1.6346909        31
----------------+-----------------------------------------
        Total   |   7.097295     1.6295446       400


                     Analysis of Variance
     Source          SS          df       MS          F      Prob > F
-------------------------------------------------------------------------
Between groups      39.50349      2     19.75174     7.69    0.0005
 Within groups    1020.00739    397      2.56929
-------------------------------------------------------------------------
        Total     1059.51087    399      2.65542


. regress bwt single divsep

     Source  |      SS         df        MS              Number of obs  =    400
------------+-------------------------------           F(2,  397)     =   7.69
      Model |   39.50349        2     19.75174          Prob > F       = 0.0005
   Residual | 1020.00739      397      2.56929          R-squared      = 0.0373
------------+-------------------------------           Adj R-squared  = 0.0324
      Total | 1059.51087      399      2.65542          Root MSE       = 1.6029


        bwt |      Coef.    Std. Err.      t      P>|t|     [95% Conf.   Interval]
------------+---------------------------------------------------------------------
     single |   -.67539      .17271     -3.91    0.000     -1.01493    -.33585
     divsep |   -.33692      .30652     -1.10    0.272      -.93953     .26568
      _cons |   7.35473      .10524     69.89    0.000      7.14784     7.56162
```

As linear regression and ANOVA are identical statistical models, the preference for one or the other is often a matter of taste. However, if the focus is on the comparison of relatively few group means, as is often the case in experimental studies, ANOVA offers the more effective presentation. On the other hand, if the model contains many interval- or ratio-level *independent* variables, regression is clearly preferable, as it can present the relationship among continuous variables in a much more parsimonious manner: a *single* slope coefficient in a regression equation can often replace numerous mean estimates assessed at *each* level of the independent variable.

EXTENSION OF THE LINEAR REGRESSION MODEL: MODIFIED FUNCTIONAL SHAPES

If applicable, linear regression models are more efficient than ANOVA models, but as always, the main issue in the choice of statistical models is the fit to the data. While linear relationships do exist, deviations from linearity are actually quite common in the medical and nursing literature. Luckily, the linear regression model is quite flexible and can accommodate a variety of different

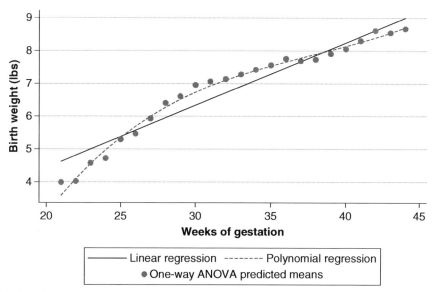

FIGURE 10.4 Birth Weights by Gestational Age (Weeks): Comparison of Linear Regression, Polynomial Regression, and ANOVA Results.

functional shapes as long as the coefficients themselves are first-power coefficients. Above, we commented on the graph in Figure 10.3 that there might be some nonlinearity in the relationship between birth weight and gestational age. Figure 10.2 also seemed to suggest a pattern deviating somewhat from strict linearity. As it turns out, we can (a) test for deviations from linearity, and (b) suggest alternative functional specifications to have a better fitting regression model. In Figure 10.4, we compare the estimated linear regression line, using the birth-weight data from 400 babies to the estimated *mean* birth-weight scores from the one-way ANOVA, which does not impose any functional shape on the sequence of means. As the means suggest a small but noticeable deviation from a strictly linear relationship between birth weights and weeks of gestation, we have also added an additional regression model. From algebra we know that the general functional shape suggested by the data is that of a polynomial function of third degree:

$$\hat{Y} = b_0 + b_1 X_1 + b_2 X_2^2 + b_3 X_3^3$$

In Table 10.5, we present the results from a regression model with X_1 = weeks of gestation, X_2 = (weeks of gestation)^2, and X_3 = (weeks of gestation)^3. This model adds the quadratic and cubic terms of the independent variable (weeks of gestation) to the equation as additional predictor variables. The results in Table 10.5 show that both the additional independent variables are statistically significant with the absolute values of the t-statistics exceeding 2.6 and the associated p-values $< .01$. In addition, compared to the linear model in Table 10.1, the R-squared value increased from 63.35% to 67.25%. This is almost as good as the fit of the unconstrained one-way ANOVA model that gives us an eta-squared value of 67.91%, a difference that is not statistically significant ($p > .997$).[7]

The graphs in Figure 10.4 confirm the very close fit of the polynomial regression model to the data (Table 10.6). The important point here is that the linear regression model is a versatile tool, which can often be employed to model relationships among variables of interest to nurses and physicians.

---

[7]This probability is based on an additional f-test (df1 = 20, df2 = 379).

TABLE 10.6 Comparison of Output From One-Way ANOVA and Polynomial Regression

Analysis of Variance

Source	SS	df	MS	F	Prob > F
Between groups	719.56533	23	31.285449	34.60	0.0000
Within groups	339.94554	376	.904110		
Total	1059.51087	399	2.655416		

Bartlett's test for equal variances: chi2(23) = 13.2461   Prob>chi2 = 0.946

. regress birthweight (bwt) gestation gest^2 gest^3

Source		SS	df	MS		Number of obs	=	400
						F(3, 396)	=	271.05
Model		712.516075	3	237.505358		Prob > F	=	0.0000
Residual		346.994799	396	.876249		R-squared	=	0.6725
						Adj R-squared	=	0.6700
Total		1059.51087	399	2.655416		Root MSE	=	.93608

bwt		Coef.	Std. Err.	t	P>|t|	[95% Conf.	Interval]
gestation		2.22638	.60222	3.70	0.000	1.04243	3.41033
gestation^2		-.05584	.01869	-2.99	0.003	-.09259	-.01909
gestation^3		.00049	.00019	2.60	0.010	.00012	.00086
_cons		-23.09928	6.31374	-3.66	0.000	-35.51192	-10.68663

In the nursing and medical literature, we find other common transformations of the linear regression model, such as logarithmic and exponential transformations (McCusker, Cole, Dendukuri, & Belzile, 2003; Mold, Lawler, Schauf, & Aspy, 2012; Stommel & Schoenborn, 2009; Suarez et al., 2004). As in all such cases, which functional shape to employ depends on theoretical reasoning as well as the actual fit to the data.

PEARSON'S *r* CORRELATION

Among the correlation coefficients found in the nursing and medical literature, the **Pearson's r correlation coefficient** is the most commonly used. As it turns out, this correlation coefficient is closely related to linear regression coefficients as well as a number of other linear statistics, such as variance and covariance. Because of this, Pearson's *r* also shares the limitations of these other statistics. Given its prominent use, it is important that we have a thorough understanding of its meaning.

Covariance

In Chapter 3, we introduced the (sample) variance of a variable X as the average squared deviation from the mean of an interval- or ratio-level variable:

$$\mathrm{Var}(X) = \frac{\sum (X_i - \bar{X})^2}{n-1} = \frac{\sum (X_i - \bar{X})(X_i - \bar{X})}{n-1}$$

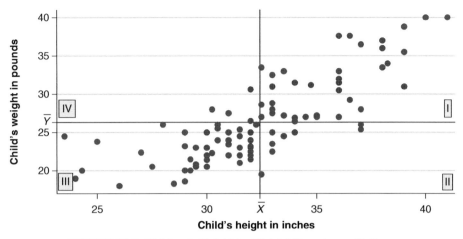

FIGURE 10.5 Children's Height by Weight Covariance Pattern.

The **covariance** between two variables X and Y is a measure of the joint variation between two interval- or ratio-level variables, and is constructed in formal analogy to the variance:[8]

$$\text{Cov}(XY) = \frac{\sum (X_i - \bar{X})(Y_i - \bar{Y})}{n-1}$$

What exactly is the covariance a measure of? In the numerator, you see the sum of all cross-products, $(X_i - \bar{X})(Y_i - \bar{Y})$. These cross-products show the deviation of an individual's value from the sample mean of X, multiplied by the deviation of the same individual's value from the sample mean of Y. As the denominator $(n - 1)$ will always be positive,[9] the covariance will be positive, if the *sum* of the cross-products is positive. For that to happen, it must be true that positive deviations of X from its mean are generally associated with positive deviations of Y from its mean and negative deviations of X are associated with negative deviations of Y.[10] On the other hand, if the predominant pattern is that positive deviations of X are associated with negative deviations of Y, and vice versa, then the sum of the cross-products will be negative and the covariance, which is nothing but the *average* cross-product, will also be negative. In short, a positive covariance implies that higher (lower) than average values on the X variable tend to be associated with the higher (lower) values on the Y variable. Figure 10.5 provides a graphical illustration of the covariance, with X being the weight and Y the height of 100 children between the ages of 6 and 30 months.

The graph in Figure 10.5 is divided into four quadrants, drawing a vertical line at the mean of the height variable, $\bar{X} = 32.42$, and a horizontal line at the mean of the weight variable $\bar{Y} = 26.34$. Thus, the first quadrant shows all the data points of toddlers with larger than average height and weight, and the third quadrant shows all the data points with smaller than average height and weight. As most babies' data lie in the first and third quadrants, the sum of the cross-products, and the covariance, are positive: $\text{Cov}(XY) = 14.55$. Had we found

---

[8]For easier recognition of this analogy, we have written out the squared term in the numerator of the variance on the previous page.

[9]The sample size n cannot be smaller than 1.

[10]The multiplication of two positive numbers or two negative numbers always yields a positive number.

most of the data points in the second and fourth quadrants, that would have meant that larger than average X values would be associated with smaller than average Y values, leading to a negative ($<$0) covariance.

Pearson's r as Standardized Covariance

While the covariance tells us whether a relationship between two variables is positive or negative, it does not give us a direct indication for how strong such a relationship is. The reason is that the specific covariance values depend on the underlying scaling units of the two variables involved. For instance, had we used centimeters instead of inches and kilogram instead of pounds, we would have obtained a different covariance estimate: $Cov(XY) = 2.59$.

This is obviously not desirable, but we can solve this problem by first *standardizing* the two variables involved. That is, if we first change X into its standardized z-score: $z_x = (X_i - \bar{X})/s_x$, and Y into its z-score: $z_y = (Y_i - \bar{Y})/s_y$, we obtain the *standardized covariance*, which is more commonly known as the **Pearson's r correlation**:

$$r_{xy} = \mathrm{Cov}\left(z_x z_y\right) = \frac{\sum (X_i - \bar{X})(Y_i - \bar{Y})}{(n-1)s_x s_y} = \frac{\sum z_x z_y}{(n-1)}$$

The standardized r_{xy} correlation has several important characteristics:

1. r_{xy} is invariant to changes in the measurement scales of either or both variables involved.

2. r_{xy} is bounded by ±1, with +1 representing a perfect positive linear relationship and −1 representing a perfect negative linear relationship.[11]

3. $r_{xy} = 0$ implies the absence of any linear relationship.

Figure 10.6 provides some examples of scatterplots of two variables and the Pearson's r correlation describing the data pattern. The upper two panels in Figure 10.6 show fairly strong linear relationships, one positive (+0.86) and the other negative (−0.81). The lower left panel shows a data pattern of essentially no correlation (neither linear nor any other functional relationship), as low values on one variable are just as likely to be paired with low and high values on the other variable, and vice versa. The final, lower-right, panel shows a well-behaved nonlinear relationship between two variables, yet the linear correlation coefficient provides an estimate of $r = +0.05$, which is close to 0. It is important to remember that Pearson's r is a linear correlation coefficient; that means it is designed to capture linear relationships. It follows that r-values close to 0 only document the absence of a linear relationship, but not the absence of all correlation patterns.

As with all sample estimates of particular statistics, we can construct 95% CIs around the sample estimate. In most applications in the literature, researchers do not report the CIs of the r-correlation coefficient, even though it would provide more precise information on the likely population value. Instead, researchers mostly report the sample estimate of the correlation and the associated p-value, which is calculated for the null hypothesis that $\rho = 0$ in the population.[12] Thus, if we see in a research report the following results: $r = 0.14$ ($p > .28$), we would conclude that the sample correlation of 0.14 does not differ significantly from the

---

[11]A "perfect" linear relationship means that all (x, y) data pairs lie on a straight line.
[12]The Greek letter ρ ("rho") refers to the population value of r.

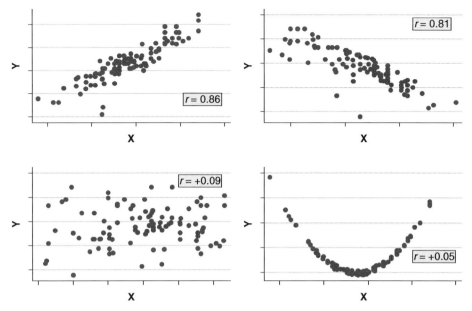

FIGURE 10.6 Pearson's r Correlations and Data Patterns.

null value of zero. In other words, there is a 28% chance that a sample correlation of this magnitude might have been the result of mere random fluctuations. Thus we do not reject the null hypothesis and conclude that it is unlikely that there is a linear relationship between two variables of interest in the population from which the sample data were obtained. By contrast, a finding of $r = 0.38$ ($p < .02$) would indicate that there is some degree of linear relationship in the population from which the sample is drawn, as the Type I error associated with the rejection of the null hypothesis of no linear relationship is less than 2%.

Alternative Versions of the Pearson's r Correlation

The Pearson's r correlation can be employed if one or both of the variables being correlated is/are dichotomous or binary measures, meaning they take on only two values. In the case of correlating two binary categorical variables, such as sex and colon cancer (having been diagnosed or not), the Pearson's r is also known as the **phi correlation**.[13] If only one of the two variables involved is binary, the Pearson's r is also known as the **point-biserial correlation**. As these two correlations can be shown to be mathematically identical to the Pearson's r and modern computers can compute the r correlation very quickly, there is no need for the simpler computational formulas of these two alternative correlations.

Pearson's r and Linear Regression

In Table 10.1, we showed the results of a simple (bivariate) linear regression model with one independent variable (weeks of gestation) predicting the birth weight of the newly born baby. We showed that the R-squared statistic equals the percentage variance in the dependent variable accounted for by the independent variable: RegSS/TSS. As the name "R-squared"

---

[13]See Chapter 15.

indicates, if we take the square root of this statistic, we obtain R. What is more, in the case of a simple regression model with one independent variable, this $R = r$. The latter is the Pearson's r correlation between the dependent and independent variable. Of course, this relationship can also be made use of the other way around. Suppose you find that the linear correlation between two variables is $r = 0.7$. Squaring this correlation yields $r^2 = 0.49$. Thus, we can conclude that, in the sample data on which this correlation was computed, one variable accounts for 49% of the variation in the other variable.

SUMMARY

In this chapter, we have explored the linear regression model with a single independent variable, also referred to as "simple linear regression." In particular, we focused on the "family resemblance" of linear regression and ANOVA, the t-test, and the Pearson's r correlation. In fact, all of these statistics are part of the general linear model (GLM), but it is important to establish that the data meet the assumptions of the model. In many cases, simple modifications in the functional shape of the independent variable(s) can be employed to meet the linearity assumption of the model. While the GLM is a flexible and versatile tool, not all types of data encountered in nursing and medical studies meet its assumptions.[14]

In the next four chapters, we explore important extensions of the linear model to accommodate more complex data. In particular, we focus on the analysis of models with multiple independent variables and their simultaneous effects on a dependent variable (factorial ANOVA and multiple regression) and on models that can accommodate repeated observations or measures on the same individuals (repeated measures ANOVA and multilevel regression). However, we will find that many of the principles governing simple linear regression and one-way ANOVA also apply to these more complex models.

LITERATURE APPLICATION

Read: Hart, S. E. (2005). Hospital ethical climates and registered nurses' turnover intentions. *Journal of Nursing Scholarship, 37*(2), 173–177.

(a) Provide a very brief (three to four sentences) summary of what this study is about.

(b) Define precisely the target population to which the statistical analysis can be generalized. Is the study sample a random sample of the target population?

(c) List all dependent/outcome variables, provide a clear definition of them, and determine their level of measurement.

(d) List the main independent/explanatory variable(s) in the study.

(e) State the null hypothesis for each Pearson's r correlation in Table 1. What do the "statistically significant" findings imply?

(f) Do the (simple) linear regressions in Tables 2 and 3 offer any additional information over the information contained in the first row of Table 1? Show how the results in Table 1 and those in Tables 2 and 3 are related.

(g) Do the authors offer evidence that the assumptions of the linear regression model and the Pearson's r correlation are met?

---

[14]Alternative statistical models for these situations will be explored in Parts III and IV of this book.

EXERCISES

1. You read that the sample covariance between X and Y equals Cov(XY) = 8.0, and the variances for X and Y are Var(X) = 9.0, Var(Y) = 16.0. What is the value of the Pearson correlation coefficient r_{xy}?

2. Given the formula for the slope regression coefficient in a simple regression, $b_1 = \sum(X_i - X)(Y_i - Y)/\sum(X_i - X)^2$, do the data provided in exercise 1 allow us to compute the sample regression coefficient? If yes, what is its value?

3. If a particular estimate of the Pearson's correlation is $r_{xy} = -0.7$, does it follow that lower than average values on X tend to be associated with lower than average values on Y? (yes/no); explain your reasoning.

4. An estimate of a linear regression model, predicting adult weight (Y, measured in lbs) from adult height (X, measured in inches) results in the following equation: $Y = -149 + 4.9X$. The standard error for the intercept coefficient is 4.8 and for the slope coefficient, it is 0.08.
   (a) Write a sentence that captures the information in this estimated regression model.
   (b) How heavy would we expect a person to be who is 6 foot 1 inch tall?
   (c) What is the significance, if any, of the intercept estimate of −149?
   (d) If the standard error for the slope coefficient had been 4.0, would that alter our inferences?

5. In the regression equation of $Y = 20 - 0.2X$, where Y = the depression score and X = age, what are the relevant null hypotheses and what do they imply?

6. In a simple linear regression model of Y on X, the regression or model sum of squares equals 80 and the residual or error sum of squares equals 420. What is the value of the correlation coefficient r between X and Y?

7. Using data from a randomly selected study sample of caregivers (N = 265), aged 35 to 85, a researcher finds the following Pearson's r correlation between the variable age and the CES-D depression score (which can vary from 0 to −60): $r = +0.14$ ($p = .435$). What precisely can we conclude? Choose *one* of the following:
   (a) The relationship between depression and age is nonlinear.
   (b) In the study sample there is a weak positive correlation of 0.14, but the p-value of .435 tells us that this positive correlation may well be the result of sampling chance.
   (c) As 43.5% of all samples of size N = 265 drawn from this same target population result in a correlation of +0.14 or larger, this indicates that, as one gets older, depression increases as well, even though by a small amount.
   (d) Had the study sample been larger (say over 1,000), we would have seen a "statistically significant" correlation between depression and age.
   (e) As $p = .435$, there is a 43.5% probability that depression increases with age among people over 34 years of age.

8. You are given the following information about the variances of two variables and the Pearson's r correlation between them: variance of Y = 64, variance of X = 100, Pearson's r = 0.5. From this, it follows that the covariance equals . . .

REFERENCES

Hardy, M. (1993). *Regression with dummy variables* (QASS 93). Newbury Park, CA: Sage.

McCusker, J., Cole, M. G., Dendukuri, N., & Belzile, E. (2003). Does delirium increase hospital stay? *Journal of the American Geriatrics Society, 51*, 1539–1546.

Mold, J. W., Lawler, F., Schauf, K. J., & Aspy, C. B. (2012). Does patient assessment of the quality of the primary care they receive predict subsequent outcomes? *The Journal of the American Board of Family Medicine, 25*(4), e1–e12.

Stommel, M., & Schoenborn, C. A. (2009). Accuracy and usefulness of BMI measures based on self-reported weight and height: Findings from the NHANES & NHIS 2001–2006. *BMC: Public Health, 9*, 421.

Suarez, J. I., Zaidat, O. O., Suri, M. F., Feen, E. S., Lynch, G., Hickman J, . . . Selman, W. R. (2004). Length of stay and mortality in neurocritically ill patients: Impact of a specialized neurocritical care team. *Critical Care Medicine, 32*(11), 2311–2317.

CHAPTER 11

Factorial Analysis of Variance and Analysis of Covariance

FACTORIAL ANOVA

In Chapter 9 we introduced the one-way ANOVA model, which can be used to analyze the relationship between one interval- or ratio-level dependent variable and a *single* nominal or categorical independent or predictor variable. In this chapter, we will extend this model to include two (or more) simultaneous predictor variables in the analysis. In both the nursing and medical literature, reports on intervention studies with two or more intervention variables are quite common (Conn et al., 2001; Gary et al., 2003; Venkateswaran et al., 2009). Such randomized clinical trials employ **factorial designs** (Stommel & Wills, 2004), which involve the *simultaneous* manipulation of two or more independent variables (or "factors"). The key advantage of such studies is that one cannot only examine the **main effects** of each separate treatment, but also their **interactions**, that is, the joint effects of the treatments on the outcome(s).

Let us look at an example of how this might play out. Here we present a **two-way factorial design** for a hypothetical (but not too far-fetched!) clinical problem in need of research. The logic underlying this example of a two-way ANOVA can readily be extended to factorial designs with more factors or more categories (treatment levels) per factor.

> Suppose a researcher has received funding to study the efficacy of two treatments (zinc inhalers and super-potent chicken broth) to shorten recovery time from viral upper respiratory infections (URIs), a commonly encountered problem in primary care settings. We assume that previous research has already provided some support for the effectiveness of either intervention in reducing recovery time, but this research was primarily based on observational studies. Furthermore, it may well be the case that the effects of the either intervention may reinforce the other, so that taking both remedies together may yield additional benefits.

A problem like this is well suited for a randomized clinical trial employing a 2×2 factorial design. The outcome variable, recovery time until the symptoms disappear, can be measured with reasonable accuracy, and exposure to the treatments can be easily manipulated. While treatment *implementation* requires cooperation of study participants in using the zinc inhaler or consuming the chicken broth, study conditions need not be "ideal." If patient cooperation

TABLE 11.1 Random Assignment of 160 Study Subjects in Two-Way Factorial Design

	NO ZINC INHALER N	ZINC INHALER N	TOTAL N
NO CHICKEN BROTH	40	40	80
CHICKEN BROTH	40	40	80
TOTAL	80	80	160

were to exceed greatly the cooperation levels during usual clinical practice, the measured study effects could be unrealistically large. In short, in this kind of study, we aim for enough subjects to adhere to the protocol so that positive *average* outcomes can be documented, *if there are some.*

In this 2 × 2 factorial design, we would *manipulate* two independent two-level factors, involving exposure or nonexposure to either chicken broth or zinc inhaler or both, and *randomly assign* study subjects to the various conditions. Given the possible combinations of the two independent factors, the study design creates four groups with different exposure levels as indicated in Table 11.1.

In the factorial ANOVA model with two experimental factors, j and k, we conceive of individual outcome scores, Y_{ijk}, as being influenced by membership in the groups formed by the two experimental variables, their possible interaction, and whatever unexplained individual differences, ε_{ijk}, remain. In our example, we have:

$$Y_{ijk} = \mu... + \delta_j + \delta_k + \delta_{jk} + \varepsilon_{ijk}$$

This equation shows an individual's outcome score as the sum of the overall mean score for all individuals in the relevant target population and various deviation terms. The effect of the intervention j is captured by the positive or negative *deviation* (δ_j) of the intervention or control group means from the overall mean score. Similarly, the main effect of intervention k is also captured as the deviation (δ_k) of the group means for exposed and nonexposed subjects from the overall mean score. The interaction effect consists of the deviation (δ_{jk}) of the mean score for doubly exposed individuals from the expected mean if no interaction is present, which would be reflected in the addition of the two main effects of δ_j and δ_k. Finally, each individual score may also have its idiosyncratic error component, ε_{ijk}.

After the experiment has been carried out with the study participants exposed to the four treatment combinations and recovery times measured, the researchers would test three major hypotheses via the rejection of three parallel null hypotheses:

1. H_{01}: $\delta_j = 0$ (recovery time for subjects exposed to chicken broth does not differ from the recovery time of subjects not exposed to chicken broth, that is, the mean outcomes in the chicken broth exposure/nonexposure groups do not differ from the grand mean)

2. H_{02}: $\delta_k = 0$ (recovery time for subjects exposed to the zinc inhaler does not differ from the recovery time of subjects not exposed to the zinc inhaler, that is, the mean outcomes in the zinc exposure/nonexposure groups do not differ from the grand mean)

3. H_{03}: $\delta_{jk} = \mu_{jk} - (\mu... + \delta_j + \delta_k) = 0$ (recovery time for subjects exposed to both chicken broth and zinc inhaler does not differ from the *addition* of the separate effects of exposure to either treatment on recovery time)

TABLE 11.2 Factorial ANOVA With One Main Effect

Means & Standard Deviations for recovery time

chicken broth	zinc inhaler yes	no	Total
yes	75.69	76.66	76.18
	3.39	3.21	3.32
no	82.90	83.53	83.22
	2.71	3.52	3.13
Total	79.29	80.09	79.69
	4.75	4.81	4.78

ANOVA recovery time chicken-broth zinc inhaler interaction: chick X zinc

Number of obs	=	120	R-squared	= 0.5553
Root MSE	=	3.22514	Adj R-squared	= 0.5438

Source	Partial SS	df	MS	F	Prob>F
Model	1506.747	3	502.249	48.29	0.0000
Chicken broth	1486.619	1	1486.619	142.92	0.0000
Zinc inhaler	19.209	1	19.209	1.85	0.1768
Chickenbr X Zinc	.919	1	.919	0.09	0.7668
Residual	1206.580	116	10.402		
Total	2713.327	119	22.801		

In Tables 11.2 through 11.4, we present three typical result patterns in a two-way ANOVA of a randomized intervention study with a 2×2 factorial design. The evidence in Table 11.2 supports the research hypothesis that only chicken broth shortens recovery time, as on the basis of the evidence we would reject H_{01}, but accept H_{02} and H_{03}. The ANOVA table shows that the sum of squares (SS) associated with chicken broth (1486.619) accounts for 98.7% of the "Model" SS (1506.749), which means that almost all between-group mean differences are accounted for by exposure or nonexposure to chicken broth. As always, we need to move beyond the description of sample statistics and ask whether the evidence is strong enough to reject the null hypothesis in question (H_{01}). The f-ratio comparing between-group variance to within-group/error variance is large, and the probability that an f-statistic with (df1 = 1/ df2 = 116) would exceed 145.92 as a result of mere random assignment is exceedingly small: $p < .00005$. Based on these study sample data, we would reject H_{01} and conclude that the observed differences in mean recovery time (76.2 hours for subjects eating the chicken broth and 83.2 hours for subjects who did not eat it) are due to the exposure to chicken broth. None of the other f-tests associated with the exposure to zinc inhalers or the interaction of the two treatments are statistically significant, which is to say their p-values exceed the usual significance criterion of 0.05.

The result shown in Table 11.3 would lead us to reject H_{01} and H_{02}, but to accept H_{03}. Thus, the research hypotheses about the **main effects** are supported: Both chicken broth and zinc inhalers separately have the effect of shortening recovery time. As in Table 11.2, the main effect of exposure to chicken broth remains the same, with a mean difference of

TABLE 11.3 Factorial ANOVA With Two Main Effects

Means & Standard Deviations for recovery time

chicken broth	zinc inhaler yes	no	Total
yes	74.79	77.56	76.18
	3.39	3.21	3.32
no	82.00	84.43	83.22
	2.71	3.52	3.13
Total	78.39	80.99	79.69
	4.75	4.81	4.78

ANOVA recovery time chicken-broth zinc inhaler interaction: chick X zinc

Number of obs	=	120	R-squared	=	0.5553
Root MSE	=	3.22514	Adj R-squared	=	0.5438

Source	Partial SS	df	MS	F	Prob>F
Model	1690.369	3	563.456	54.17	0.0000
Chicken broth	1486.619	1	1486.619	142.92	0.0000
Zinc inhaler	202.831	1	202.831	19.50	0.0000
Chickenbr X Zinc	.919	1	.919	0.09	0.7668
Residual	1206.580	116	10.402		
Total	2896.949	119	24.344		

$76.18 - 83.22 = -7.04$. However, the main effect of exposure or nonexposure to zinc inhalers has changed: A mean difference of $78.39 - 80.99 = -2.6$ in Table 11.3 replaces a difference of -0.8 in Table 11.2, with SS, MS, and f-statistic all larger, resulting in a p-value of $p < .00005$. Given this evidence, we would reject H_{02}: $\delta_k = 0$ and conclude that exposure to zinc has an independent effect on shortening recovery, independent, that is, of the effect of exposure to chicken broth.

Table 11.4 shows results, which support all three research hypotheses, as the evidence would lead us to reject H_{01}, H_{02}, and H_{03}. However, the main story in the results pattern we see in Table 11.4 is the new **interaction effect**, which posits an effect on recovery time that goes beyond the main effects. A good way to grasp the meaning of the interaction effect is to look back at the sample means in Table 11.3 and compare them to those in Table 11.4. Focusing on the right-hand column in Table 11.3, we see that the chicken broth effect is captured as the overall sample mean difference of $76.18 - 83.22 = \underline{-7.04}$. The mean differences *within* the *separate* groups, defined by exposure or nonexposure to a zinc inhaler, are also quite similar: $77.56 - 84.43 = \underline{-6.87}$ and $74.79 - 82.00 = \underline{-7.21}$. In fact, the nonsignificant interaction effect ($p > .7668$) in Table 11.3 tells us that these differences are well within the margin of sampling chance alone. In other words, the *absence* of an interaction effect tells us that *the effect of chicken broth on recovery time is the same, regardless of exposure or nonexposure to a zinc inhaler.*[1]

---

[1]Readers should convince themselves from the results in Table 11.3 that the effect of exposure to zinc inhalers is also essentially the same, whether or not a person also consumes chicken broth.

TABLE 11.4 Factorial ANOVA With Two Main and One Interaction Effect

```
Means & Standard Deviations for recovery time

     chicken  |     zinc inhaler
      broth   |    yes        no  |  Total
    ----------+-------------------+------
        yes   |   71.59     79.36 |  75.48
              |    3.39      3.21 |   5.11
    ----------+-------------------+------
         no   |   82.70     85.13 |  83.91
              |    2.71      3.52 |   3.34
    ----------+-------------------+------
       Total  |   77.15     82.25 |  79.69
              |    6.38      4.42 |   6.04

ANOVA recovery time chicken-broth zinc inhaler interaction: chick X zinc

            Number of obs   =     120    R-squared      =  0.5553
            Root MSE        = 3.22514    Adj R-squared  =  0.5438

            Source |  Partial SS    df       MS         F      Prob>F
         ----------+-----------------------------------------------------
             Model |   3131.760      3   1043.920   100.42   0.0000
     Chicken broth |   2136.732      1   2136.732   205.42   0.0000
      Zinc inhaler |    780.360      1    780.360    75.02   0.0000
    Chickenbr X Zinc|   214.668      1    214.668    20.64   0.0000
          Residual |   1206.580    116     10.402
         ----------+-----------------------------------------------------
             Total |   4338.340    119     36.457
```

Now contrast these results to those in Table 11.4. For persons not exposed to the zinc inhaler, the effect of chicken broth consumption on recovery time is captured in the following mean difference: $79.36 - 85.13 = \underline{-5.77}$; for those using the zinc inhaler, the effect of chicken broth consumption is $71.59 - 82.70 = \underline{-10.56}$, which is to say almost twice as large. Clearly, in this hypothetical example, a **synergistic effect** is present, that is, *the two treatments mutually reinforce each other*. To say this in another way: The effect of one treatment variable depends on the level of the other treatment variable. It should now be apparent why it does not make much sense to talk of a "main effect," if an interaction effect is present: Its existence implies that there are no uniform effects across the levels of the other exposure variables. By contrast, a main effect is simply the effect of a single independent variable or factor on a dependent variable, which remains the same, *regardless of the level of exposure to the other factor(s)*.

Figure 11.1 offers a graphical depiction of the different effect patterns shown in Tables 11.2 through 11.4. The left-hand panel corresponds to the results in Table 11.2: The steep decline in mean recovery time associated with exposure (yes) as opposed to nonexposure (no) to chicken broth is evident for both the groups exposed to the zinc inhaler (solid line) and the group not exposed to the zinc inhaler (dashed line). On the other hand, the very small vertical difference between the parallel lines for the two zinc exposure groups indicates a nonsignificant difference based on this exposure. The parallel lines in the middle panel again indicate that exposure to chicken broth has a strong and similar effect on reducing recovery time in both zinc exposure groups. However, the much larger distance between the parallel lines indicates that exposure to the zinc inhaler at all levels of exposure to chicken broth reduces

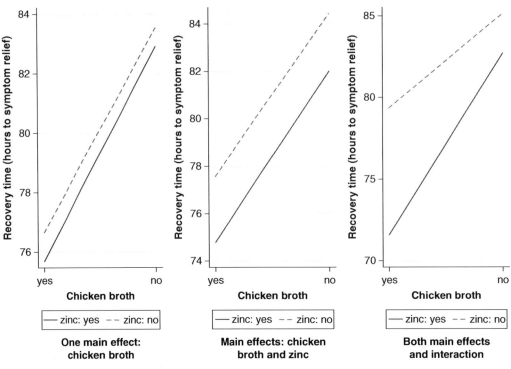

FIGURE 11.1 Patterns of Main Effects and Interactions in Two-Way ANOVA.

recovery time. The third panel (on the right) is a graphical depiction of the interaction effect shown in the results of Table 11.4: While exposure to chicken broth reduces mean recovery time among persons not exposed to the zinc inhaler (dashed line), the reduction in recovery time is steeper for persons exposed to both treatments (solid line).

GENERAL INTERPRETATION OF INTERACTION EFFECTS

What statisticians call "interaction effects" or "moderator effects" (Whisman & McCelland, 2005) are common phenomena in health care and clinical practice. To assert that one treatment interacts with another treatment is to say that the generality of the treatment's effect is limited to specific conditions under which the intervention works better or worse. In short, the effect on a dependent variable is "moderated" by another independent variable.[2] The classic medical example is that of drug interactions, as when the simultaneous intake of a second drug might either enhance ("synergistic") or reduce ("antagonistic") the effects of a given drug.[3] However, interaction effects do not only occur as a result of the interplay of multiple interventions or treatments. They are also common in the interplay of interventions and certain population subgroups. For instance, a particular nursing educational intervention may work with adults, but not necessarily with adolescents (Pbert, 2011). The call for cultural sensitivity in providing nursing and medical care implies that the same approach to care may not work as well among all ethnic or religious groups in society (Chang, 2007). In short, care interventions

---

[2]The terms "moderation" and "statistical interaction" are used interchangeably.

[3]For a quick overview, see the Wikipedia article on "drug interactions": en.wikipedia.org/wiki/Drug _interaction

"interact" with patient characteristics such as ethnic or religious affiliations. To test the effectiveness of care interventions empirically, a study employing a factorial design would allow one to test explicitly whether the effectiveness of an intervention differs, depending on certain patients' ethnic, religious, educational, or other cultural backgrounds.

DECOMPOSITION OF VARIANCE IN FACTORIAL ANOVA WITH ORTHOGONAL/BALANCED DESIGNS

One of the intuitively attractive features of ANOVA is that it often allows us to decompose the variation in the outcome variable and *attribute it to the various factors*. However, the ability to attribute variation in outcomes *uniquely* to independent factors requires data with **orthogonal**[4] independent factors.

The ANOVA example of the chicken broth and zinc inhaler interventions we introduced rests on such an orthogonal study design. The study is deliberately designed, so that exposure to the chicken broth and the zinc inhaler treatment are *independent* from each other (uncorrelated). Recall from Chapter 4 that two events A and B are considered independent, if the probability of event A remains the same, regardless of the occurrence of event B. In the intervention study discussed here, the probability of being assigned to the zinc inhaler intervention is 0.5, regardless of whether a person is or is not also assigned to the chicken broth intervention. That makes these events independent, with the important consequence that the SSs and variances associated with each of the effects do not overlap and can be added, regardless of the order in which the independent factors appear. Thus, in Table 11.4, the Model SS is simply the sum of the separate SSs attributed to chicken broth, zinc inhaler, and their interaction, and we would get the same numbers, if we changed the order, for example, computing the SS for zinc inhaler first, and so forth. This allows us to attribute a unique percentage of variance to each separate factor and the model as a whole. As a consequence, with an orthogonal study design the decomposition of variance in an ANOVA model gives us an estimate of the *relative effectiveness or contribution* that several factors make to variation in the dependent variable. As we will see in the next chapter on multiple regression analysis, when we analyze *observational* data, we have no control over whether or not two or more independent variables are correlated; consequently, *with observational data it is no longer possible to assign explained variance uniquely to each independent variable*.

ANALYSIS OF COVARIANCE (ANCOVA)

In our discussion of factorial ANOVA, we chose as our example the simplest possible factorial design: the simultaneous manipulation of two treatments, each with only two levels (presence or absence) of treatment. Factorial designs and factorial ANOVA are not limited to treatments with only two levels, nor are they limited to only two simultaneous treatments. While adding to the complexity in the analysis, the main principles of distinguishing between main and interaction effects remain the same. Factorial designs may also be used to analyze data from **randomized block designs**. In such study designs, researchers undertake the random assignment to treatment and control groups *within* blocks, with the blocks defined by variables that have a known effect on the dependent variable in question (Friedman et al., 2010; Polit & Beck, 2003). For example, in a study designed to test learning abilities of schoolchildren, age

---

[4]The term "orthogonal" refers to the geometric representation of variables and means literally "right-angled." It is used synonymously with "uncorrelated," as the geometric representation of two vectors representing uncorrelated variables is the right angle.

would certainly be an important predictive factor. To separate the age effect from the comparison of the treatment and control groups, one would create age blocks consisting of *pairs* of children of the same age. The random assignment to either the treatment or control group would then proceed *within* each pair of age peers, *guaranteeing* the same age distribution in the treatment and control groups. In this way, researchers can make certain that age cannot account for group differences (as it is uncorrelated with group membership), and, in the analysis stage, they can separate out the variance associated with age from the outcome variable.

The **ANCOVA** is yet another way of dealing with possible nuisance variables in the analysis stage of a study. ANCOVA extends the ANOVA model by including continuous interval- or ratio-level variables into the model. In effect, ANCOVA combines ANOVA and linear regression into a single model.

Here is how it works: Let us go back to the example of chicken broth and zinc inhaler. We know from clinical experience that a person's age is likely to affect recovery time, such that older people, on average, take longer in their recovery from viral URIs. Knowing this, we would collect information on the age of all study participants. Why? Wouldn't the fact that we randomly assign study participants to the four treatment conditions (exposure to chicken broth only, to zinc inhaler only, to both, or to neither) take care of possible age differences between the comparison groups, as long as the study samples are sufficiently large? True, but random assignment of sufficiently large comparison groups would only lead to roughly equal *mean* ages in the comparison groups. Within-group variation in age would remain and, if age is a strong predictor of recovery time, this would add to the individual within-group variation in recovery time. Now recall, that our statistical tests concerning group mean differences in the dependent variable are based on the *f*-ratio, which compares the relative magnitude of between-group variance in outcome scores (BGSS/$k - 1$) to within-group variance (WGSS/$n - k$). If we could reduce the size of the within-group individual, that is, error variance, we would increase the magnitude of the *f*-ratio, resulting in greater power to detect differences in outcomes between the experimental and control groups. In short, our tests would become more efficient.

In the ANCOVA model with two experimental factors, j and k, we conceive of individual outcome scores, Y_{ijk}, as being influenced by membership in the groups formed by the two exposure variables as well as their covariate attribute X_{ijk}, and whatever unexplained error variance remains ε_{ijk}. In our example, we have:

$$Y_{ijk} = \mu... + \delta_j + \delta_k + \delta_{jk} + \beta(X_{ijk} - \bar{X}...) + \varepsilon_{ijk}$$

This equation is modeled after the factorial ANOVA and shows that an individual's score on the outcome variable is the sum of the overall mean score for all individuals in the relevant target population, the effect of the intervention j as captured by the deviation (δ_j), the effect of intervention k as captured by the deviation (δ_k), the interaction effect as captured in the deviation (δ_{jk}), and a term that captures all other, unaccounted for influence ε_{ijk}. What is new here, compared to the factorial ANOVA, is the regression term, $\beta(X_{ijk} - \bar{X}...)$. It captures the linear effect of the nuisance or control variable on the outcome variable. If we now compare the error terms in the ANCOVA to the error terms in ANOVA model without the covariate, it is easy to see that the former is smaller than the letter, as long as $\beta \neq 0$:

$$\varepsilon_{ijk} = Y_{ijk} - \mu... - \delta_j - \delta_k - \delta_{jk} - \beta(X_{ijk} - \bar{X}...) \text{ [ANCOVA]}$$
$$\varepsilon_{ijk} = Y_{ijk} - \mu... - \delta_j - \delta_k - \delta_{jk} \text{ [ANOVA]}$$

Again, if the covariate is related to the outcome variable, removing its effect on the dependent variable will lead to a more efficient *f*-test. For illustration, we present a numerical

TABLE 11.5 ANCOVA With Two Main, One Interaction Effect and a Continuous Covariate

```
. correlation: recovery-time age
(obs=120)

              |  recovery~    age
-----------+----------------
recovery-time |   1.0000
         age  |   0.4170     1.000
                (0.0000)


ANOVA recovery time chicken-broth zinc inhaler interaction: chick X zinc

              Number of obs =    120        R-squared     =  0.5553
              Root MSE      =  3.22514      Adj R-squared =  0.5438

          Source  |  Partial SS    df       MS        F      Prob>F
       ---------+-------------------------------------------
           Model |   3646.706     4      911.676   151.59   0.0000
             age |    514.945     1      514.945    85.62   0.0000
   Chicken broth |   2033.604     1     2033.604   338.13   0.0000
    Zinc inhaler |    672.925     1      672.925   111.89   0.0000
  Chickenbr X Zinc |  198.139     1      198.139    32.95   0.0000
        Residual |    691.635   115        6.014
       ---------+-------------------------------------------
           Total |   4338.340   119       36.457
```

example of a covariance analysis for the randomized two-way experiment involving chicken broth and zinc inhaler as treatments and age as the continuous covariate factor: We started with the interaction model in Table 11.4, but added age as the covariate. The information in Table 11.5 tells us that the linear correlation between recovery time and age (in years) is 0.417 ($p < .00005$); thus, we use age in the ANCOVA as a control variable (covariate).

As mentioned before, ANCOVA can be thought of as a two-step procedure: linear regression of the within-group error terms on the covariate, followed by a regular ANOVA on the remaining error terms after the covariate effect has been subtracted. Comparing the output in Table 11.5 to the output in Table 11.4, notice that there is no change in the total SS (4338.34), but age is now part of the "Model" SS (3646.706) and the unexplained or error SS has shrunk from 1206.58 in the ANOVA model of Table 11.4 to 691.635 in the ANCOVA model of Table 11.5. Dividing the error SS by its degrees of freedom (df), we get an error variance of 6.014 compared to 10.402 in the ANOVA model of Table 11.4. With the remaining random error about 40% smaller in the ANCOVA, every f-ratio comparing systematic to error variances test is now larger, increasing the probability that an intervention effect will be found statistically significant, if there is such an effect. In this example, even without the covariate adjustment, the interventions were found to be statistically significant; in other cases, that may not be so. In short, covariate adjustments in randomized clinical trials can increase their efficiency and reduce the required sample size to find an effect, if there is one.

ASSUMPTIONS OF ANOVA AND ANCOVA

None of the assumptions are new: Like factorial ANOVA, ANCOVA assumes multivariate normal distributions of the individual error terms within each population group formed by the treatment factor combinations. And like linear regression, the covariate is thought to have a linear relationship to the dependent variable. The F-test is quite robust in the face of deviations from the normality assumption about the error terms, as long as the samples are sufficiently large and heteroskedasticity[5] is not a major problem. The model is not robust with respect to deviations from the assumption of a linear relationship between the outcome variable and the covariate; however, as in regression analysis, algebraic transformations of the covariate (e.g., logarithmic, exponential, and so forth) can sometimes "linearize" the relationship between the covariate and the dependent scores.

SUMMARY

In this chapter, we have discussed two common extensions of the simple one-way analysis of variance: factorial ANOVA and ANCOVA. The discussion was limited to data from (hypothetical) randomized experiments, instead of observational data. ANOVA models were originally developed for experimental studies, but they can be applied to observational data, even though this adds a number of complications to be considered when interpreting the results. In particular, when the independent factors or variables are correlated, as is usually the case with observational data, the decomposition of variance becomes more complicated as well.

As the ANOVA model is mathematically identical to the linear regression model, and regression analysis was originally designed to deal with observational data, we will take up the issue of how to interpret ANOVA tables based on observational data in the next chapter on multiple (linear) regression models.

LITERATURE APPLICATION

Read: Gary, T. L., Bone, L. R., Hill, M. N., Levine, D. M., McGuire, M., Saudek, C., & Brancati, F. L. (2003). Randomized controlled trial of the effects of nurse case manager and community health worker interventions on risk factors for diabetes related complications in urban African Americans. *Preventive Medicine, 37*(1), 23–32.

(a) Provide a very brief (3–4 sentences) summary of what this study is about.

(b) Define the target population to which the statistical analysis can be generalized. What were the eligibility and exclusion criteria for study participants? Is the study sample a random sample of the target population?

(c) The researchers used a randomized block design, blocking on sex and clinic site. What is the purpose of this?

(d) List all dependent/outcome variables, provide a clear definition of them, and determine their level of measurement.

(e) List the main independent/explanatory factor(s) in the study. Do the authors control for covariates?

(f) Do the comparison groups differ according to baseline characteristics?

(g) State the null hypotheses for each of the effects shown in Figure 1. Is the evidence strong enough to reject the null hypotheses?

(h) Do the authors provide evidence that the data meet the assumptions of their statistical tests?

(i) Summarize the main findings in your own words: Are the conclusions of the authors consistent with the evidence presented?

---

[5] Heteroskedasticity refers to the existence of unequal within-group variances across comparison groups.

EXERCISES

1. The following output shows the ANOVA results from a randomized intervention study, exposing study participants to a physical exercise (yes or no) and/or a nutrition (yes or no) intervention in a 2 × 2 factorial design. The outcome measure is the body mass index (BMI) measured after 6 months of the ongoing interventions.

Factorial ANOVA With Two Main and One Interaction Effect

Means and Standard Deviations of BMI 6 months after continuous nutrition & exercise intervention

Exercise Intervention vs. Control Group	Nutrition Intervention vs. Control Group		Total
	control-gp	intervention-gp	
control group	26.46(n=23) 5.01	24.74(n=23) 3.58	25.60(n=46) 4.39
intervention group	24.14(n=23) 5.13	19.05(n=23) 3.83	21.60(n=46) 5.16
Total	25.30(n=46) 5.15	21.90(n=46) 4.66	23.60(n=92) 5.17

anova BMI ExGroup NutGroup ExGroup x NutGroup

	Number of obs = 92		R-squared = 0.2876		
	Root MSE = 4.43925		Adj R-squared = 0.2633		
Source	Partial SS	df	MS	F	Prob >
Model	700.193	3	233.398	11.84	0.0000
ExGroup	368.433	1	368.433	18.70	0.0000
NutGroup	266.538	1	266.538	13.53	0.0004
ExGroup#NutGroup	65.222	1	65.222	3.31	0.0723
Residual	1734.211	88	19.707		
Total	2434.404	91	26.752		

Answer the following questions about the results in the table:
(a) Does exposure to physical exercise have an effect on the BMI? (Write a short paragraph incorporating all the relevant information in the table.)
(b) Does exposure to the nutrition intervention have an effect on the BMI? (Write a short paragraph incorporating all the relevant information in the table.)
(c) Do the two interventions/treatments interact to provide a synergistic effect?
(d) Why is the df associated with each intervention effect equal to one?
(e) Why does the model SS equal the sum of the SSs associated with the individual interventions?
(f) Show how the f-ratio associated with the effect of the nutrition intervention (13.53) is computed from the available results.
(g) How much variation in BMI scores is accounted for by the two main effects?
(h) Which one is more effective, the exercise or the nutrition intervention?

2. Researchers are interested in the relative effectiveness of physical exercise and medication on reducing hypertension among sedentary individuals. They devise a randomized intervention study in which different subjects are exposed to three levels of exercise graded in terms of strenuousness (minimal, moderate, strenuous) and four dosages of an antihypertensive drug (placebo, 10 mg, 20 mg, 30 mg). The study design is a fully crossed, 3 × 4 balanced design, with each of the 12 groups containing 12 subjects.

    (a) Construct the df table for all main and interaction effects, as well as the model and error components.

    (b) Assuming the *p*-values associated with each of the effects are all $p < .01$, can we conclude from this information that 20 mg of the drug has a bigger effect on reducing hypertension than 10 mg?

    (c) Given the information provided, can we conclude that the interaction effect is synergistic, for example, that exercise and drug exposures together produce a bigger reduction in hypertension than the sum of the two main effects?

    (d) If the total SS of the hypertension measure equals 840 and the interventions together account for 30% for the variation in blood pressure scores, how large is the error or residual SS?

3. Give three examples of "interaction effects" you are familiar with or may have observed in clinical practice.

4. The following data are a small subset of data from a study comparing the adherence to a healthy nutrition regimen after exposure to written material provided only once (control group) or weekly written material plus biweekly phone contacts over 3 months (intervention group). Subjects were split into men and women, with random assignment to intervention and control groups within the gender groups. The outcome measure is an adherence scale score ranging from 0 to 20. Here are data from eight cases:

DATA FOR ADHERENCE TO INTERVENTION STUDY

INTERVENTION/CONTROL	Ctrl. gp	Ctrl. gp	Ctrl. gp	Ctrl. gp	Int. gp	Int. gp	Int. gp	Int. gp
Sex	Male	Male	Female	Female	Male	Male	Female	Female
Adherence score	12	13	11	13	14	16	19	20

    (a) Compute all separate SSs adding up to total sum of squares.

    (b) Construct the df table associated with the SSs.

    (c) Compute the *f*-ratio and compare it to the appropriate critical *f*-value in the *f*-distribution table for a significance level of $\alpha = 0.05$ (Appendix E).

    (d) Write a short paragraph summarizing your findings.

    (*Tip*: At first, use a hand calculator to get the results before employing any statistical program to check your results.)

REFERENCES

Chang, M., & Kelly, A. E. (2007). Patient education: Addressing cultural diversity and health literacy issues. *Urologic Nursing, 27*(5), 411–417.

Conn, V. S., Rantz, M. J., Wipke-Tevis, D. D., & Maas, M. L. (2001). Designing effective nursing interventions. *Research in Nursing & Health, 24*(5), 433–442.

Gary, T. L., Bone, L. R., Hill, M. N., Levine, D. M., McGuire, M., Saudek, C., & Brancati, F. L. (2003). Randomized controlled trial of the effects of nurse case manager and community health worker interventions on risk factors for diabetes related complications in urban African Americans. *Preventive Medicine, 37*(1), 23–32.

Pbert, L., Druker, S., DiFranza, J. R., Gorak, D., Reed, G., Magner, R., Sheetz, A. H., & Osganian, S. (2011). Effectiveness of a school nurse–delivered smoking-cessation intervention for adolescents. *Pediatrics, 128*(5), 926–935.

Polit, D. F., & Beck, C. T. (2003). *Nursing research: Principles and methods* (7th ed.). Philadelphia, PA: Lippincott Williams & Wilkins.

Stommel, M., & Wills, C. (2004). *Clinical research.* Philadelphia, PA: Lippincott Williams & Wilkins.

Venkateswaran, R. V., Steeds, R. P., Quinn, D. W., Nightingale, P., Wilson, I. C., Mascaro, J. G., . . . Bonser, R. S. (2009). The haemodynamic effects of adjunctive hormone therapy in potential heart donors: A prospective randomized double-blind factorially designed controlled trial. *European Heart Journal, 30*(14), 1771–1780.

Whisman, M. A., & McClelland, G. H. (2005). Designing, testing, and interpreting interactions and moderator effects in family research. *Journal of Family Psychology, 19*(1), 111–120.

CHAPTER 12

Multiple Linear Regression

In the previous chapter, we introduced factorial analysis of variance (ANOVA) and analysis of covariance (ANCOVA) as extensions of one-way ANOVA, adding additional independent or predictor variables to the model. In this chapter, we discuss a parallel extension of the simple linear regression model: **multiple regression** analysis. Such models involve at least two, sometimes many more, independent variables used to predict variation in one dependent interval- or ratio-level variable. We already showed in Chapter 10 that the one-way ANOVA model can be expressed as a regression model with dummy-coded independent variables providing identical results. Similarly, factorial ANOVA and ANCOVA models can also be expressed as multiple regression models. Again, there is no difference in the mathematical underpinnings and assumptions about the data in ANOVA and linear regression models; however, historically, ANOVA models were developed for the analysis of data from experimental studies, and regression models were originally developed independently for the analysis of data from observational studies (Snedecor & Cochran, 1989). While both ANOVA and the regression models can be used to analyze either experimental or observational data, in practice, it is important never to lose sight of the fact what types of data one deals with. There are two major reasons for this:

1. Just because we use statistical models that make a distinction between dependent and independent variables, this does not mean that we have already established causality. Rather, the statistical models *assume* it, and we must look elsewhere for justifications to draw causal inferences.[1]

2. With observational data, we cannot guarantee that the multiple independent variables are uncorrelated. As we will see in this chapter, this has consequences for how we can decompose variance and attribute it to various independent variables.

Beyond the question of whether or not we should interpret associations between a dependent and independent variable in causal terms, the choice of ANOVA/ANCOVA or linear regression models to analyze data is largely a matter of personal preference. However, the regression model is generally more efficient and easier to handle in the presentation, whenever a particular analysis involves many continuous or interval-/ratio-level *independent* variables.

---

[1]Primarily, the justification for causal inference depends on the strengths of the research design and theoretical rationale(s).

GENERAL FORM OF THE MULTIPLE LINEAR REGRESSION MODEL

The general form of the multiple linear regression looks like this:

$$Y_i = \beta_0 + \beta_1 X_{i1} + \beta_2 X_{i2} + \beta_3 X_{i3} + \cdots + \beta_k X_{ik} + \varepsilon_i$$

where Y_i refers to the dependent variable score of an individual i, β_0 is the intercept (or "constant") in the equation, and the $\beta_k X_{ik}$ terms refer to k independent variables, X_{ik}, multiplied by their respective regression coefficients, β_k. Finally, we use ε_i to refer to the residual or error term, which captures the difference between the actual score of individual i and the predicted score based on the regression equation. Employing the Greek letters for the coefficients indicates that we are referring to the **population parameters**. When estimating the regression coefficients based on available *sample* data, we make several assumptions about the data, which are already familiar from the simple linear regression model. They are summarized in Box 12.1.

BOX 12.1	ASSUMPTIONS OF MULTIPLE LINEAR REGRESSION MODEL

1. Interval/ratio level of measurement for outcome/dependent variable
2. Linearity of relation between dependent and independent (interval/ratio-level) variables
3. Independence of individual observations (uncorrelated error terms)
4. Normally distributed error terms with mean 0, that is, normally distributed error terms around the estimated regression line, that is, for all the categories defined by the independent variables
5. Equal variances (or standard deviations) within *all* comparison populations defined by the independent variables: σ = constant
6. Randomly drawn study sample for population inferences

As with simple linear regression, we use the same *least squares* criterion to calculate the sample estimates of the regression coefficients: We choose the values for the coefficient estimates so as to minimize the squared error terms, which is to say, we minimize the squared deviations of the observed dependent variable scores from the scores predicted by the regression equation: $\min(\Sigma e_i^2 = \Sigma(Y_i - \hat{Y}_i)^2)$.

EMPIRICAL EXAMPLE OF A MULTIPLE LINEAR REGRESSION ANALYSIS

For an example of a multiple regression analysis, we go back to the birth-weight data of Chapter 10. For the simple regression model presented in Table 10.1, we only used gestational age (measured in weeks) as a single predictor variable of birth weight. This time, we add the smoking status of the mother, the mother's age at the baby's birth, and the mother's years of formal education as additional predictors of the baby's birth weight. The results from the multiple regression analysis with data on 400 births are shown in Table 12.1. In this table, we see the estimates for the regression coefficients (column labeled "Coef."), their standard errors ("Std. Err."), and p-values for the t-tests ("P > |t|"). We are also provided summary statistics like the overall f-test for the equation as a whole, and R-squared, the measure of explained variance.

TABLE 12.1 Multiple Linear Regression: Birth Weights on Gestational Age, Mother's Age, Mother's Education, and Mother's Smoking Status

```
regress birthweight(bwt) gestation, smoking[Y/N](smoke), mother's age(mage), years of
formal education(educyrs)
```

Source	SS	df	MS		Number of obs	=	400
					F(4, 395)	=	207.34
Model	717.689	4	179.422		Prob > F	=	0.0000
Residual	341.821	395	.865		R-squared	=	0.6774
					Adj R-squared	=	0.6741
Total	1059.511	399	2.655		Root MSE	=	.93025

bwt	Coef.	Std. Err.	t	P>|t|	[95% Conf.	Intervl]	Beta
gestation	.17126	.00738	23.20	0.000	.15674	.18577	.71630
smoke	-.65882	.11960	-5.51	0.000	-.89396	-.42369	-.16268
mage	.02188	.00751	2.91	0.004	.00711	.03664	.08648
educyrs	.05537	.01987	2.79	0.006	.01631	.09443	.08325
_cons	.12542	.34322	0.37	0.715	-.54934	.80019	

With the information provided in Table 12.1, we can write out the estimated regression equation:

Estimated equation[2]: $$\hat{Y} = 0.125 + 0.171X_1 - 0.659X_2 + 0.022X_3 + 0.055X_4$$

Standard error of coefficients: (0.343) (0.007) (0.120) (0.008) (0.020)

p-values: $>0.715 \le 0.001 \quad \le 0.001 \quad \le 0.004 \quad \le 0.006$

Summary statistics: $R^2 = 0.667, F(4/395) = 207.34, p < 00005$

In the estimated equation, $\hat{Y}$ is the predicted birth weight, based on the equation and the values substituted for the independent variables; 0.125 is the estimated value of the intercept or constant coefficient $(\hat{b}_0)$; 0.171 is the estimated regression coefficient $(\hat{b}_1)$ associated with X_1, the measure for weeks of gestation; −0.659 is the estimated regression coefficient $(\hat{b}_2)$ associated with X_2, the dichotomous measure of a mother's smoking status (1 = smoker, 0 = nonsmoker); 0.022 is the estimated regression coefficient $(\hat{b}_3)$ associated with X_3, the measure of the mother's age (in years) at the baby's birth; and 0.055 is the estimated regression coefficient $(\hat{b}_4)$ associated with X_4, the measure of formal education (in years) achieved by the mother. Note that three of the predictor variables (weeks of gestation, mother's age and education) are ratio-level variables, and one predictor (smoking status) is a dummy-coded categorical variable.

Before we interpret the estimated regression equation, let us briefly review the summary statistics: The model R-squared[3] equals $R^2 = 0.667$, which means that the independent

---

[2] All coefficients in the book have been rounded to the third decimal.

[3] Recall that R^2 is also the ratio of Model SS over total SS; in Table 12.1, we have: 717.689/1059.511 = 0.6774. R^2 in a multiple regression model can also be interpreted as the square of the linear correlation (Pearson's r) between the observed, Y_i, and predicted, $\hat{Y}$, values of the dependent variable, with the prediction based on the estimated equation.

variables *together* account for 66.7% of the variation in birth weights among the 400 sample babies. The null hypothesis for the *f*-test is that *none* of the independent variables account for any variation in birth weights *in the target population*. An observed *f*-ratio of 207.34 is extremely unlikely ($p < .00005$) to occur in a sample, if the null hypothesis is actually true. Thus, we reject the null hypothesis for the *f*-test and conclude that *at least some* of the independent variables predict variation in birth weights. The summary statistics also include the root mean square error (MSE) of 0.93. This statistic is a measure of the standard deviation of the residuals,[4] which can be thought of as the average error associated with this regression model.

Now we turn to the estimates of the individual regression coefficients. In each case, the null hypothesis stipulates that the coefficient does not differ from zero in the population, as this would imply that the predicted $\hat{Y}$ does not change, regardless of the values or levels of the associated independent variable (X_k). The results in Table 12.1 show that, with the exception of the intercept term, all regression coefficients are statistically significant, as their *p*-values are substantially smaller than the usual significance criterion of $\alpha = 0.05$. These significance tests are based on the relevant *t*-distributions, with the *t*-values calculated as the ratios of the estimated regression coefficients and their associated standard errors. For instance, the regression coefficient for mother's age (0.02188) and its associated standard error (0.00751) yield a *t*-value of $t = 0.02188/0.00751 = 2.91$. The probability that a sample regression coefficient differs from zero by 2.91 standard errors, even though the population coefficient is zero, is very small indeed: A *t*-value as large or larger than 2.91 on a *t*-distribution with 395 degrees of freedom (df)[5] has a *p*-value of less than .0045, that is, less than 5 in 1,000 samples would return such a value as a result of mere sampling fluctuation. Thus, we reject the null hypothesis and infer that the true regression coefficient for mother's age differs from zero. Similar inferences can be made about the other regression coefficients, except for the intercept: We would *not* reject the null hypothesis that the intercept coefficient differs from zero, as the sample evidence is consistent with the null hypothesis; the chance of observing a sample intercept of 0.125, even though the null hypothesis is true, is quite large—it is 71.5%.

INTERPRETING A LINEAR REGRESSION EQUATION

As we have shown that the regression coefficients are "statistically significant," we are now ready to interpret the regression equation.

1. The intercept or "constant" is an indicator of the expected average value of birth weights, if *all* independent variables are equal to zero. Because of the lack of statistical significance, we would infer that the true population intercept equals zero. However, it is often the case—and this example is no exception—that the intercept coefficient does not have a meaningful interpretation. In the example of Table 12.1, it would not make much sense to ask: What is the mean birth weight of babies, born after *zero* weeks of gestation to mothers, who are *zero* years old, and have *no* education?

---

[4] Root MSE $= \sqrt{\dfrac{\Sigma(Y_i - \hat{Y})^2}{n - k - 1}}$.

[5] The df for the *t*-test of regression coefficient equal $n - k - 1$, with $n =$ sample size and $k =$ number of regression coefficients associated with the independent variables.

2. The estimate for the first regression coefficient, $\hat{b}_1 = 0.171$, tells us that, for every additional week of gestation, we can expect the average baby weight to increase by 0.171 pounds. Thus, a 10-week difference in the length of the pregnancy would result in an average difference in birth weight of 1.7 pounds, *independent of the effects that the other predictor variables have on the outcome*. As with all regression predictions, they retain validity only for the range of tested values in the predictor variable. As the data on which the estimates are based include a range of 22 to 44 weeks of gestation, one should not extrapolate beyond this existing range and "predict" average birth weights for babies born, for instance, after 14 weeks of gestation. Such a prediction assumes that the same linear relationship between gestation and birth weight continues outside the covered range; an assumption for which there is no empirical evidence.

3. The estimate for the second regression coefficient is: $\hat{b}_2 = -0.659$. As X_2 is a categorical variable coded (0, 1), we can say that the average expected birth weight for babies of smoking mothers should be lower, by more than half a pound, than the average expected birth weight for babies of nonsmoking mothers.

4. The estimates for the last two regression coefficients are: $\hat{b}_3 = 0.022$ and $\hat{b}_4 = 0.055$. The estimate for the regression coefficient associated with X_3 indicates that older mothers tend to give birth to heavier babies, such that for each additional year of the mothers' age babies' average birth weight is 0.022 pounds higher. Similarly, for additional year of a mother's formal education (X_4), her baby's birth weight increases by 0.055 pounds on average. As with gestational age, these predictions should be limited to the actual ranges of mothers' ages (17–44 years) and educational levels (8–20 years), on which the prediction is based.

When we look at the magnitudes of the estimated regression coefficients, we should be careful not to compare them directly. For instance, the coefficient estimates for $\hat{b}_4 = 0.055$ and $\hat{b}_3 = 0.022$ do *not* imply that years of mother's formal education have more than twice the effect on birth weights than her age. Similarly, the regression coefficient for smoking status (−0.659) is almost four times as large as that for weeks of gestation (+0.171), but this does not imply anything about their relative importance as predictors. One reason for this noncomparability of the *unstandardized* estimates of regression coefficients is simply that they are measured in different units. Years of education are not equivalent to years of life, not to speak of weeks of gestation. In addition, we could easily change the units of measurement (e.g., months of gestation), which would also change the magnitude of the regression coefficient estimates, as they show the change in the dependent variable *for a one-unit change in the independent variable*. In the nursing and medical literature, results from multiple regression models are often reported in terms of *standardized regression coefficients*, sometimes called *betas* as opposed to *bs* for the unstandardized coefficients. Standardized coefficients are obtained by converting all variables in the regression model from the original to standardized scores, using the familiar z-score transformation: $z_i = (x_i - \bar{x})/s$. This is done in order to make the effects of independent variables, measured in different measurement units, more comparable. The standardized coefficients provide estimates of how many standard deviations the dependent variable changes for a one-standard-deviation change in the independent variable(s). In Table 12.1 we see, for instance, that the magnitudes of the betas (regardless of sign) show the following rank order: gestation > smoking > mother's age > years of education. The unstandardized coefficients, on the other hand, show this rank order: smoking > gestation > years of education > mother's age. According to the standardized regression coefficients, it seems clear that "weeks of gestation" has a bigger effect on birth weight than smoking; but that conclusion would be too hasty. For a number of reasons, standardized regression coefficients ("betas") do not provide an unambiguous measure of the relative magnitude of the effects of various independent variables on the dependent variable. One reason for this is that standard deviations of independent variables are sensitive to the skew of these variables, with more heavily skewed independent variables having comparatively larger standard deviations. Thus, standard deviations may not provide an unambiguous metric for comparisons of effects. Another reason for this is the presence of confounding.

CONFOUNDING AND DECOMPOSITION OF VARIANCE IN DATA FROM OBSERVATIONAL STUDIES

In the last chapter on ANOVA and ANCOVA, we used data from a randomized intervention study. Such studies are deliberately designed so that the exposure and nonexposure to simultaneous treatments are independent of each other, that is, the independent factors' variables are *uncorrelated* with each other. In observational studies, we do not have this luxury. It is rarely the case that one gathers information on several variables in a particular target population, and these variables turn out to be completely uncorrelated. As an illustration of this point, for the multiple regression model in Table 12.1, we display the sample (Pearson's r) correlations, and their p-values, in Table 12.2.

Notice that all *sample* correlations differ from zero and, with the exception of the correlation between the mother's age and her smoking status, all are statistically significant at the α-level of 0.05. This means that the predictor variables in this multiple regression model do not vary independently: their variation partially overlaps (see Figure 12.1 for a graphical illustration). Consequently, when we talk about "accounting for" variance in the dependent

TABLE 12.2 Pearson's *r* Correlations Among Variables in Multiple Regression of Table 12.1: Birth Weights on Gestational Age, Mother's Age, Mother's Education, and Mother's Smoker Status

correlations birthweight(bwt), gestation, smoking[Y/N](smoke), mother's age(mage), years of formal education(educyrs)

	bwt	gestation	smoke	mage	educyrs
bwt	1.0000				
gestation	0.7959	1.0000			
	0.0000				
smoke	−0.3431	−0.4204	1.0000		
	0.0000	0.0000			
mage	0.2988	0.2584	−0.0968	1.0000	
	0.0000	0.0000	0.0530		
educyrs	0.3074	0.2576	−0.1704	0.1379	1.0000
	0.0000	0.0000	0.0006	0.0058	

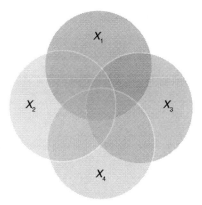

FIGURE 12.1 Overlapping Variances.

variable, there is no longer a straightforward answer. For instance, X_1, which is our measure of weeks of gestation is correlated with X_3, the age of the mother. Thus, part of the variance accounted for in the dependent variable is explained *jointly* by these two predictor variables (see overlapping circles for X_1 and X_3 in Figure 12.1). That poses the question: Should this overlapping area be attributed to X_1 or X_3, when we apportion "explained" variance in the dependent variable?

In fact, when we hierarchically, or sequentially, decompose the sums of squares (SSs), it matters in which order the predictor variables are entered into the model. This is so, because, with hierarchical decomposition of variance, we attribute to the first predictor variable all the variance in the dependent variable it can account for; predictor variables entered later into the model each explain the *remaining* variance,[6] not yet accounted for by the previous independent predictor(s). In terms of the graph in Figure 12.1, the variance attributed to X_1 would be represented by the whole X_1 circle, the variance attributed to X_3 would be represented by the circle of X_3 *minus* its overlapping areas with X_1 and X_2, and so forth. For a numerical example, see Table 12.3.

In Table 12.3, we revisit the multiple regression model in Table 12.1, but show two more detailed ANOVA tables comparing the hierarchical decomposition of the variance after entering weeks of gestation as the first predictor variable (Model 1, as in Table 12.1) and after entering it as the last predictor variable (Model 2). Notice that the overall Model SS remains the same: The variance accounted for by all predictor variables combined remains the same, regardless of the order of the independent variables in the model. However, in Model 1, weeks of gestation account for 63.35% (671.226/1,059.511 = 0.6335) of the variation in birth weights, while in Model 2, the same variable accounts for only 43.95% (465.632/1,059.511) of the variation in birth weights. This difference of about 20% points is the result of the fact that the variable "weeks of gestation" is correlated with the other predictor variables, and *it is not possible* to attribute this joint variation uniquely to one or the other independent predictors.

If independent variables in a multivariate model are correlated, we witness the presence of **confounding** effects. Usually, researchers focus on one or a few potential predictor variables whose relationship to the outcome variable they want to explore or test. In our example, the primary interest of a researcher may be to obtain estimates of the strength of the association between gestational age and birth weight. However, the existing literature has already shown that mothers' age, education, and smoking also affect birth weight (Cogswell & Yip, 1995).

---

[6]The SSs associated with the remaining, uniquely attributable variance are also called *partial SS*.

TABLE 12.3 Two Hierarchical Decompositions of Variance in Multiple Linear Regression: Birth Weights on Gestational Age, Mother's Age, Mother's Education, and Mother's Smoker Status

Model 1: Gestational Age as 1st Predictor Variable:

regress birthweight(bwt) gestation, smoking[Y/N](smoke), mother's age(mage), years of formal education(educyrs)

Number of obs = 400   R-squared   = 0.6774
Root MSE   = .930253   Adj R-squared = 0.6741

Source	Seq. SS	df	MS	F	Prob > F
Model	717.689	4	179.422	207.34	0.0000
gestation	671.226	1	671.226	775.65	0.0000
smoke	31.311	1	31.311	36.18	0.0000
mage	8.431	1	8.431	9.74	0.0019
educyrs	6.721	1	6.721	7.77	0.0056
Residual	341.821	395	.865		
Total	1059.511	399	2.655		

Model 2: Gestational Age as last Predictor Variable:

regress birthweight(bwt) smoking[Y/N](smoke), mother's age(mage), years of formal education(educyrs), gestation

Number of obs = 400   R-squared   = 0.6774
Root MSE   = .930253   Adj R-squared = 0.6741

Source	Seq. SS	df	MS	F	Prob > F
Model	717.689	4	179.422	207.34	0.0000
smoke	124.735	1	124.735	144.14	0.0000
mage	75.418	1	75.418	87.15	0.0000
educyrs	51.905	1	51.905	59.98	0.0000
gestation	465.632	1	465.632	538.07	0.0000
Residual	341.821	395	.865		
Total	1059.511	399	2.655		

Thus, these confounding variables cannot be ignored. Even though confounding variables may not be of primary interest, controlling for them changes the estimates of the relationship between the dependent and the focal independent variable. If you go back to Chapter 10, you will find an estimate of the regression coefficient associated with weeks of gestation that differs from the one in the multiple regression model: $\hat{b}_1 = 0.1903$ (Table 10.1) versus $\hat{b}_1 = 0.171$ (Table 12.1). This is the result of the fact that the model in Table 10.1 is a *simple* regression model with "weeks of gestation" as the only predictor variable. After accounting for the mothers' age, education, and smoking status, we see that the *remaining* effect of gestational age on birth weights is a bit smaller than originally estimated.

From our discussion of confounding, it should be apparent that estimates of supposed "effects," which are based on observational data, are always subject to the critique that they may have omitted important confounding variables, which would have modified the reported estimates. For instance, in the current example, it is likely that the mothers' nutrition and alcohol consumption as well as family income, with its attendant social consequences, all have the potential to modify the regression coefficient estimating the relationship between gestational age and birth weight. It follows that the reader of a study using observational data should always ask whether the analysis has properly controlled for already known confounders. These would be other variables, whose effects on the dependent variable have been demonstrated in the literature and which are correlated with the primary predictor variable of interest. While one can never rule out for certain that there are no unrecognized confounders, the credibility of an empirical investigation, using observational data, depends on the care with which the researchers address confounding variables in the analysis.

CONFOUNDING AND MULTICOLLINEARITY

Confounding can pose technical problems in the estimation of a regression model, if the independent variables are correlated too highly. This so-called **multicollinearity** problem arises because highly correlated independent or predictor variables imply that we cannot separate out the independent contribution that each of these predictor variables makes toward accounting for variation in the dependent or outcome variable. For example, suppose an epidemiologist is studying physical fitness among school-age students. The study sample contains students from grades 1 to 12. The data set contains a variable for the grade a student is in and a variable with information on the student's age. The correlation between these two variables can be expected to be larger than 0.9, as most students advance both in school grades and age at the same pace. It would not make any sense to use both variables as predictors in the same regression equation, as their *independent* effects could not be determined. Take an even more extreme example: Suppose you had data on only Black women and White men, but no Black men and White women. In that case, race and sex would be completely confounded ($r = 1.0$); as a result, it would be impossible to distinguish a "race effect" from a "sex effect." In short, when multicollinearity is present, there is not enough independent information, that is, variation among some or all independent variables, so that separate effects can be estimated. In terms of Figure 12.1, just imagine that the circle for X_4 almost completely overlaps with those of X_1 to X_3 leaving only a tiny sliver representing independent variation.

How does a reader recognize the presence of a multicollinearity problem in a published analysis? The telltale sign is the combination of a highly significant *f*-test with insignificant *t*-tests for the individual regression coefficients, whose standard errors would be comparatively large. This makes sense, because *jointly* the independent variables do predict variation in the dependent variable, but we cannot separate out the independent contributions. If multicollinearity is present, the analyst must drop one or more of the problematic variables from the model equation. However, statistics alone does not offer an answer as to which of the highly correlated independent variables should be dropped; that is a question of theory and the objectives of the analysis. For instance, in the example of student age and school grades, it depends on the primary research question as to which variable to highlight and which to drop. In the case of the race–sex confounding example, only additional data collection, such as including Black men and White women, could help disentangle race from sex effects.

A NOTE ON CONFOUNDING AND STANDARDIZED REGRESSION COEFFICIENTS

We wrote earlier that standardized regression coefficients do not necessarily provide unambiguous measures of the relative magnitude of multiple predictor variables in a regression model. While it is true that standardization ignores the original measurement units, it also needs to be remembered that regression coefficients, whether standardized or not, only capture the *unique* associations of independent variables with the dependent variable, that is, independent of the effects of all other variables in the equation. Thus, variables with smaller betas may well have larger overall associations with the dependent variable. In addition, some of the independent variables in a model may be intervening or *mediating* variables (Bennett, 2000). In our example of smoking and weeks of gestation, there is little doubt that the mother's smoking has an indirect effect on weeks of gestation: As the negative correlation in Table 12.2 shows ($r = -0.42$), the smoking mothers tend to have shorter gestation periods. Thus, comparing the magnitudes of betas does not necessarily provide a simple answer to the question—which independent variable has the biggest effect on or association with the dependent variable?

INTERACTIONS IN MULTIPLE REGRESSION MODELS

The linear regression equation associated with the estimates in Table 12.1 is a so-called main-effects model. Just as in ANOVA, interaction effects can also occur in regression models, and they have the same general interpretation. The regression model based on Table 12.1 contained the following estimates for the regression coefficients:

$$\hat{Y} = 0.123 + 0.171X_1 - 0.659X_2 + 0.022X_3 + 0.055X_4$$

where all coefficients, except the intercept, differ significantly from the null value of zero. If this model were a true reflection of reality, it would lead us to the conclusion that, for every additional week of gestation, baby weights can be expected to increase by 0.171 pounds on average, regardless of whether or not the mother is a smoker, whether or not she is younger or older, or what educational achievements she has. Similarly, the absence of all interaction effects would posit that the effect of age on birth weights is the same, regardless of whether the mother is a smoker or not, and so forth. These are *assumptions*, which the researcher needs to *test* against the data before presenting the main-effects model as the proper representation of the reality.

Interaction effects in multiple linear regression (and ANOVA) models are modeled as additional independent predictors consisting of multiplicative terms involving two or more independent variables already in the model. For example, let us test the assumption that the effect of the mother's age on birth weights is the same, regardless of whether the mother is a smoker or not. The expanded model would look like this:

$$Y_i = \beta_0 + \beta_1 X_{i1} + \beta_2 X_{i2} + \beta_3 X_{i3} + \beta_4 X_{i4} + \beta_5 X_{i5} + \varepsilon_i$$

where $X_{i5} = X_{i2} X_{i3}$.

Table 12.4 shows the results of estimating this regression model with the interaction term: Overall, this model has a better explanatory power than the main-effects model, as shown by the significant coefficient for the interaction effect (Mother's Age × Smoking Status) or $\hat{b}_5 = -0.046$ ($p \leq .008$) as well as the somewhat improved R^2 estimate of 0.6831. To see how we can interpret the interaction effect, we show first the estimated equation for the

TABLE 12.4 Multiple Linear Regression With Interaction: Birth Weights on Gestational Age, Mother's Smoking Status, Age and Education, and Mother's Age × Smoking Status

```
regress birthweight(bwt), gestation, smoking (Y/N)(smoke), mother's age (mage),
years of formal education (educyrs)

      Source |       SS     df       MS              Number of obs =     400
-------------+--------------------------------       F( 5, 394)    =  169.89
       Model |   723.799      5   144.760            Prob > F      =  0.0000
    Residual |   335.712    394      .852            R-squared     =  0.6831
-------------+--------------------------------       Adj R-squared =  0.6791
       Total |  1059.511    399    2.655             Root MSE      =  .92307


         bwt |     Coef.   Std. Err.      t     P>|t|     [95% Conf.   Interval]
-------------+-----------------------------------------------------------------
   gestation |    .16950     .00736    23.04    0.000      .15504      .18396
       smoke |    .51224     .45316     1.13    0.259     -.37867     1.40315
        mage |    .03283     .00850     3.86    0.000      .01611      .04954
     educyrs |    .05552     .01971     2.82    0.005      .01676      .09428
 mage x smoke|   -.04624     .01727    -2.68    0.008     -.08018     -.01229
       _cons |   -.10736     .35149    -0.31    0.760     -.79839      .58367
```

total population and simplify the model, by listing separate models for smoking and nonsmoking mothers:

$$\hat{Y} = -0.107 + 0.170X_1 + 0.512X_2 + 0.033X_3 + 0.056X_4 - 0.046X_5$$

Recall that the variable indicating smoking status, X_2, is coded 0 for nonsmoking mothers and 1 for smoking mothers. As the interaction term involving smoking status and mother's age is $X_5 = X_2X_3$, it follows that $X_5 = 0$, if $X_2 = 0$. Thus, for nonsmoking mothers the equation simplifies to:

$$\hat{Y} = -0.107 + 0.170X_1 + (0)(0) + 0.033X_3 + 0.056X_4 - 0.046(0)X_3$$

(We substitute (0) for the regression coefficient of X_2 because it is *not* statistically significant [$p > .259$] and we cannot reject the null hypothesis; we substitute (0) for X_3, which is one component of X_5, as $X_5 = X_2X_3$.)

The final equation for nonsmokers becomes:

$$\hat{Y} = 0.107 + 0.170X_1 + 0.033X_3 + 0.056X_4$$

For smoking mothers, this equation will be simplified as follows:

$$\hat{Y} = -0.107 + 0.170X_1 + (0)(1) + 0.033X_3 + 0.056X_4 - 0.046(1)X_3$$

(As before, we substitute (0) for the regression coefficient of X_2 and (1) for X_2; as $X_5 = X_2X_3$, it become X_3, if $X_2 = 1$; combining the two terms involving X_3 yields (0.033 − 0.046) $X_3 = -0.013X_3$.)

The final equation for smokers becomes:

$$\hat{Y} = 0.107 + 0.170X_1 - 0.013X_3 + 0.056X_4$$

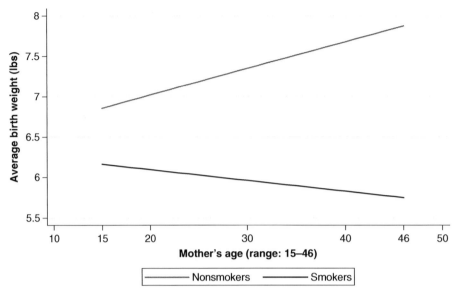

FIGURE 12.2 Change in Average Birth Weight by Mother's Age: Interaction of Mother's Age and Smoking Status.

Now we can better see what the meaning of the interaction term is: Among nonsmoking mothers, greater age is associated with higher average birth weight; for each additional year of age, average birth weights increase by 0.033 pounds. By contrast, among smoking mothers, higher age is associated with *declining* average birth weight: For each additional year of age, average birth weights are 0.013 pounds lighter. Figure 12.2 offers a visual representation of this interaction. Again, as in ANOVA, an interaction effect in a regression model indicates that the effect of one predictor variable on the outcome changes, depending on the level of another predictor variable.

CHECKING THE ASSUMPTIONS OF THE MODEL

As mentioned in Box 12.1, the multiple linear regression model assumes interval/ratio levels of measurement for the dependent variable; linearity of relations between dependent and independent (interval/ratio-level) variables; uncorrelated error terms; normally distributed error terms around the estimated regression line with mean zero and equal variances or standard deviations across different levels of the predicted outcome: σ = constant (homoskedasticity assumption).

A simple way to test these assumptions is to plot the error terms against the predicted value of Y in a scattergram, as depicted in Figure 12.3.

As can easily be seen, the mean of these residuals is indeed close to zero; the variances appear to be constant across different levels of the predicted dependent variable, that is, visually the spread of data points is about the same regardless of the level of the predicted dependent variable. There is only one major outlier with a standard deviation larger than 3, and there appears to be no discernible nonlinear pattern in the distribution of these error terms around the predicted regression line. Thus, we conclude that the multiple regression model with the age and smoking-status interaction term provides a reasonable fit to the data at hand.

When reading the empirical literature in the clinical journals, the reader will notice that information on whether the data meet the assumptions of the statistical model chosen is often missing or incomplete. While many careful researchers do check the assumptions, it cannot

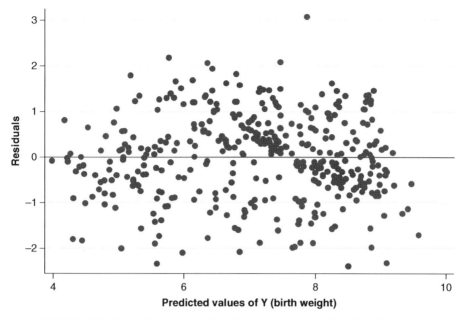

FIGURE 12.3 Plot of Regression Residuals Against Predicted Birth Weight.

always be taken for granted. As a reader, your trust in research results should increase, if the researchers provided you with the information necessary to assess the adequacy of the statistical model.

SUMMARY

In this chapter we reviewed multiple linear regression models, which are among the most frequently employed analysis models in the clinical literature. While mathematically equivalent to ANOVA and ANCOVA models, linear regression models are more often employed in the analysis of observational data, such as data from health surveys. The most important issue in the statistical analysis of observational data is the ever-present problem of confounding: If a correlated predictor is omitted from the regression model, this can lead to substantial biases in the estimates of regression coefficients, as the omission of confounders will have the effect of attributing accounted for variance to variables in the model, which should have been attributed to the confounding variable(s). While the linear regression model is quite versatile and can be employed with many types of data, successful use requires care in checking the assumptions: Chief among them is testing for interactions and nonlinearity of relationships as well as violations concerning homoskedasticity and, particularly in small data sets, normality of error terms.

So far, all statistical models we have discussed dealt with cross-sectional data, that is, data collected once and referring to a particular point in time. However, clinicians are often interested in longitudinal data, as when they follow up patients recovering from an illness or want to know about the trajectory of growth and decline patterns in aging human beings. In the next chapter, we will discuss repeated-measures ANOVA, which is a statistical model that is often appropriate for the analysis of clinical trials with repeated measures. The last chapter in this section (Chapter 14) will then provide a brief overlook of newer statistical models, which have become common in the clinical literature, that can be used to analyze many kinds of longitudinal data.

LITERATURE APPLICATION

Read: Andrews, M. E., Stewart, N. J., Morgan, D. G., & D'arcy, C. More alike than different: A comparison of male and female RNs in rural and remote Canada. *Journal of Nursing Management*, *20*(4), 561–570.

(a) Provide a very brief (three to four sentences) summary of what this study is about.

(b) Define the target population to which the statistical analysis can be generalized. What were the eligibility and exclusion criteria for study participants? Is the study sample a random sample of the target population?

(c) The researchers used a randomized block design, blocking on sex and clinic site. What is the purpose of this?

(d) Provide a clear definition of the outcome/dependent variable and a short description of the instrument used to measure it. Is the level of measurement likely to be interval level?

(e) In table 6 of the article, the authors show the results of a multiple regression analysis for male and female nurses as well as both groups combined ("full model"). In a sentence or two, interpret the regression coefficients associated with age and gender. What do they mean?

(f) Calculate the *t*-values for the "colleague support in medicine" variable across all three regression models and look up the associated *p*-values in the appropriate *t*-distribution table of Appendix B.

(g) What appears to be the main reason why many more regression coefficients for the male regression model are not statistically significant?

(h) Do the authors provide evidence that the data meet the assumptions of their statistical tests?

(i) Comparing the results from the regression models for male and female nurses, do you suspect interaction effects between gender and some of the other independent variables? If yes, how should one test an interaction hypothesis involving gender?

(j) State in your own words, what an interaction effect involving gender means.

(k) The regression models in table 6 contain a binary predictor variable answering the question: Have you looked for other employment opportunities in the past year? When considering the dependent or outcome variable, would you classify the potential causal status of this variable? What does it suggest to you about the interpretation of the regression model?

(l) Summarize the main findings in your own words: Are the conclusions of the authors consistent with the evidence presented?

EXERCISES

1. In Table 12.1, the R-squared estimate is given as 0.6774. Show how this value is derived from the ANOVA table accompanying the regression output.

2. A study of 450 randomly selected community hospitals in the United States predicts annual turnover rates among hospital nurses (as percentage of the nursing labor force in a hospital). The predictor variables are: X_1 = deviation of nurses' average earnings in

a hospital (measured in $1,000) from the median earnings of active RNs in the United States ($64,000), X_2 = deviation of average age of nursing labor force in a hospital from the mean age (46) of active U.S. nurses, and two dummy variables indicating location of the hospital: X_3 = rural (1) versus nonrural (0), X_4 = urban (1) versus nonurban (0), with the reference category being suburban location of the hospital. The estimated regression equation (with standard error in parentheses) is as follows:

$$\hat{Y} = 17.70 - 0.70X_1 + 0.50X_2 - 0.85X_3 - 2.23X_4$$
$$(1.82) \quad (0.25) \quad (0.18) \quad (0.38) \quad (0.76)$$

(a) Write a short paragraph summarizing the essential information contained in this equation.
(b) What is the expected annual turnover rate among nurses in a hospital that is located in the suburbs, has a nursing staff with mean age = 46 and pays its nurses, on average, $3,000 more than the U.S. median earnings?
(c) Are all regression coefficients statistically significant at the α-level 0.05? Provide the reasoning for your answer.
(d) What is the meaning of the intercept coefficient (17.7)?

3. Suppose a researcher studies predictors of the frequency of emergency department visits in an urban area, with $[X_1]$ race (1 = African American, 0 = other ethnic groups), $[X_2]$ family income (measured in $1,000), and $[X_3]$ having health insurance (1 = yes, 0 = no) as predictors. The researcher reports the results from three (hierarchical) regression equations, in which the additional predictors are entered successively:

1. $\hat{Y} = 2.7 + 0.90X_1$
2. $\hat{Y} = 3.3 + 0.50X_1 - 0.10X_2$
3. $\hat{Y} = 3.5 + 0.10X_1 - 0.05X_2 - 2.85X_3$

In all three equations, the intercept coefficient is significant at the 0.05 level, but the race coefficient declines in size and is no longer statistically significant ($p > .46$) in the third equation. The coefficients for family income and health insurance status in the second and third equations are all statistically significant ($p < .05$). Explain, why this pattern might occur.

REFERENCES

Bennett, J. A. (2000). Focus on research methods: Mediator and moderator variables in nursing research: Conceptual and statistical differences. *Research in Nursing & Health, 23*(3), 415–420.

Cogswell, M. E., & Yip, R. (1995). The influence of fetal and maternal factors on the distribution of birthweight. *Seminars in Perinatology, 19*(3), 222–240.

Snedecor, G. W., & Cochran, W. G. (1989). *Statistical methods* (8th ed.). Ames, IA: Iowa State University Press.

CHAPTER 13

Repeated-Measures Analysis of Variance

Suppose you are interested in the effectiveness of a physical activity intervention to reduce obesity among mobile residents of assisted-living facilities. You devise two programs for group activities: a three-times-a-week walking program for the intervention group and a three-times-a-week social club for the control group, which involves a variety of physically undemanding social activities. You enroll 92 volunteers, who agree to be randomly assigned to either the intervention or control (social club) group. At the start of the programs, each subject's height and weight are measured (pretest) using standardized procedures. After 6 months of enrollment in the study, you again obtain each subject's height and weight measures (posttest). Your primary outcome measure to gauge the success of the physical activity intervention is the body mass index (BMI), which is obtained by dividing a person's weight (in kilograms) by his or her squared height (in meters): $BMI = kg/m^2$. Table 13.1 shows the mean BMI scores of the pretest and posttest measures for both comparison groups: There appears to be a noticeable decline in the mean BMI within the intervention group, but not the control group. However, we need a statistical test to determine whether this decline is "statistically significant" and not just a sampling fluke due to random assignment or due to the inevitable random measurement error.

We might be tempted to employ a series of t-tests, each of which could be used to test for mean differences between a particular pair of measures. Table 13.2 shows the four relevant t-tests: using the two sample t-test to compare the intervention and control groups at Time 1 (pretest) and Time 2 (posttest) and using the paired t-test to compare the change in means within the intervention and the control group. The results confirm a pattern that could have been expected based on the description of the intervention study:

1. After random assignment, but before the start of the intervention programs, we would not expect statistically significant differences in the BMI pretest scores between intervention and control groups. In fact, the test confirms this: The observed sample mean difference is $-.1858$ ($p > .844$).

2. Six months later after participation in either of the two programs, we would anticipate statistically significant differences in the BMI posttest scores between the intervention and control groups. The results again confirm this: The observed sample mean difference is -4.002 ($p < .001$).

TABLE 13.1 Mean BMI Scores for 92 Subjects in Physical Activity/ Walking-Intervention Study

Means, Standard Deviations of BMI and No. of Subjects				
Intervention vs. Control Group	Time: Pretest	Posttest	Total	
control group (social club)	25.87 4.50 46	25.60 4.39 46	25.73 4.42 92	
intervention group (exercise)	25.68 4.54 46	21.60 5.16 46	23.64 5.25 92	
Total	25.77 4.49 92	23.60 5.17 92	24.69 4.95 184	(BMI Means) (BMI St.Dev's) (n)

3. Considered separately, we would not necessarily expect a statistically significant change of BMI scores in the control group. However, the observed change in sample means is -0.2261 ($p < .148$); thus, while the change may be small, we do observe a statistically significant decline in mean BMI scores, using the conventional significance level of $\alpha = 0.05$ as the criterion.

4. In the intervention group, we would definitely expect a statistically significant decline in BMI scores. The results again confirm this: The observed change in sample means is -4.0827 ($p < .001$).

There are a number of issues with an analysis such as this. To begin with, there is the sheer cumbersomeness of having to use four separate tests to confirm that the intervention had an effect. If possible, we would prefer to incorporate all this information into a single omnibus test that answers the question about the effectiveness of the intervention. Alternatively, we could have just ignored the pretest scores and concentrated on the posttest results alone, comparing the BMI scores in the intervention and control groups after random assignment. This would be a valid test of the intervention's effectiveness; and, in this example, we did find a statistically significant difference in the posttest scores with lower mean BMI scores in the intervention compared to the control group. However, by not incorporating the information contained in the pretest scores, the power of the posttest only comparison is lower than it would have been otherwise. Particularly with smaller study samples, we might have been unable to show statistically significant differences. In addition, a posttest only comparison does not provide a direct estimate of how much mean BMI scores *change* as a result of the physical activity intervention.

Relying on separate paired t-tests in either the intervention or the control group does give us estimates of mean changes in BMI scores, but these tests entirely ignore what is happening in the other comparison group(s). For instance, we found that participants in the control group exposed to a social club program experienced a small, but statistically significant decline in BMI scores. Whatever the reasons for this decline, we could not adequately

TABLE 13.2 Four *t*-Tests of Mean BMI Scores in Physical Activity Intervention Study

Two-sample t test with equal variances for Time 1 (pretest):
```
--------------------------------------------------------------------
            |    Obs     Mean      Std. Err.           [95% Conf. Interval]
---------+----------------------------------------------------------
Group diff  |    92     -.1858      .9418             -2.0568      1.6851
--------------------------------------------------------------------
```
Group diff = mean(intervention) – mean(control)   t = 0.1973
Ho: diff = 0,   deg. of freedom = 90,   Ha: diff ≠ 0,   Pr(|T| > |t|) = 0.8440

Two-sample t test with equal variances for Time 2 (posttest):
```
--------------------------------------------------------------------
            |    Obs     Mean      Std. Err.           [95% Conf. Interval]
---------+----------------------------------------------------------
Group diff  |    92     -4.002      .9990             -5.9871     -2.0176
--------------------------------------------------------------------
```
Group diff = mean(intervention) – mean(control)   t = 4.0063
Ho: diff = 0,   deg. of freedom = 90,   Ha: diff ≠ 0,   Pr(|T| > |t|) = 0.0001

Paired t test (Time 2 – Time 1) in Control Group:
```
--------------------------------------------------------------------
            |    Obs     Mean      Std. Err.    Std. Dev.    [95% Conf. Interval]
---------+----------------------------------------------------------
Time diff   |    46     -.2661      .1304        .8844       -.5288      -.0035
--------------------------------------------------------------------
```
    mean(diff) = mean(BMI2 – BMI1)   t = -2.0411
Ho: mean(diff) = 0,   deg. of freedom = 45,   Ha: diff ≠ 0,   Pr(|T|>|t|) = 0.0471

Paired t test (Time 2 – Time 1) in Intervention Group:
```
--------------------------------------------------------------------
            |    Obs     Mean      Std. Err.    Std. Dev.    [95% Conf. Interval]
---------+----------------------------------------------------------
Time diff   |    46     -4.0827     .2723       1.8467       -4.6311     -3.5343
--------------------------------------------------------------------
```
    mean(diff) = mean(BMI2 – BMI1)   t = -14.9945
Ho: mean(diff) = 0,   deg. of freedom = 45,   Ha: diff ≠ 0,   Pr(|T|>|t|) = 0.0000

gauge the intervention effect of exposure to the walking program, unless we acknowledge that changes/declines in BMI scores could occur even without any walking intervention. What we need is a way to incorporate all the information contained in the data into a single test.

THE ANCOVA APPROACH TO ANALYZING DATA FROM PRETEST/POSTTEST STUDY DESIGNS

One possible way to take advantage of all the information collected in a pretest/posttest randomized intervention study is to employ an analysis-of-covariance (ANCOVA) model, with the pretest scores used as a continuous covariate, that is, as an additional independent control variable. The results of such an analysis are shown in Table 13.3.

As was discussed in Chapter 11, the ANCOVA combines the between-group analysis-of-variance (ANOVA) approach with the linear regression approach, controlling for at least one independent continuous variable. Using this approach, we can compare the mean BMI

TABLE 13.3 ANCOVA Approach to Testing Mean BMI Scores for 92 Subjects in Physical Activity Intervention Study

```
ancova BMI2(posttest) c.BMI1(pretest) Walking, seq

                    Number of obs =     92          R-squared     = 0.9226
                      Root MSE = 1.4551             Adj R-squared = 0.9209

        Source  |    Seq. SS     df        MS        F      Prob > F
    ------------+-------------------------------------------------------
         Model  |   2245.975      2    1122.988   530.42    0.0000
                |
   Pretest BMI1 |   1911.474      1    1911.474   902.84    0.0000
   Walking(Y/N) |    334.501      1     334.501   157.99    0.0000
                |
      Residual  |    188.429     89       2.117
    ------------+-------------------------------------------------------
         Total  |   2434.404     91      26.752
```

score at the time of the posttest between the intervention and the control group, after removing the variation in individual posttest BMI scores that are accounted for by the BMI pretest scores. In effect, this test would be equivalent to a between-group test on the change scores of BMI posttest minus BMI pretests. In Table 13.3, the f-test associated with the comparison of BMI-posttest scores in the walking-intervention and control group yields: f(df1 = 1/df2 = 89) = 157.99, $p < .00005$, a much more powerful f-test than that from one-way ANOVA: f(df1 = 1/df2 = 90) = 16.05, $p \leq .0001$, which is equivalent to the two-sample t-test on the posttest only data in Table 13.2.[1]

REPEATED-MEASURES ANOVA

While the ANCOVA approach works with data from a randomized controlled pretest/posttest study and is commonly employed in the literature (Good et al., 2013; Tsay & Hung, 2004; Tseng et al., 2010), it cannot handle more complex study designs with additional repeated measures. For instance, researchers may decide to continue the study for another 6 months and collect information on a second posttest to gauge the longer-term effects of the intervention. Furthermore, while the ANCOVA approach offers valid and efficient tests of the mean differences between intervention and control groups at the time of the posttest, it does not offer direct comparisons of the magnitudes of average *changes* in the intervention and control group scores. This can be accomplished more easily with a model that treats the BMI scores at the different times of measurement as dependent outcomes and models the change explicitly.

One approach to analyzing such data is the **repeated-measures ANOVA**. It combines the traditional ANOVA approach of comparing mean outcomes in different groups of individuals, defined by the "between-subjects" factor(s), with comparing mean outcomes among the same set of individuals at different times, defined by the "within-subjects" factor.

To understand how this works, we reuse the previous example of the Physical Activity/Walking-Intervention Study, but extend it to a second follow-up observation of the participants'

---

[1]Recall from Chapter 9 that in a single two-group comparison, the one-way f-test and the t-test are related: $f = t^2$.

TABLE 13.4 Mean BMI Scores for 92 Subjects in Physical Activity/Walking-Intervention Study

Means, Standard Deviations of BMI and No. of Subjects					
Intervention vs. Control Group	Pretest (baseline)	Posttest 1 (6 months)	Posttest 2 (12 months)	Total	
control group (social club)	25.87 4.50 46	25.60 4.39 46	25.42 4.47 46	25.63 4.43 138	
intervention group (walking)	25.68 4.54 46	21.60 5.16 46	20.55 5.37 46	22.61 5.47 138	
Total	25.77 4.49 92	23.60 5.17 92	22.99 5.49 92	24.12 5.19 276	(BMI Means) (BMI St.Dev's) (n)

BMI at 12 months after the baseline enrollment. Table 13.3 shows the descriptive information for the three observation times in both the intervention and control groups.

The data in Table 13.4 represent summaries of individual BMI scores for 92 individuals, split into 46 individuals in the intervention and 46 individuals in the control group at three different occasions: pretest, posttest at 6 months, and posttest at 12 months. Thus, the design involves one between-group factor with two levels and one within-group factor with three levels. As the 92 study individuals were measured at three different occasions, we have a total of 276 individual BMI scores with an overall mean of 24.12. When considering the decomposition of variance in an ANOVA model like this, we start, as usual, with the total sum of squares (TSS) as the measure of how much overall variation there is among all 276 BMI scores. This TSS is obtained in the familiar fashion: by subtracting from each individual BMI score the overall mean, squaring the differences, and summing them: $\Sigma(Y_{igt} - \overline{\overline{Y}}_{..})^2 = \Sigma(Y_{igt} - 24.12)^2$.[2] From the results shown in Table 13.5, we see that this TSS equals 7,408.223.

With a repeated-measures design, we need to distinguish two basic types of variations in outcome scores: variation across different individuals ("between-subjects") and variation across different measurement occasions (time) within individuals ("within-subjects"). When we compute the between-subjects sum of squares (SS), we disregard the within-subjects variation by averaging the scores of each individual at the different measurement occasions (such as baseline, 6 months, and 12 months). With the current data, this will yield 92 timed-averaged BMI scores. The total between-subjects SS would thus be $\Sigma(Y_{igt} - \overline{\overline{Y}}_{..})^2 = \Sigma(Y_{igt} - 24.12)^2 = 6,571.446$. This particular number for the total between-subjects SS can easily be recovered from the ANOVA table in Table 13.4: It is the sum of the between-group SS associated with membership in either the walking treatment or the control group and the residual SS, which is a measure of the squared deviations of individual

---

[2]*Note*: i (1...92) is the subscript for individual study participants, g (1, 2) indicates a study participant's group assignment (experimental vs. control), and t (1, 2, 3) indicates the time a particular BMI score was measured.

TABLE 13.5 Mean BMI Scores for 92 Subjects in Physical Activity/Walking-Intervention Study

```
. anova BMI Walking / id|walking time walking*time, repeated(time)

                              Number of obs = 276       R-squared     = 0.9789
                              Root MSE      = .932369   Adj R-squared = 0.9677

               Source  |   Partial SS    df        MS         F       Prob > F
          ------------+-------------------------------------------------------
                Model  |    7251.747      95      76.334     87.81     0.0000
                       |
          Walking(Y/N) |     629.512       1     629.512      9.53     0.0027
   Btw-Subject Residual|    5941.934      90      66.021
          ------------+-------------------------------------------------------
                 time  |     394.361       2     197.180    226.82     0.0000
         Walking*time  |     285.941       2     142.970    164.46     0.0000
                       |
    Within-Subj. Residual|   156.476     180       .869
          ------------+-------------------------------------------------------
                Total  |    7408.223     275      26.939
```

```
Between-subjects error term:   id|walking
                   Levels:     92          (90 df)
      Lowest b.s.e. variable:  id
      Covariance pooled over:  walking     (for repeated variable)

Repeated variable: time
                                              Huynh-Feldt epsilon      = 0.6301
                                         Greenhouse-Geisser epsilon    = 0.6188
                                         Box's conservative epsilon    = 0.5000
                                         ------------- Prob > F -------
               Source  |   df       F      Regular    H-F      G-G      Box
          ------------+-------------------------------------------------------
                 time  |    2    226.82    0.0000    0.0000   0.0000   0.0000
         Walking*time  |    2    164.46    0.0000    0.0000   0.0000   0.0000
              Residual |  180
          ------------+-------------------------------------------------------
```

time-averaged BMI scores from the mean group scores[3]: 629.512 + 5,941.934 = 6,571.446. By contrast, the within-subjects variation in BMI scores only captures the individual variation of BMI scores over time as they differ from each individual's time-averaged BMI score: $\Sigma(Y_{igt} - \overline{Y}_{.t})^2$. This sum of squared deviations can be thought of as a one-way ANOVA with all 276 BMI measures as the only outcome variable and *id* as the only independent factor with 92 levels. In effect, the *id* variable creates 92 comparison groups, each one representing a single study participant, and the outcome is each participant's mean BMI score over the three measurement occasions. This SS equals 836.777, and can be recovered from the ANOVA table in Table 13.4 as the sum of the time effect, the time-by-group interaction effect, and the remaining individual over-time variation captured by the residuals: 394.361 + 285.941 + 156.476 = 836.777. Adding the SSs for between-subjects and within-subjects variation yields the TSS: 6,571.446 + 836.777 = 7,408.223.

---

[3]This residual SS would be considered the within-group or error SS in a one-way ANOVA.

In order to obtain the relevant variance estimates for the f-test, we must divide these SSs by their associated degrees of freedom (df; see Box 13.1). Adding up the df for the between-subjects and within-subjects components, we get: $(n - 1) + (N - n) = N - 1$;[4] in the example, we have: $91 + 184 = 275$.

BOX 13.1	DEGREES OF FREEDOM FOR REPEATED-MEASURES ANOVA MODEL WITH A TWO-GROUP X THREE-OCCASION DESIGN

Total between-subjects degrees of freedom: $df_i = n - 1 = 92 - 1 = 91$

Between-group degrees of freedom: $df_g = g - 1 = 2 - 1 = 1$

Remaining residual degrees of freedom between subjects: $df_{bs\text{-}res} = (n - 1) - (g - 1) = 91 - 1 = 90$

Total within-subjects degrees of freedom: $N - n = 276 - 92 = 184$

(N = total number of observations [276] consisting of 92 triplets, each containing three within-subjects observations)

Within-time degrees of freedom: $df_t = t - 1 = 3 - 1 = 2$

Within time-by-group degrees of freedom: $df_g \times df_t = (2 - 1)(3 - 1) = 2$

Remaining residual degrees of freedom within subjects: $df_{ws\text{-}res} = N - n - (t - 1) - (g - 1)(t - 1) = 180$

From the previous discussion of ANOVA and ANCOVA models, we know that the f-test compares the systematic variance attributable to differences in experimental exposure to the variance of the error terms. As we have both between-subjects and within-subjects effects, we also have two separate residual or error terms. For example, the output in Table 13.4 shows that the f-ratio for the averaged between-groups effect compares the between-group variance (629.512) to the residual between-subjects/within-group variance (66.021), yielding an f-statistic of $629.512/66.021 = 9.53$. By contrast, the f-ratio for the within-subjects effects of time is $f = 197.18/0.869 = 226.82$.

Now we are finally in a position to address the hypotheses associated with this study. It is obvious that the main purpose of this physical activity/walking-intervention study is to show that regular walking programs, instituted at assisted-living facilities, will lead to a reduction in average BMI and associated obesity rates. Looking at the specific study design with a two-group comparison of intervention and control group, and BMI measures obtained at baseline and two follow-up occasions (6 months and 12 months), we can formulate three *null* hypotheses:

1. Averaged over all three measurement occasions, the intervention and control groups do not differ in mean BMI: H_0: $\mu_{1.} = \mu_{2.}$. This is the test for a *main group* effect. In Table 13.3, this effect is represented by the two averaged sample group means in the right-hand column: 25.63, 22.61.

2. Averaged over the two comparison groups, the mean BMI scores do not differ over time: H_0: $\mu_{.1} = \mu_{.2} = \mu_{.3}$. This is the test for a *main time* effect. In Table 13.3, this effect is represented by the three average sample group means in the bottom row: 25.77, 23.60, and 22.99.

---

[4]In the current context, n refers to the number of subjects, and N refers to the number of observations.

3. Changes in mean BMI scores over time do not differ between the intervention and control groups. This is the test for the *group-by-time interaction* effect. In Table 13.3, this effect is represented by the comparison of the three time-related group means in the intervention and the three parallel group means in the control group: 25.87, 25.60, 25.42 versus 25.68, 21.60, 20.55.

The reader might ask whether we should consider all three null hypotheses (and their complementary research hypotheses) equally important. For this study, the answer would be "no." For instance, the first null hypothesis involves differences between the intervention and the control group concerning the *time-averaged* BMI scores. This means the test also includes the *baseline* BMI scores as one of the three time-averaged scores. But that implies that this between-group test is not a pure measure of the intervention effect, as we would not expect any mean differences in BMI after randomization and before the intervention programs get started. The second null hypothesis does test whether or not there are any changes in mean BMI scores over time; but, because this test does not separate out the intervention and control groups, it too is not a pure measure of the intervention effect. That leaves us with the third null hypothesis (and associated research hypothesis). This is clearly the one of highest interest: If we cannot reject this null hypothesis, then we are essentially saying that the intervention has no effect, as over-time *changes* in mean BMI scores do not *differ* in the intervention and control groups.

The results in Table 13.4 show that we would reject all three null hypotheses; however, as just discussed, it is the rejection of the third null hypothesis that is of the greatest interest here. To see what a statistically significant interaction of the group-by-time effect looks like, take a look at the graph in Figure 13.1. As we saw earlier, there is, in fact, a small but still significant ($p < .02$) decline of mean BMI scores in the control group from 25.87 to 25.42, but the statistically significant ($p < .00005$) decline in the intervention group from 25.68 to 20.55 is substantially larger.[5] Further tests reveal that, while the rate of decline in mean BMI

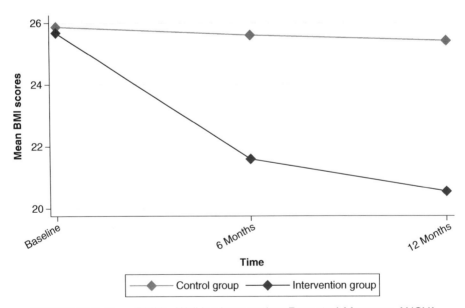

FIGURE 13.1 Mean BMI by Walking Intervention: Repeated-Measures ANOVA. Between-Subjects Factor: Walking Versus no Walking; Within-Subjects Factor: Time.

---

[5]The *p*-values for the separate within-group changes are not shown in Table 13.4.

scores is greater in the intervention than the control group for both time periods (baseline to 6 months and 6 months to 12 months), the decline in the intervention group slows for the second period.

The Sphericity Assumption and the Appropriate *f*-Test

Using the ANOVA approach to analyzing data from repeated-measures designs should only be done if the data are consistent with the assumptions of the model. If not, the statistical tests have to be modified. While independence of observations across different individuals remains a reasonable assumption, the assumptions of independence are not reasonable with respect to repeated measures obtained from the same individuals. If one were to apply the ANOVA model without modification to such repeated-measures data (see Box 13.2), the data must at least meet the assumption of sphericity, which posits that the covariances between any two different time measures of the same individuals must be equal. While this assumption is often violated with repeated measures, there exist a number of modified *f*-tests that provide corrected *p*-values. Table 13.5 shows three modified tests by Huynh–Feldt, Greenhouse–Geisser, and Box, all of which adjust the *f*-tests by modifying the df based on the epsilon statistic. If epsilon equals one, no adjustments are necessary. If epsilon is less than 1, the *p*-values associated with the modified *f*-tests for the within-subjects effects should be used, instead of the *p*-values associated with the original *f*-test. As a general rule, Box's epsilon adjustment is the most conservative (minimizing the Type I error), followed by Greenhouse–Geisser and Huynh–Feldt, and the uncorrected *f*-test. In the above example, we get the same results with or without modifications of the *f*-test.

BOX13.2	ASSUMPTIONS OF THE ANOVA MODEL APPLIED TO DATA FROM REPEATED-MEASURES DESIGNS

1. Interval/ratio level of measurement for outcome/dependent variable
2. Independence of observations across individuals (uncorrelated between-subjects error terms)
3. Normally distributed dependent variable in populations defined by the within- and between-group factors
4. Equal variances (or standard deviations) within population groups defined by the between-group factor(s) and the measurement occasions or within-group factor(s)
5. Equal covariances for all pairs of within-subjects measures at time *j* with time *k*; this is known as the *sphericity* assumption
6. Randomly drawn/assigned study sample

ATTRITION AND ITS EFFECTS ON STATISTICAL TESTS

When you look back at the data in Table 13.4, you see information on 92 individuals, split into 46 treatment and 46 control group subjects, all providing information on their measured height and weight, three times over a 12-month period. In "real life" it would be highly unusual to conduct a clinical intervention study and obtain information on *all* outcome measures for all study participants during the follow-up data collections. Even with the best study management, it is usually impossible to avoid all dropouts, especially if the follow-up periods are lengthy, spanning weeks, months, and even years. There are many reasons for this: Over extended periods of time, study participants may become weary of continued participation and refuse to be contacted further, even if they originally agreed; they may become sicker or healthier, both of which can become a reason for dropping out; sometimes it is family members who pressure the participants to cease participation, and sometimes study participants move and can no longer be found, and some may even die. This type of subject attrition can wreak havoc with the random assignment process. In turn, statistical tests, which are based on the assumption that the data represent randomized comparison groups, may become invalidated.

Traditionally, some researchers have simply ignored this problem and analyzed only cases with complete data ("complete case analysis"); such approaches are still common enough in the clinical literature (Anderson et al., 2005). One alternative for clinical trial data has been to conduct an "intent-to-treat" (ITT) analysis. The main principle of ITT analysis is to include all cases in the analysis that were originally randomized to the various treatment and control groups. To accomplish this, one must impute values for the missing outcome measures, usually following the principle of "last observation carried forward" (LOCF). This is still a widely practiced principle in the analysis of randomized clinical trial data, and, for a long time, it was thought that this was a "conservative" approach.[6] However, as the example of the walking-intervention study in this chapter shows, LOCF need not be conservative: For instance, if a control group subject had dropped out after 6 months, we would assume that the 12-month BMI score is unchanged from the 6-month score, even though the control group also shows a significant decline in BMI scores. In this case, the LOCF could actually widen the difference between the intervention and control groups (Salim et al., 2008). There are now better imputation methods available, but they are beyond the scope of this book (Olsen et al., 2012). However, it is important to realize that the repeated-measures ANOVA and ANCOVA models can only be used to analyze cases with complete information on all variables involved in the model. If information is missing on some outcome variables, ANOVA and ANCOVA, as well as linear regression models, either are performed only on cases with complete data, which often generates a sampling bias, or the analyst must have used some imputation method to substitute for missing values. As a reader of clinical research, you should expect a clear accounting of all cases originally enrolled in the study; likewise there should be clear explanations as to how the attrition problem in an intervention study was addressed, lest there remain biases in the estimates of the effects.

SUMMARY

In this chapter we discussed repeated-measures ANOVA, which is a statistical model that can be used to explore longitudinal data with continuous outcome variables. While commonly employed to analyze data from randomized clinical trials or intervention studies, there is no principal reason why it could not also be used with observational data. However, some of the assumptions underlying the correct application of repeated-measures ANOVA are restrictive as, for example, the sphericity assumption. Other problems arise, when data are incomplete, as is often the case with longitudinal data. In the next chapter, which will conclude our survey of linear models predicting continuous outcome variables, we provide a brief introduction into alternative regression models that can be used to analyze longitudinal data. Such "mixed method" models are now commonly seen in the clinical literature.

---

[6] If one carries the last observation over to later outcome measures, for example, the pretest scores are substituted for missing posttest sores, one is implicitly assuming there is no change.

EXERCISES

1. In your own words: What is the advantage of a repeated-measures pretest/posttest design over a posttest only design?

2. Formulate the null hypothesis for a time-by-group interaction.

3. In a the analysis of data from a pretest/posttest randomized design with one treatment and one control group, researchers find no significant difference for the main between-group effect, no significant difference for the time-by-group effect, but a significant change for the time effect. Does this pattern of results suggest that the intervention is effective? If yes, why? If no, why not?

REFERENCES

Anderson, R. M., Funnell, M. M., Nwankwo, R., Gillard, M. L., Oh, M., & Fitzgerald, J. T. (2005). Evaluating a problem-based empowerment program for African Americans with diabetes: Results of a randomized controlled trial. *Ethnicity & Disease, 15*(3), 671–678.

Good, M., Albert, J. M., Arafah, B., Anderson, G. C., Wotman, S., Cong, X., . . . Ahn, S. (2013). Effects on postoperative salivary cortisol of relaxation/music and patient teaching about pain management. *Biological Research for Nursing, 15*(3), 318–329.

Olsen, M. K., Stechuchak, K. M., Edinger, J. D., Ulmer, C. S., & Woolson, R. F. (2012). Move over LOCF: Principled methods for handling missing data in sleep disorder trials. *Sleep Medicine, 13*(1), 123–132.

Salim, A., Mackinnon, A., Christensen, H., & Griffiths, K. (2008). Comparison of data analysis strategies for intent-to-treat analysis in pre-test–post-test designs with substantial dropout rates. *Journal of Psychiatry Research, 160*(3), 335–345.

Tsay, S.-L., & Hung, L.-O. (2004). Empowerment of patients with end-stage renal disease—A randomized controlled trial. *International Journal of Nursing Studies, 41*(1), 59–65.

Tseng, Y.-F., Chen, C.-H., & Lee, C.-S. (2010). Effects of listening to music on postpartum stress and anxiety levels. *Journal of Clinical Nursing, 19*(7–8), 1049–1055.

CHAPTER 14

Introduction to Mixed-Effects Regression Models

In this chapter, we provide a short overview of mixed-effects regression models, introducing some of the basic ideas and vocabulary underlying these models. A full treatment of **mixed-effects models** is beyond the scope of this book. As statistics is a multidisciplinary effort with models developed by biostatisticians, psychometricians, econometricians, and so forth, it is no surprise that there is a lack of unified terminology in the field. For instance, you may encounter such terms as **multilevel models**, **hierarchical linear models**, **linear mixed-effects models**, and **generalized estimating equations**, all of which start with relaxing the assumptions in classical analysis-of-variance (ANOVA) and linear regression models that individual observations are assumed to vary independently of each other. Here we aim at a basic understanding of the principal ideas that differentiate these models from the classical linear models, as the employment of such models has become increasingly common in the nursing and medical research literature (Marion, Finnegan, Campbell, & Szalacha, 2009; van Weert, Jansen, Spreeuwenberg, van Dulmen, & Bensing, 2011; Woods-Giscombe, Lobel, & Crandell, 2010). There exist several good, fairly nontechnical articles in the literature that the interested reader might want to consult for deeper understanding (Atkins, 2005; Hayat & Hedlin, 2012).

The basic idea underlying mixed-effects regression models is that there are two kinds of independent or predictor variables: those whose levels are fixed, and those whose levels vary depending on the study sample in question. The classic example of a **fixed factor** is the intervention variable in a drug trial, which defines the different dosages of the drug to be administered, including the placebo condition. In this situation, the researcher is interested in inferences about the relative effectiveness of the *given* treatments, but not in inferences about *other* dosages not administered in the trial. By contrast, when we study the effects of a behavioral intervention, such as standard protocol of telephone reminders, on adherence to a specific drug regimen, the particular nurses in the randomized intervention study may vary in their personal effectiveness. From the point of view of the effectiveness of the intervention *protocol* in another clinical setting, the variation due to personal differences among local study personnel would be a random effect. As **random effects** do affect the variance of the outcome variable, it is sometimes important to take them explicitly into account in the analysis.

A second related principle about mixed-effects models is that they involve multiple levels (thus the term "multilevel analysis") in which individual observations are thought to be *nested* within larger contexts, with the consequence that the nested observations can no longer be assumed to be independent of each other. This idea of nested observations actually fits well with the concerns and experiences of health care providers: While clinicians are primarily concerned with the health outcomes of individual patients, these patients live lives that are *nested* within families, institutional settings, or particular communities. As such, the factors that affect their health outcomes or recovery from an illness are not only individual-level factors (e.g., a patient's education, income, access to health insurance, patient mobility, and so forth); their health outcomes are also partially determined by the environment in which they live. For instance, geographic neighborhoods differ by the availability of public transportation (a possible factor contributing to obesity), pollution (a possible lung disease impact), or the proximity to an emergency room (a possible factor in stroke or heart disease outcomes). Similarly, hospitals differ in their organizational procedures designed to reduce infection rates; nursing schools differ in terms of per-student resources, affecting learning behavior beyond the individual's efforts; families differ by nutrition patterns or emphasis on health behaviors. In all those cases, individuals are *nested* within these macro units and tend to share characteristics and outcomes they do not share with individuals located in different macro units. As a result, we should expect that many variables of interest are correlated *within* the macro units, but *not across* the macro units, violating the assumption of classical linear models of uncorrelated error terms.

Longitudinal data share the same basic structure, except that we conceive of the individual as the "macro unit" and the repeated observations about the individual as *nested* within the individuals. Again, we would expect that multiple observations of the same individuals taken at different occasions are, in part, caused by unique characteristics of the individual. Thus, within-subjects observations should share common antecedents not shared by observations from different individuals. Either way, multilevel models put the nesting of particular observations in a common context at the center of the modeling process. This has consequences for how we think about variance decomposition and different sources of variation.

In the last chapter, we introduced repeated-measures ANOVA as a model to analyze repeated measures of a continuous outcome variable from a randomized experiment. As we discussed, in addition to the need for adjustments to the *f*-test, if the sphericity assumption is not met, ANOVA models also require complete data on all the variables involved. Yet the reality of following patients over time shows that complete data for all study participants are often impossible to obtain. In particular, extended follow-up of patients with chronic diseases often results in data with complex missing patterns, with some individuals dropping out, others skipping a particular repeated measure only to participate again at a later data (Stommel, Kurtz, Kurtz, Given, & Given, 2004). In short, longitudinal data are rarely balanced.[1] ANOVA models are also not well suited in analyzing repeated-measures data, if time differences between any pair of two observations show substantial individual variation. Again, such variations are not uncommon in **panel studies** with long-term follow-up.

To get a handle on data with repeated observations, we will look at two ways of formatting such data. In the traditional "wide" format, each row represents an individual case and the columns represent variables, including both repeated and one-time measures on these individuals. For instance, the data in wide format in Table 14.1 show four cases (IDs 1–4), their ages at the time of the study, their sex (1 = female, 2 = male), and up to three diastolic

---

[1]In experimental studies, a balanced study design is one in which each comparison group contains an equal number of subjects. In a repeated-measures study, balanced data would mean an equal number of observations on all subjects.

TABLE 14.1 Two Data Formats for Longitudinal Data

WIDE FORMAT					
ID	AGE	SEX	DBP1	DBP2	DBP3
1	21	1	81	76	77
2	46	2	84		81
3	34	1	80	82	82
4	28	2	87	85	

LONG FORMAT				
ID	TIME	AGE	SEX	DBP
1	1	21	1	76
1	2	21	1	81
1	3	21	1	77
2	1	46	2	84
2	3	46	2	81
3	1	34	1	80
3	2	34	1	82
3	3	34	1	82
4	1	28	2	87
4	2	28	2	85

blood pressure readings (DBPi) taken at different times. As is apparent, for ID No. 2, the second DBP measure is missing, and, for ID No. 4, the third is missing. The same data have been transformed to "long" format in the lower part of Table 14.1. All of the data contained in the wide format are also contained in the long format, but in the long format, each row represents only a single DBP observation, while time-invariant variables like ID, Age,[2] and Sex remain the same and are repeated in each row. Notice also that the long format shows the unbalanced design, with unequal numbers of observations per study participants. Still, we can analyze such data with mixed-effects models, whereas an analysis of the data in wide format would have excluded any case with missing observations on any of the relevant variables. We can also take explicit account of the time between the observations, if that is important for the analysis. Suppose we recode all the dates at which the DBP measures are made, then, instead of simply using a categorical/ordinal Time variable with three categories (first to third observations), we could count the number of days since the baseline measure for the second and third observations on each individual. That way we could explicitly model the time effect on the dependent variable and would be able to accommodate different time intervals for different individuals.

Here is how this looks. We start with an equation that models the within-subjects changes in individual scores over time. Here, we choose the simplest model, using a linear equation:

$$Y_{ti} = \beta_{0i} + \beta_{1i}t_{1i} + \varepsilon_{ti},$$

---

[2] As age is measured in years, it appears as a time-invariant variable, but over longer time periods, this variable could certainly change.

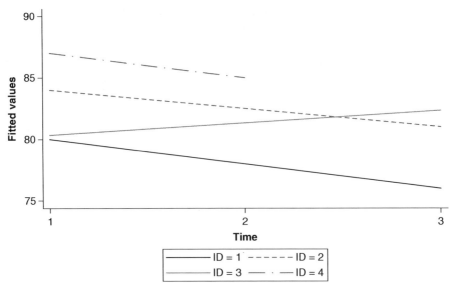

FIGURE 14.1 Within-Subjects Linear Regression Lines of DBP on Time.

where Y_{ti} refers to the within-subjects DBP scores of individual i over time, β_{0i} is the intercept (or "constant") in the equation for the ith individual, and t_{1i} is the time variable, either coded 1, 2, 3 for each observation period or, more precisely, indicating the actual time between the observations for individual i. The symbol β_{1i} refers to the regression coefficient for individual i, indicating how the observed scores of Y for individual i change over time; and finally, we use ε_{ti} to refer to the residual or error term, which captures the deviation of observed scores from the linear model. Figure 14.1 shows the fitted regression lines for the four *individual* cases in Table 14.1.

In a second step, we can now model the between-subjects effects. Remember that for each individual case we have a linear equation modeling the over-time change. Thus we get n intercepts[3] and n slope coefficients from step one, which are subsequently modeled as part of the separate between-subjects equation:

$$\beta_{0i} = \gamma_{00} + \gamma_{10}B_{10} + \gamma_{20}B_{20} + \rho_{00i}$$

$$\beta_{1i} = \gamma_{01} + \gamma_{11}B_{11} + \gamma_{21}B_{21} + \rho_{01i}$$

As the intercept and slope coefficients vary across individuals, we can treat them as outcome variables, whose variation across different groups of individuals can be predicted based on any between-subjects difference of interest. In the example, one between-subjects variable is age (B_1), the other is sex (B_2), and they can be used to predict individual variation in the intercept and slope coefficients associated with all individuals in the within-subjects models. If one substitutes the equations in step two into the equation in step one, one gets a more complicated model, which contains both within-subjects (ε_{ti}) and between-subjects error terms (ρ_{01i}). How one proceeds now depends on one's interest and hypotheses. We may not be interested in the subject-specific random-effects per se, but may instead average these effects across population groups of interest. Nonetheless, the estimation must take account of the correlation among within-subjects scores.

---

[3] In our example: 4.

To illustrate the general idea, we use an example of a data set of 20 primary care patients, for whom we have *up to* three repeated DBP measures taken one week apart. On 15 subjects we have all three measures, on 2 subjects we have only the first two DBP readings, and on 3 subjects we have only the first and the third DBP reading, resulting in a total of 55 sample observations with an unbalanced distribution of the observations across individuals. The data are organized in long format, as illustrated in Table 14.1, with each DBP observation occupying a separate row.

Table 14.2 presents summary statistics for the variables of interest. Note that the outcome measure (DBP readings) varies over time, while subjects' age and gender are fixed over the time period in question. Any differences in mean age scores and in the percentage distribution of male and female patients over time are due to the fact that not all patients participated in all measurements over time.

Ignoring the fact that the DBP measures involve both readings from different individuals and repeated readings of the same individuals, we could run a regular linear regression model with time, age, and sex as independent predictors of the DBP readings. Table 14.3 gives the results. Based on this model, we would conclude that average DBP readings declined by

TABLE 14.2 Summary Statistics for DBP Readings Over Three Occasions (Sample *N* = 20)

```
. sum DBP if time==1
Variable      |   Obs      Mean    Std. Dev.   Min    Max
--------------+------------------------------------------
DBP(time 1)   |    20     86.85    4.05586      79     93
DBP(time 2)   |    17  84.82353    4.111498     76     90
DBP(time 3)   |    18  83.11111    3.802304     77     88

Age(time 1)   |    20      30.3    6.883237     21     46
Age(time 2)   |    17  29.35294    6.194162     21     41
Age(time 3)   |    18      30.5    7.245688     21     46

Sex(time 1)   |  Freq.   Percent      Cum.
--------------+------------------------------
Male          |    10     50.00     50.00
Female        |    10     50.00    100.00
--------------+------------------------------
Total         |    20    100.00

Sex(time 2)   |  Freq.   Percent      Cum.
--------------+------------------------------
Male          |     8     47.06     47.06
Female        |     9     52.94    100.00
--------------+------------------------------
Total         |    17    100.00

Sex(time 3)   |  Freq.   Percent      Cum.
--------------+------------------------------
Male          |     9     50.00     50.00
Female        |     9     50.00    100.00
--------------+------------------------------
Total         |    18    100.00
```

TABLE 14.3 Linear Regression Model of 55 DBP Observations on Time (Three Occasions), Sex, and Age of Subjects (Sample of Observations: *N* = 55)

```
. regress DBP time age sex

    Source |       SS        df       MS                    Number of obs =      55
-----------+------------------------------------           F(3, 51)      =    7.34
     Model | 288.237956       3   96.0793186                Prob > F      = 0.0000
  Residual | 673.762044      51   13.2110205                R-squared     = 0.2996
-----------+------------------------------------           Adj R-squared = 0.2584
     Total |        962      54   17.8148148                Root MSE      = 3.6347


       DBP |    Coef.    Std. Err.      t      P>|t|     [95% Conf.    Intervl]
-----------+----------------------------------------------------------------------
      time | -1.892998   .5902226    -3.21    0.002     -3.077919    -.7080764
       age |  .2535532   .0739647    -3.43    0.001      .1050629     .4020434
       sex | -.0716446   .9813029     0.07    0.942     -2.041692    1.898403
      cons |  81.20024   2.895136    28.05    0.000      75.38801    87.01247
```

1.89 ($p \leq .002$) after each month and increased by 0.25 ($p \leq .001$) for each additional year of age. There appears to be no significant difference in average DBP readings by sex. However, this conclusion would be erroneous, as our statistical model ignores (a) the uneven number of observations per subject (giving more weight to between-subjects factors like age to subjects with complete observations), and (b) the fact that the repeated measures of the same subjects are correlated; in other words, that multiple observations are *nested* within the same individuals.

Instead of the regression model that treats each outcome observation as independent, we can run a mixed-effects linear regression model that includes both fixed effects and random effects. The focus is still on the fixed effects of time, age, and sex, but we allow for randomly varying intercepts of the within-subjects regressions of DBP on time. As Figure 14.2 shows, for the most part the decline in DBP over 2 months is nearly linear among the individuals, with little variation in the slopes but larger variation in the intercepts. That is, the random individual variation primarily involves inter-individual differences in the level of DBP resulting in parallel lines, but not differences in the decline over time, which would indicate different slopes.[4]

Table 14.4 shows the output from the mixed-effects linear regression model. At first, we review some basic information: The number of total DBP observations is 55 obtained from 20 "groups," which in this panel study are the 20 individuals in the sample. We also learn that there are at least two observations and a maximum of three observations per individual/group, with an average of 2.8 observations per individual/group. The estimation method employed is known as **restricted maximum likelihood (REML)**, but we ignore the specifics here and move on to the regression coefficient estimates for the fixed effects predictors. The estimate for the time effect is very similar to the one from the previous linear model without a random effect component: -1.87 ($p \leq .0005$); however, age is no longer a significant predictor: 0.21 ($p \geq .081$), while sex remains insignificant: -0.33 ($p \geq .839$). Table 14.4 also provides some

---

[4]An alternative model specification allowing for individual slope variation showed no significant improvement over a model with only a random intercept.

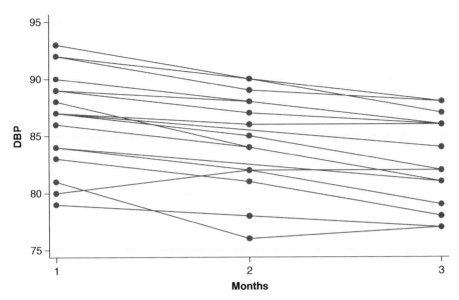

FIGURE 14.2 Within-Subjects Changes in DBP for 20 Individuals for Data Summarized in Table 14.2. (Note: Individuals With the Same DBP Trajectory Overlap.)

TABLE 14.4 Mixed Effects Linear Regression Model of 55 DBP Observations on Time (Three Occasions), Sex, and Age of Subjects (Sample of Observations: N = 55)

```
. xtmixed DBP time age sex, || ID:, covariance(identity)
```

Mixed-effects REML regression

Group variable: ID

Log restricted-likelihood = −115.87402

Number of obs	=	55
Number of groups	=	20
Obs per group: min	=	2
avg	=	2.8
max	=	3
Wald chi2(3)	=	105.00
Prob > chi2	=	0.0000

DBP	Coef.	Std. Err.	z	P>|z|	[95% Conf.	Interval]
time	−1.866109	.184719	−10.10	0.000	−2.228151	−1.504066
age	.2132989	.1223018	1.74	0.081	−.0264082	.453006
sex	−.333784	1.64027	−0.20	0.839	−3.548653	2.881086
_cons	82.72779	4.386016	18.86	0.000	74.13135	91.32422

Random-effects Parameters		Estimate	Std. Err.	[95% Conf.	Interval]
ID: Identity	sd(_cons)	3.592632	.6383852	2.536065	5.089384
	sd(Residual)	1.124235	.1362756	.886498	1.425728

LR test vs. linear regression: chibar2(01) = 62.67 Prob >= chibar2 = 0.0000

Likelihood-ratio test   LR chi2(1) = 1.46

(Assumption: randint nested in randslope)   Prob > chi2 = 0.2277

information on the random intercept effect: The individual intercepts or constants from the 20 individual (for each ID) linear regressions of DBP on time have an estimated standard deviation of 3.59 with a 95% confidence interval of 2.54 to 5.09. The output also shows an additional residual standard deviation [sd(Residual)], which is the estimated standard deviation of the overall error associated with the 55 observations. Finally, the likelihood ratio test at the bottom compares this mixed-effects model to the ordinary regression model in Table 14.3; the test indicates a significant difference between the two models: In short, the mixed-effects model offers an improvement over the ordinary linear regression model, which ignores the distinction between within- and between-subjects effects. On the basis of these sample data, we cannot confidently conclude that the mean DBP levels differ by age for individuals 21 to 46 years old, as the ordinary linear regression model would have suggested.

SUMMARY

In this chapter, we have provided some rudimentary description of the mixed-effects regression model. The focus here was on linear models, but the basic principles of mixed-effects models apply to all regression models, including the regression models addressed in later chapters of this book (logistic and survival regression models). Multilevel modeling is an attractive tool, because the data of interest to nurses and other health professionals often involve clusters of individuals in different institutions or longitudinal panel data with multiple measures on the same individuals. In either case, the number of observations within clusters or individuals may vary. Classical repeated-measures ANOVA cannot deal with such complexities. We have provided only a very brief introduction to mixed-effects models; the interested reader may want to consult a more comprehensive, but accessible treatment in Kreft and Leeuw (1998).

This chapter concludes Part II of the book, in which we discussed linear models for interval-level outcome variables. These models are versatile and robust, and they continue to be frequently employed in the health care literature; still, many data of interest to nursing and medical researchers do not even approximately meet the assumptions of measurement level and normally distributed error terms. Thus, in Part III of this book, we turn to the statistical models that can be employed in the analysis of categorical outcome data, followed by models for censored data in Part IV.

REFERENCES

Atkins, D. C. (2005). Using multilevel models to analyze couple and family treatment data: Basic and advanced issues. *Journal of Family Psychology, 19*(1), 98–110.

Hayat, M. J., & Hedlin, H. (2012). Modern statistical modeling approaches for analyzing repeated-measures data. *Nursing Research, 61*(3), 188–194.

Kreft, I., & de Leeuw, J. (1998). *Introducing multilevel modeling.* London, UK: Sage Publications.

Marion, L. N., Finnegan, L., Campbell, R. T., & Szalacha, L. A. (2009). The Well Woman Program: A community-based randomized trial to prevent sexually transmitted infections in low-income African American women. *Research in Nursing & Health, 32*(2), 274–285.

Stommel, M., Kurtz, M. E., Kurtz, J. C., Given, C. W., & Given, B. A. (2004). A longitudinal analysis of the course of depressive symptomatology in geriatric patients with cancer of the breast, colon, lung, and prostate. *Health Psychology, 26*(6), 564–576.

van Weert, J. C. M., Jansen, J., Spreeuwenberg, P. M. M., van Dulmen, S., & Bensing, J. M. (2011). Effects of communication skills training and a Question Prompt Sheet to improve communication with older cancer patients: A randomized controlled trial. *Critical Reviews in Oncology/Hematology, 80*(1), 145–159.

Woods-Giscombé, C. L., Lobel, M., & Crandell, J. L. (2010). The impact of miscarriage and parity on patterns of maternal distress in pregnancy. *Research in Nursing & Health, 33*(3), 316–328.

PART III. MODELS FOR CATEGORICAL OUTCOME MEASURES

CHAPTER 15

Nonparametric/Ordinal Statistics

So far in this book we have discussed only parametric statistics. The *t*-test, analysis of variance (ANOVA), linear regression as well as the Pearson's *r* correlation all share the assumption that at least the dependent variable (in the case of ANOVA and *t*-test) or sometimes both the dependent and independent variables (in the case of linear regression and the Pearson correlation coefficient) are continuous and measured at an interval or ratio level. The reason for the assumption of continuous outcome variables is obvious: All of these statistical models assume that one can calculate means and distances from means, that is, deviation scores, which are the basic components of the variance and standard deviation. In addition, statistical inference based on these linear models relies heavily on the normality assumption, meaning, these models assume that error terms, that is, deviations of observed values from predicted values within the categories of the independent variable(s), are normally distributed in the target populations.

Even though the linear models perform well (are "robust") in the presence of minor deviations from the assumptions about the normality of the distribution of error terms and homoskedasticity, that is, equal variances across comparison groups, they can lead to wrong inferences in cases of pronounced nonlinearity of relationships, substantial skew, outliers, lack of sufficient numbers of categories/values, and the presence of purely ordinal rankings. As we have seen in the previous chapters, there are several "fixes" available for skewed distributions and nonlinearity of relationships, but dependent variables consisting of ordinal rankings with few categories present a challenge for linear models. So do dependent variables with large outliers. Yet in health-related research we often use rating scales—as do nurses and physicians in clinical practice (Brunelli et al., 2010; Wong, Holroyd-Leduc, Simel, & Straus, 2010)—which do not meet the assumptions of interval-level measurement. Outliers are also a common occurrence in health care data, as, for example, systolic blood pressure readings above 160 or extreme obesity levels with a body mass index (BMI) greater than 40 (Ogden et al., 2006).

As we discussed in Chapter 2, ordinal levels of measurement represent rankings or rank orders. Strictly speaking, for such variables the distances between two values or categories are not defined. Table 15.1 provides an example of a frequency distribution showing 360 self-rated responses to the question: "How often do you exercise?"

TABLE 15.1 Survey Responses to the Question: "How Often Do You Exercise?"

```
tab exercise

    exercise  |    Freq.    Percent    Cum.
--------------+---------------------------------
   1. Rarely  |     102      28.33     28.33
2. Sometimes  |     142      39.44     67.78
   3. Often   |      71      19.72     87.50
4. Routinely  |      45      12.50    100.00
--------------+---------------------------------
       Total  |     360     100.00
```

The labels for the four categories clearly indicate a rank order of more or less frequent exercising, but computing the mean for this variable (it is 2.16) is problematic: We would have to assume that the distance between 1 and 2 is the same as between 3 and 4. Yet, we cannot be sure that the difference in frequency of exercising between "rarely" and "sometimes" is the same as between "often" and "routinely," nor can we be sure that all respondents use a similar "internal" frequency scale. Furthermore, this frequency distribution takes on only four distinct values/categories. As we can see from the following graph (Figure 15.1), such a distribution will never be smooth enough to approximate a normal or *t*-distribution. While there are no absolute rules about how many categories a dependent variable in a linear regression or ANOVA model ought to have, when there are fewer than 10 categories, it will often be the case that the normality assumptions about error terms are substantially violated, in particular, as the skew of a distribution of few categories cannot easily be remedied with any algebraic transformation.

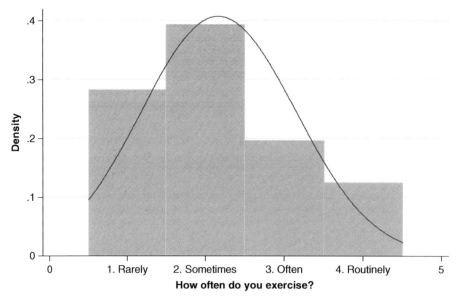

FIGURE 15.1 Distribution of Responses to an Exercise Frequency Question: Four Ordinal Responses With Normal Distribution Superimposed.

TABLE 15.2 BMI Data for 30 Individuals: 1–15 (Female), 16–30 (Male)

Female ID:	1	2	3	4	5	6	7	8	9	10	11	12	13	14	15
BMI:	20	28	23	26	22	19	25	22	25	22	23	27	19	21	33
Male ID:	16	17	18	19	20	21	22	23	24	25	26	27	28	29	30
BMI:	28	25	23	26	30	29	34	27	18	26	29	23	24	28	54

t test bmi, by(sex) unequal welch

Two-sample t test with unequal variances

Group	Obs	Mean	Std. Err.	Std. Dev.	[95% Conf. Interval]	
1. female	15	23.66667	.9742722	3.77334	21.57706	25.75627
2. male	15	28.26667	2.07127	8.021994	23.82423	32.7091
combined	30	25.96667	1.20295	6.588827	23.50636	28.42698
diff		−4.6	2.288966		−9.363665	.1636647

diff = mean(1.female) − mean(2.male)   t = −2.0096

Ho: diff = 0   Welch's degrees of freedom = 20.7497

Ha: diff ≠ 0; Pr($|T| > |t|$) = 0.0577

Outliers in interval-level variables can also have a substantially distorting effect on summary statistics, particularly in smaller data sets. Suppose you have BMI data on 30 individuals (15 women and 15 men) as shown in Table 15.2. Notice that one man has a very high BMI score of 54 and the range of BMI scores among these men is 18 to 54. Among the women, the range of the BMI scores is 19 to 33. The *t*-test shows a great disparity in the standard deviations (or variances) of BMI scores between the men and women, but even after Welch's adjustments to the degrees of freedom (df) for unequal within-group variances, the overall *t*-test for the mean differences is not significant ($p > .057$). The reason for this is that large outliers can substantially inflate the sample variances and standard deviations, which, in turn, affects the estimates of the standard errors. As we know by now, large standard errors make it less likely that we find significant differences between the means of the groups compared.

It is in cases like these, of ordinal scales with only a few categories or highly skewed variables with outliers, that we look for alternative statistical models that are impervious to the impact of outliers or do not assume a measurement level beyond ordinal ranking.

THE WILCOXON RANK-SUM TEST AND THE MANN–WHITNEY U TEST

The Wilcoxon rank-sum test and the Mann–Whitney U test are essentially the same test. They are used instead of the independent sample *t*-test to answer the question: Is the average rank in the two populations, from which the study sample is drawn, the same or different?

In Table 15.2 we saw the output from the *t*-test: Based on these results, we could not reject the null hypothesis that the mean BMI scores are equal between the men and women. We may doubt, however, that the distribution of BMI scores meets the *t*-test assumptions. In this situation, we may want to use the Wilcoxon rank-sum test (or its "cousin," the Mann–Whitney U test).

To show how the test works, we turn again to the BMI data. In Table 15.3 the data are displayed again, but this time rank scores are added. Proceeding from the lowest to the highest, the rankings are applied to all study participants in the total sample based on their BMI scores (18 is the lowest score, so it gets the rank no. 1.0; 54 is the highest score, so it gets rank no. 30.0). For individuals with the same BMI score ("ties"), we use the convention of assigning an average rank associated with that group. For instance, there are three individuals with a BMI score of 22. Five others have a lower score. Thus, the three individuals occupy ranks 6, 7, and 8, and the average rank for individuals in this group equals 7. At the bottom of

TABLE 15.3 BMI Data for 30 Individuals With Ranks Added

BMI scores (Total)	BMI ranks (Total)	BMI scores (women)	BMI ranks (women)	BMI scores (men)	BMI ranks (men)
18	1.0			18	1.0
19	2.5	19	2.5		
19	2.5	19	2.5		
20	4.0	20	4.0		
21	5.0	21	5.0		
22	7.0	22	7.0		
22	7.0	22	7.0		
22	7.0	22	7.0		
23	10.5	23	10.5		
23	10.5			23	10.5
23	10.5			23	10.5
23	10.5	23	10.5		
24	13.0			24	13.0
25	15.0	25	15.0		
25	15.0	25	15.0		
25	15.0			25	15.0
26	18.0			26	18.0
26	18.0	26	18.0		
26	18.0			26	18.0
27	20.5	27	20.5		
27	20.5			27	20.5
28	23.0	28	23.0		
28	23.0			28	23.0
28	23.0			28	23.0
29	25.5			29	25.5
29	25.5			29	25.5
30	27.0			30	27.0
33	28.0	33	28.0		
34	29.0			34	29.0
54	30.0			54	30.0
Sums: 779	465.0	355	175.5	424	289.5
Means: 25.97	15.5	23.67	11.7	28.27	19.3

Table 15.3, the *rank* sums and *rank* means are displayed. Focus first on the *sum* of ranks for the total sample: For any given sample size, the sum of ranks will always be equal to $n(n + 1)/2$, where n = total sample size. Thus, with a sample size of $n = 30$, we get here: $30(30 + 1)/2 = 30 \times 31/2 = 465$. By the same token, the mean rank for the total sample is always equal to the sum of all ranks divided by the number of cases. In our case the mean rank is $465/30 = 15.5$. As we do not change the ranks, when splitting up the sample into the two comparison groups of men and women, the rank sums for women (175.5) and men (289.5) must add up to the total sample rank sum. Under the assumption that there is no difference between the two comparison groups, the null hypothesis states that the mean *ranks* in the two groups are the same. If both comparison groups are of equal size, we would also expect that, if the null hypothesis is true, the rank sums in both groups would be of equal size. As the two comparison groups may not always be of equal size, the actual test statistic used in the Wilcoxon test is slightly different: It is the *sum* of ranks in the comparison group with the *smaller* sum, which, in our example, is the female group.

Now, we are ready to construct our test statistic: We compare W_1, the sum of observed ranks in the group with the smaller rank sum, to W_e, the expected sum of ranks in that group. The latter is computed under the assumption that the null hypothesis (*mean* ranks in the comparison groups are equal) holds. It turns out that W_e can be computed as follows:

$$W_e = n_1(n_1 + n_2 + 1)/2,$$

where n_1 = the sample size of the first comparison group (here: women) and n_2 = sample size of the second comparison group (here: men). As there are both 15 men and women, we get:

$$W_e = n_1(n_1 + n_2 + 1)/2 = 15(15 + 15 + 1)/2 = 15 \times 31/2 = 465/2 = 232.5$$

Again, when the comparison groups are equal in size, their rank sums should be equal as well, if the null hypothesis holds, as the rank sums are nothing but the product of the average rankings times the number of cases in each group. With a total sample rank sum of 465, the *expected* rank sum of either of two equal-sized groups should be equal to 232.5. As Table 15.3 shows, the actual rank sum in the female group is 175.5. This leaves us with the final question: Is the difference of $175.5 - 232.5 = -57$ between the observed rank sum and the expected rank statistically significant under the null hypothesis?

This question can only be answered, if we have an estimate of the appropriate standard error for this statistic. Without providing the (somewhat involved) proof, here is the way we estimate the standard error for the W statistic from the sample data: $\mathrm{SE}_w\sqrt{(n_1n_2s^2)/n}$. The variance expression in this formula, $s^2 = \frac{1}{n-1}\Sigma(r_i - \bar{r})^2$, is nothing but the ordinary variance computed on the *rankings*, while n_1 refers to the sample size of the first comparison group and n_2 to the sample size of the second comparison group, with n representing the combined sample size.

For the data in Table 15.3, we can calculate a total sample variance of the rankings of 77. Thus we get: $\mathrm{SE}_w = \sqrt{(n_1n_2s^2)/n} = \sqrt{(15 \times 15 \times 77)/30} = \sqrt{577.5} = 24.03$. With this estimate of the standard error of the W statistic, we then convert the W statistic into a standardized z-score (observed W_1 minus expected W_e under the null hypothesis) using the standard error: $(175.5 - 232.5)/24.03 = -2.372$. This is the value shown in Table 15.4. We know from the normal distribution that a z-score of -2.372 differs significantly from 0 (it is more than 1.96 SE away from the null value of zero). Thus we would reject the null hypothesis ($p < .018$) and conclude that the mean rank orders of BMI scores are indeed different from each other in the population from which they were drawn.

TABLE 15.4 Wilcoxon Rank-Sum Test for Ranked BMI Data Comparing 15 Women and 15 Men

```
. ranksum bmi, by(sex)

Two-sample Wilcoxon rank-sum (Mann-Whitney) test

      sex |    obs    rank sum    expected
 ---------+--------------------------------
 1. female |    15      175.5        232.5
 2. male   |    15      289.5        232.5
 ---------+--------------------------------
 combined |    30        465          465

 unadjusted variance     581.25
 adjustment for ties      -3.75
                         -------
 adjusted variance       577.50    Ho: bmi(sex=1.female) = bmi(sex=2.male)

                           z =  -2.372    Prob > |z| =  0.0177
```

In sum, if we want to compare two group means in independent population groups, but the outcome variable is either measured at an ordinal level of measurement, or it is an interval-level variable that is highly skewed with large outliers, then we can employ the Wilcoxon rank-sum test instead of the *t*-test. Often, the *t*-test and the rank test will give us the same results, but in the case of divergent outcomes, that is, one test shows statistical significance while the other does not, then we should trust the Wilcoxon test over the *t*-test, because it makes fewer assumptions (see Box 15.1) about the data.

BOX 15.1	ASSUMPTIONS OF WILCOXON RANK-SUM TEST

- Interval/ratio *or* ordinal level of measurement for single dependent variable
- Independent/predictor variable is categorical and limited to two groups
- Outcome observations are independent of each other (uncorrelated)
- Randomly drawn study sample for population inferences

THE WILCOXON SIGNED-RANK TEST

Just like the paired *t*-test is a test of mean differences between paired variable scores, for example, pulse rates of the same individuals before and after an exercise intervention, we can also construct a test based on the *rankings* of the paired differences. When we rank difference scores, the ranks are based on the absolute value of the differences $|d_i|$, that is, the rankings are performed on the magnitude of the differences, disregarding whether they are positive or negative. Then we can test whether the average rank of the paired differences is positive (implying an average increase in paired scores) or negative (decrease in paired scores), or if positive or negative differences are roughly balanced (null hypothesis of no change). This test, known as the Wilcoxon signed-rank test, should be used as a substitute for the paired *t*-test,

TABLE 15.5 Paired *t*-Test to Examine 10-Year Changes in BMI Among 16 Individuals

Paired t test

Variable	Obs	Mean	Std. Err.	Std. Dev.	[95% Conf. Interval]	
bmi2	16	27.4375	.9352751	3.741101	25.44401	29.43099
bmi1	16	25.8125	.8476376	3.390551	24.0058	27.6192
diff	16	1.625	.7295832	2.918333	.0699302	3.18007

mean(diff) = mean(bmi2 − bmi1)   t = 2.2273
Ho: mean(diff) = 0   degrees of freedom =   15

Ha: mean(diff) ≠ 0   Ha: mean(diff) > 0
Pr(|T| > |t|) = 0.0417   Pr(T > t) = 0.0208

if the assumption that the actual differences between the original scores, or change scores, are roughly normally distributed does not hold. Notice however, that this test differs from the rank-sum test in that it *does* make the assumption of interval-level measurement for the original scores, as the rankings are performed on the original *difference* or *change* scores, whose magnitudes can only be compared if the numbers reflect comparable distances. Still, the test is useful if the normality assumption cannot be maintained.

Suppose we have data on 16 adults, whose initial BMI scores are based on measured height and weight at the ages 28 to 33. After a period of 10 years, we obtain a second set of measurements for the same group of adults, now aged 38 to 43. As the BMI is a ratio-level variable, we initially analyze the data using the paired *t*-test (see Chapter 8) to examine possible changes in the mean BMI over time. Table 15.5 shows the results.

The data show a mean increase in the BMI of 1.6 units from 25.8 at Time 1 to 27.4 at Time 2. Testing the null hypothesis that no change occurred over the 10 years, that is, H_0 = mean change = 0, the paired *t*-test results in a *p*-value of .0417, which would normally lead us to reject the null hypothesis and accept the research/alternative hypothesis that a change in mean BMI occurred. In fact, the *p*-value for the one-sided *t*-test with the alternative hypothesis that the mean BMI score increased is .0208, providing seemingly stronger evidence of an increase in weight. However, the paired *t*-test assumes normally distributed change scores within the target population (see Box 8.3). Yet, the following histogram (Figure 15.2) of the 16 change scores throws doubt on this assumption.

As an alternative to the paired *t*-test, we may employ the Wilcoxon signed-rank test. The results are shown in Table 15.6. The test is based on the following logic. There are 16 Time 1 BMI measures and 16 Time 2 BMI measures. Between them, we have 16 pairs of Time 2–Time 1 difference scores. For each pair of BMI scores, we compute the difference or change score d_i and rank all pairs from smallest to largest, while disregarding the sign during the ranking process. Table 15.6 shows that among the 16 paired change scores, 11 have a positive sign (BMI2 > BMI1), 4 have a negative sign (BMI2 < BMI1), and one difference score remains unchanged (BMI2 = BMI1).

As there are 16 change scores, ranked from smallest (1) to largest rank (16), the sum of all ranks must be 136: $n(n + 1)/2 = 16(16 + 1)/2$. Table 15.6 shows that the rank sum for the 11 pairs with an increase in BMI scores over 10 years is equal to 104, the rank sum for the 4 pairs

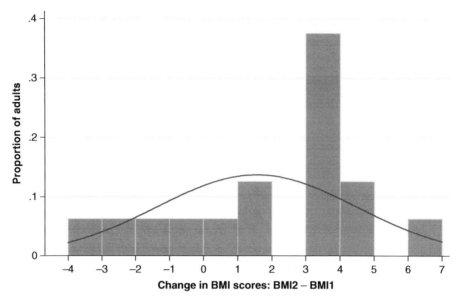

FIGURE 15.2 Changes in BMI Scores During One Decade: 16 Adults Measured at Ages 28 to 33 and Again at Ages 38 to 43.

showing a decline in the BMI is 31, and the rank sum for the pair showing no change is 1.[1] If there is no systematic tendency toward change as asserted under the null hypothesis, we would expect the same rank sum for increases (positive changes) as for decreases (negative changes) in BMI scores over the 10-year period. Thus, the basic test statistic can be expressed as the difference of the *observed* rank sum for positive changes minus the *expected* rank sum for positive changes. Under the null hypothesis, this difference would be equal to zero:

$$H_0 : \sum r_{i+} - \mathrm{Exp}\left(\sum r_{j+}\right) = 0$$

The variance needed to compute the relevant standard error is estimated using the formula:

$$\mathrm{Var(Test\ Statistic)} = n(n + 1)(2n + 1)/2$$

This is the unadjusted variance formula, which assumes that all change scores are different and thus have a unique rank. When ranks are tied, this reduces the variance; similarly a zero change in the original score reduces this variance. Table 15.6 shows the adjusted variance, and we get our test statistic expressed as a z-score: $z = (104 - 67.5)/\sqrt{366.68} = 1.907$. The associated *p*-value is .0565, which is larger than .05. Given the evidence from just 16 cases, we *cannot* reject the null hypothesis that no change occurred in the mean BMI values over the 10 years.

THE SIGN TEST

As we have seen, the Wilcoxon signed-rank test still makes the assumption that the *change scores* or paired differences can be ranked in terms of their magnitude, thus assuming that the underlying original measurement of the variable involved is at least an interval-level

---

[1] Why 1? Recall that we rank the absolute value of changes; thus a zero change is the smallest possible "change," which gets rank 1.

TABLE 15.6 Wilcoxon Signed-Rank Test to Examine 10-Year Changes in BMI Among 16 Individuals

```
Wilcoxon signed-rank test

    sign  |   obs    sum ranks    expected
----------+------------------------------
 positive |    11         104         67.5
 negative |     4          31         67.5
     zero |     1           1            1
----------+------------------------------
      all |    16         136          136

unadjusted variance        374.00
adjustment for ties         -7.38
adjustment for zeros        -0.25
                          -------
adjusted variance          366.38

Ho: bmi2 = bmi1
           z = 1.907,   Prob > |z| = 0.0565


Sign test

    sign  |  observed   expected
----------+--------------------
 positive |     11         7.5
 negative |      4         7.5
     zero |      1           1
----------+--------------------
      all |     16          16

Two-sided test:
   Ho: median of bmi2 – bmi1 = 0 vs. Ha: median of bmi2 – bmi1 ≠ 0
   Pr(#positive >= 11 or #negative >= 11) =
   min(1, 2*Binomial(n = 15, x >= 11, p = 0.5)) = 0.1187
```

measurement. For the BMI data, this assumption is valid. However, if both the earlier and later measurements in a pair are truly ordinal, as in the responses to the exercise frequency question shown in Table 15.1, we should not rank the change scores based on the *magnitude* of the change. For instance, if the responses of one individual are "rarely" (=1) at Time 1 and "sometimes" (=2) at Time 2, while another individual's responses are "sometimes" (=2) at Time 1 and "routinely" (=4) at Time 2, we would get a change score of $2 - 1 = 1$ for the first individual and a change score of $4 - 2 = 2$ for the second individual. Yet, it is problematic to assume that the first individual's change over time (from "rarely" to "sometimes") is smaller than the second individual's (from "sometimes" to "routinely"). We can, however, legitimately say whether an individual chooses a higher or lower ranking response, or whether the response remains the same at the second data collection time. This leads to a very simple test statistic: We ask how many pairs of individual responses show an increase (+), a decrease (−), or no change in the rankings over time. Under the null hypothesis, increases and decreases should balance each other out, that is, if there is no systematic change in individuals' ordinal ratings over time, then the probability of a positive or negative change is .5. After making some adjustments for ties (no change in the ordinal responses of an individual), we can employ the binomial probability distribution to estimate the probability that a sample of paired responses shows positive (or negative) changes that exceed a certain number.

Even though the data underlying the test in Table 15.6 do meet the interval-level requirements of the Wilcoxon signed-rank test, we can use these data to show how the sign test works. We already know that there are 16 paired BMI scores, of which 11 show an increase, 4 a decrease, and 1 no change. As we have 15 change scores, and observe 11 increases and 4 decreases, we can ask: What is the probability of observing an increase in 11 or more change scores or the reverse, a decrease in 4, or fewer of them? If that probability is less than the conventional .05 level, we would say that the sample evidence is inconsistent with the assumption that increases and decreases in change scores are equally likely. In short, we reject the null hypothesis that there is no systematic trend in the change scores.

The binomial distribution, $p = \frac{n!}{k!(n-k)!}\pi^k(1-\pi)^{n-k}$, can be used to estimate the probability that 0, 1, 2, 3, or 4 of the paired difference scores show a decline and that 11, 12, 13, 14, or 15 of the change scores show an increase, for example:

$$p_{(1)} = \frac{15!}{0!15!}0.5^0 0.5^{15} = .0000305, \quad p_{(1)} = \frac{15!}{1!14!}0.5^1 0.5^{14} = .0004578$$

$$p_{(2)} = \frac{15!}{2!13!}0.5^2 0.5^{13} = .0032044, \quad p_{(3)} = \frac{15!}{3!12!}0.5^3 0.5^{12} = .0138855$$

$$p_{(4)} = \frac{15!}{4!11!}0.5^4 0.5^{11} = .0416565$$

$$p_{(11)} = \frac{15!}{11!4!}0.5^{11} 0.5^4 = .0416565, \quad p_{(12)} = \frac{15!}{12!3!}0.5^{12} 0.5^3 = .0138855$$

$$p_{(13)} = \frac{15!}{13!2!}0.5^{13} 0.5^2 = .0032044, \quad p_{(14)} = \frac{15!}{14!1!}0.5^{14} 0.5^1 = .0004578$$

$$p_{(15)} = \frac{15!}{0!15!}0.5^{15} 0.5^0 = .0000305$$

Adding up the probabilities of observing 11 or more increases in the paired difference scores, we get: .0416565 + .0138855 + .0032044 + .0004578 + .0000305 = .05935. As the probability of having fewer than 5 increases among the 15 paired difference scores is also .05935, the two-sided probability of observing more than 10 increases or more than 10 decreases (fewer than 5 increases) is .1187 (see Table 15.6). Thus, according to the sign test, we again come to the conclusion, that the sample evidence is not strong enough for us to conclude with at least 95% confidence that there has been a general weight gain over the 10-year observation period.

KRUSKAL–WALLIS TEST

Just as one-way ANOVA is a generalization of the independent sample t-test to the comparison of more than two groups, the Kruskal–Wallis test is a generalization of the Wilcoxon rank-sum test. The Kruskal–Wallis test is designed to test the hypothesis that median outcomes

TABLE 15.7 Kruskal–Wallis Test to Compare Average Rank Orders in Three Groups

```
kwallis exer if age>19 & age<60, by(newsmoke)

Kruskal-Wallis equality-of-populations rank test

+------------------------------------+
| newsmoke |  Obs  |  Rank Sum  |
|----------+-------+------------|
|        0 |  182  |  27480.00  |
|        1 |   78  |  12211.50  |
|        2 |   37  |   4561.50  |
+------------------------------------+

chi-squared = 4.019 with 2 d.f.
probability = 0.1340

chi-squared with ties = 4.418 with 2 d.f.
probability = 0.1098
```

in several samples come from the same population and thus do not vary significantly from each other. Going back to the self-rated exercise question of Table 15.1, we may want to know whether people with different smoking history (nonsmoker, former smoker, or current smoker) differ in their median response to this question. As the outcome variable is a rank-order variable with few categories asking respondents to rate the frequency of their exercise using four categories, there is some doubt as to whether one-way ANOVA is appropriate in comparing mean scores (as strictly speaking, neither means nor distances from the means are defined here). Table 15.7 shows the results from this test applied to data from 297 respondents between the ages of 20 and 59. With 297 cases, the total rank sum equals $[297 \times (297 + 1)]/2 = 44{,}253$ and an average rank of 149. The test compares the observed rank sum in each comparison group to the one expected under the null hypothesis. For instance, with an average rank of 149 among 37 current smoker, the expected rank *sum* under the null hypothesis for this group would be $149 \times 37 = 5513$, while the observed rank sum of 4561.5 (implying an average rank of 123.3) appears to indicate that current smokers rate their exercise activities as less frequent. However, with three comparison groups, the chi-squared test with ties in the rankings and $3 - 1 = 2$ df results in a *p*-value of .1098. Thus, based on the available evidence, we would not reject the null hypothesis that the median self-rated exercise frequency rankings differ among the three groups of smokers and nonsmokers.

FRIEDMAN TEST

The Friedman test can be considered a generalization of the Wilcoxon signed-rank test, as it can be used to test for changes in median ranks over time at more than just two occasions. In short, just as repeated-measures ANOVA is a generalization of the paired *t*-test, the Friedman test allows for the comparison of more ordinal measures taken at more than two occasions among the same group of people. The test can also be used with interval- or ratio-level data as an alternative to ANOVA, in case the assumption of normally distributed error terms is substantially violated, as would be the case with large outliers (see Box 15.2).

BOX 15.2	ASSUMPTIONS OF FRIEDMAN TEST

- Interval/ratio *or* ordinal level of measurement for single dependent variable
- Single group/sample measured at three or more occasions (correlated measures)
- Randomly drawn study sample for population inferences

As with other ordinal statistics, we start with converting the original scores into rankings; but this time we rank-order the responses of each subject over time. For example, Table 15.8 shows the health self-ratings of eight patients on an ordinal scale with 5 points: 1 = poor, 2 = fair, 3 = good, 4 = very good, 5 = excellent. Each of these patients rated their own health one day before surgery (pretest), 1 week after surgery (Posttest 1), and 3 months after surgery (Posttest 2). Rather than using the original ratings, we convert them to *within-subjects rankings* such that the lowest of the three rankings receives a 1, the second lowest a 2, and the highest a 3.[2] Under the null hypothesis, we assume that the mean rankings do not change over the three measurement occasions. Friedman's statistic amounts to comparing observed rank sums for each measurement occasion to expected rank sums under the null-hypothesis of no difference. The test statistic has a chi-square distribution with df equal to the number of measures $-$ 1. As the results show, the Friedman test is significant with $p < .002$; thus we reject the null hypothesis that self-rated health does not change over time.

TABLE 15.8 Friedman Test to Compare Average Rank Orders Over Three Occasions

```
        Original Subject Ratings:  |   Within-Subject Ranks:
      +------------------------------------------------------------+
  N   | pre    post1    post2  |   Rpre    Rpost1    Rpost2  |
  --- |------------------------------------------------------------|
  1   |  3       3        5    |   1.5      1.5        3     |
  2   |  2       2        4    |   1.5      1.5        3     |
  3   |  3       3        3    |    2        2         2     |
  4   |  1       2        2    |    1       2.5       2.5    |
  5   |  2       4        4    |    1       2.5       2.5    |
  6   |  1       2        4    |    1        2         3     |
  7   |  1       3        5    |    1        2         3     |
  8   |  3       4        5    |    1        2         3     |
      +------------------------------------------------------------+
 Sums:  16      23       32    |   10       16         22
 Means:  2     2.875      4    |  1.25       2        2.75
```

Friedman's Chi-squared statistics: 12.0, df.: 2, p<0.002

Wilcoxon signed-rank test

Ho: Rpre = Rpost1	Ho: Rpost1 = Rpost2	Ho: Rpre = Rpost2
z = –2.191	z = –2.206	z = –2.487
Prob > |z| = 0.0285	Prob > |z| = 0.0274	Prob > |z| = 0.0129

---

[2] In the case of ties, the same rules apply as for the Wilcoxon rank-sum test; see Table 15.3.

As we used the Friedman test in the example to test for significant changes in the average rankings over *three* occasions, it is a multivariate test. If the test is significant ($\alpha < 0.05$), it usually makes sense to follow up with three Wilcoxon signed-rank tests, each of which compares pairs of rankings from two rating occasions at a time. At the bottom of Table 15.8, we see that all rating pairs exhibit significant increases in the average rankings between the two time points.[3]

SPEARMAN'S RANK-ORDER CORRELATION AND KENDALL'S TAU-B

When we discussed the Pearson's r correlation in Chapter 10, we emphasized two important assumptions concerning its usage: Pearson' r is designed as a correlation coefficient between two interval- or ratio-level variables, because the actual formula assumes one can compute mean and distance values for the two variables involved. Pearson's r also assumes that two variables are *linearly* related. Ordinal correlation coefficients do not make such assumptions; thus, they turn out to be more appropriate correlations in many situations. As is the case for other ordinal statistics, Spearman's rank-order correlation rho (ρ) can be used with variables measured at the ordinal, interval, or ratio level. In fact, Spearman's ρ is equivalent to the Pearson's r correlation computed on the rank scores, instead of the original scores. Like Pearson's r, and many other correlation coefficients, Spearman's ρ is bounded by -1 and $+1$ with zero indicating the absence of any correlation between the two rank-order variables compared. The simplified computational formula for Spearman's ρ is:[4]

$$\rho = 1 - \frac{6\sum d_i^2}{n(n^2 - 1)},$$

where d_i refers to the differences in paired rankings and n equals the number of pairings (sample size).

The example data in Table 15.9 show diastolic blood pressure (DBP) readings for eight individuals taken within 10 minutes. Notice the big outlier of 126 mmHg: It influences both the mean and the standard deviation (and variance) of the Time 1 measure, all of which are sensitive to outliers.

The same can be said about the Pearson's r correlation: It too is sensitive to outliers and nonlinearity in the relationship between the two variables involved. As Spearman's ρ is calculated on the ranks, the existence of outliers does not necessarily reduce the fit of the correlation model to the data, as shown in Figure 15.3. As long as there is a largely monotone increasing (decreasing) relationship between the two variables involved—higher ranks on one variable are associated with higher (lower) ranks of the other variable—Spearman's ρ will be large, even if the relationship is not linear. On the other hand, outliers often have a disproportionate impact on the linearity of a relationship. As a result, in the example of Table 15.9 we have a Pearson's r correlation of 0.58 versus 0.88 for Spearman's ρ. The two graphs in Figure 15.3 confirm the better fit of ρ compared to r. This suggests a quick useful test for correlations based on interval-level variables: If Spearman's ρ exceeds Pearson's r by a substantial margin, there is likely to be some nonlinearity in the relationship involved. In that situation, we would graph the relationship and see whether a better fitting function can be found through transformations of one or the other variable.

---

[3] The negative z-scores are a result of the fact that the later higher ranking is subtracted from the earlier lower ranking in each pair.

[4] A more detailed discussion can be found in Siegel, *Nonparametric Statistics*.

TABLE 15.9 Diastolic Blood Pressure Data for Spearman's Rank-Order Correlation ρ

ID	DBP READINGS TIME 1	DBP READINGS TIME 2	DBP RANKINGS TIME 1	DBP RANKINGS TIME 2	DIFFERENCE IN PAIRED RANKINGS d_i	d_i^2
1	75	1	1	1	0	0
2	84	3	3	3	0	0
3	91	4	6	4	2	4
4	126	7	8	7	1	1
5	87	5	5	5	0	0
6	95	8	7	8	−1	1
7	86	6	4	6	−2	4
8	83	2	2	2	0	0
	$\bar{x}_1 = 90.875$ $SD_1 = 15.36$	$\bar{x}_2 = 87.625$ $SD_2 = 5.40$				$\sum d_i^2 = 10$

$$\text{Spearman's } \rho = 1 - \frac{6\sum d_i^2}{n(n^2-1)} = 1 - \frac{6 \times 10}{8(8^2-1)} = 1 - \frac{60}{8(63)} = 1 - 0.119 = 0.881$$

$$\text{Pearson's } r = 0.5751$$

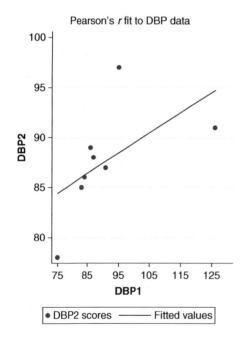

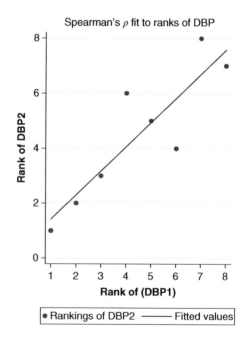

FIGURE 15.3 Fit of Pearson's r and Spearman's ρ to Data With Outliers.

SUMMARY

In this chapter, we discussed several ordinal statistics as alternatives to the *t*-test, one-way ANOVA, repeated-measures ANOVA, and the Pearson's *r* correlation coefficient. The statistics discussed in this chapter may all be applied to original ordinal variables as well as interval- or ratio-level variables. In the latter case, comparing the results of the parametric to the nonparametric statistics is often instructive in shedding light on the effects of violations of the underlying assumptions of the parametric models.

While ordinal statistics are often encountered in the clinical literature (Nathanson et al., 2011; Prendergast, Jakobsson, Renvert, & Hallberg, 2012), statistics used to analyze nominal categorical data that cannot be rank-ordered are even more important. Many data sets relevant to clinical problems involve simply counting the number of patients, who fall into one or another diagnostic category or who do or do not experience a clinical outcome of interest. It is to the analysis of such categorical outcomes that we will turn next.

LITERATURE APPLICATION

Read: Prendergast, V., Jakobsson, U., Renvert, S., & Hallberg, I. R. (2012). Effects of a standard versus comprehensive oral care protocol among intubated neuroscience ICU patients: Results of a randomized controlled trial. *Journal of Neuroscience Nursing, 44*(3), 134–146.

(a) Provide a very brief (three to four sentences) summary of what this study is about.

(b) Define the target population to which the statistical analysis can be generalized. What were the eligibility and exclusion criteria for study participants? Is the study sample a random sample of the target population?

(c) Provide a clear definition of the outcome/dependent variables and a short description of the instrument used to measure them.

(d) Provide a clear definition of all independent/predictor variables and a short description of the instruments used to measure it.

(e) Describe the study design: How many comparison groups? How many observations per subjects? Randomization? Attrition?

(f) On page 139, the authors mention the specific statistical models used to compare subjects in the intervention and control groups and over time. List each of the ordinal tests and provide a rationale for why they were used. Why did the authors use a Bonferroni adjustment for the Wilcoxon signed-rank test, and why did they set the α-level for this adjustment to 0.017?

(g) In tables 4 and 5, the authors associate specific tests with specific variables tested. Provide rationales for the authors' choices.

(h) Summarize the main findings in your own words. Are the conclusions of the authors consistent with the evidence presented?

EXERCISES

1. Compute the Pearson's *r* correlation for the *rankings* of the DBP1 and DBP2 measures in Table 15.9 and verify that this sample correlation is identical to the Spearman's ρ correlation. You may either use software or a hand calculator using the Pearson's *r* formula from Chapter 10.

2. The following data show the rankings of 12 hospitals by two independent inspection teams in terms of a safety score. The safety score is a composite measure that takes into account infection risks, surgical errors, other bodily harm attributable to interventions, and so forth, with a theoretical range of 0 to 100.

Hospital:	A	B	C	D	E	F	G	H	I	J	K	L
Team A Score:	95	87	74	93	96	88	99	86	85	92	94	81
Team B Score:	93	90	78	96	94	89	97	90	89	90	93	88

(a) What test would you use to determine whether the two teams report similar safety rankings for the 12 hospitals?
(b) State the null hypothesis for the test statistic.
(c) Report your results.

3. The following safety rankings compare two groups of 10 hospitals each, randomly chosen from two states.

Hospital:	A	B	C	D	E	F	G	H	I	J
State A Score:	94	85	74	94	91	86	95	85	83	89
State B Score:	93	90	78	96	90	84	92	90	89	90

(a) What test would you use to compare the safety of the hospitals in the two states?
(b) State the null hypothesis for the test statistic.
(c) Can we conclude that the safety records of hospitals in State B are better than those in State A?

4. When comparing *mean* outcomes on an *interval-level* variable, would it ever be preferable to use the Kruskal–Wallis test over ANOVA? If yes, why? If no, why not?

5. In a study of several thousand adults, the Pearson's r correlation between two variables (age and the BMI) is $+0.28$ ($p < .046$) and the Spearman's ρ correlation between the same two variables is $+0.47$ ($p < .001$). What could be the reason for the difference in the magnitude of the correlations?

REFERENCES

Brunelli, C., Zecca, E., Martini, C., Campa, T., Fagnoni, E., Bagnasco, M., . . . Caraceni, A. (2010). Comparison of numerical and verbal rating scales to measure pain exacerbations in patients with chronic cancer pain. *Health Quality Life Outcomes, 8*, 42.

Nathanson, B. H., Henneman, E. A., Blonaisz, E. R., Doubleday, N. D., Lusardi, P., & Jodka, P. G. (2011). How much teamwork exists between nurses and junior doctors in the intensive care unit? *Journal of Advanced Nursing, 67*(8), 1817–1823.

Ogden, C. L., Carroll, M. D., Curtin, L. R., McDowell, M. A., Tabak, C. J., & Flegal, K. M. (2006). Prevalence of overweight and obesity in the United States, 1999–2004. *The Journal of the American Medical Association, 295*(13), 1549–1555.

Prendergast, V., Jakobsson, U., Renvert, S., & Hallberg, I. R. (2012). Effects of a standard versus comprehensive oral care protocol among intubated neuroscience ICU patients: Results of a randomized controlled trial. *Journal of Neuroscience Nursing, 44*(3), 134–146.

Wong, C. L., Holroyd-Leduc, J., Simel, D. L., & Straus, S. E. (2010). Does this patient have delirium? Value of bedside instruments. *The Journal of the American Medical Association, 304*(7), 779–786.

CHAPTER 16

Frequency Cross-Tabulations: 2 × 2 Tables

In the last chapter, we discussed some commonly encountered ordinal statistics. While nurses and physicians often employ rating scales, one example being visual analog scales for pain measurement (Hjermstad et al., 2012), even more important is the "simple" classification of patients for both clinical practice and research. Examples include knowing a patient's blood type, clinical diagnosis, presence or absence of a certain genetic trait, family situation, and so forth. All of this information may trigger different courses of clinical actions, making classification a fundamental component of clinical work.

In our general discussion of levels of measurement in Chapter 2, we emphasized that a good classification system only requires the establishment of mutually exclusive categories. For convenience in the statistical analysis of data sets, we usually assign numerical labels to the *nominal* categories; yet, as illustrated in Table 16.1, such numerical labels are completely arbitrary. This implies we cannot use them in our mathematical calculations at all: For instance, to say that the "average blood type" among U.S. residents is 3.4 would be a nonsensical statement.

This begs the question: How should we analyze categorical data? The answer at its most basic level is simply that we can *count* the number of people, cases, or observations that fall into certain categories of interest. As it turns out, that does not prevent us from using sophisticated statistical models to explore the relationships among categorical variables, but they are different from both the parametric and ordinal models we have dealt with so far.

Looking at the eight blood types listed, one might want to know whether the prevalence[1] of particular blood types is the same across ethnic or gender groups. Or one might be interested in establishing whether the risk[2] of leukemia is the same or differs across blood types. These kinds of comparisons involve counts and proportions as the basic staple of describing clinical phenomena.

In this chapter, we will start our discussion of statistical models for categorical data with an exposition on the 2 × 2 frequency table. This table format is used to display the simplest

---

[1] The prevalence is simply the proportion of cases in a well-defined population at a given time that has the trait or disease in question.

[2] The *absolute* risk is a measure of the rate of (new) occurrence of a disease or adverse event in a population over a specified period of time. It is also known as the incidence rate. The *relative* risk (RR) is the ratio of the incidence rates in two comparison groups. See the discussion of RR below.

TABLE 16.1 Alternative Numerical Codes for Blood Types

BLOOD TYPE	CODING SCHEME 1	CODING SCHEME 2	CODING SCHEME 3
A+	1	8	1
A–	2	7	3
B+	3	6	8
B–	4	5	6
AB+	5	4	2
AB–	6	3	4
O+	7	2	7
O–	8	1	5

possible example of a bivariate distribution, that is, the simultaneous distribution of cases across two variables, each having two categories. Not only are such tables frequently encountered in health care research, but they can be used to demonstrate the calculation of many statistical measures commonly found in the health care literature.

(*Caution*: Do *not* confuse the 2 × 2 *frequency* table with the 2 × 2 factorial analysis-of-variance (ANOVA) table. In the case of a factorial ANOVA with two factors, the tables show the *mean scores* for the outcome variable within the categories created by crossing two factor variables. That is, in a two-factor ANOVA we are dealing with *three* variables, including the two independent factors and the outcome variable, which is measured at the interval level).[3]

Going back to the 2 × 2 frequency table, the capitalized letters in Table 16.2 are used to indicate the *numbers* of cases or study subjects in each of the cells. These letters can then be employed to define various statistical measures.

In Table 16.2, both variables are examples of nominal/categorical variables forming a 2 × 2 table, in which each variable has only two categories: One variable represents the gender of a subject, the other the absence or presence of (a diagnosis of) diabetes. In this situation, the data entries in the various cells (represented here by the letters) refer to frequency counts. For instance, A represents the number of female subjects who have been diagnosed with diabetes and D represents the number of male subjects who do not have diabetes, and so forth. Overall, a 2 × 2 table has four (inner) cells denoted here by their frequency counts: A, B, C, and D. There are also four marginal cells: E, F, G, and H, which contain sums of the number of cases in their respective rows or columns. Thus, the number of cases in the first row (=G) equals the

TABLE 16.2 2 × 2 Table Showing Joint Distribution of Study Subjects Across Two Variables: Gender and Diabetes Status

		DIABETES STATUS		ROW MARGINAL FREQUENCIES
		HAS DIABETES	NO DIABETES	
Gender	Women	A	B	G = A + B
	Men	C	D	H = C + D
Column marginal frequencies		E = A + C	F = B + D	Totals I = E + F = G + H = A + B + C + D

---

[3]Recall the nutrition and exercise data introduced in Chapter 11, in which the outcome measure is the body mass index (BMI), and study participants are exposed to two types of interventions designed to reduce persons' BMI. In such a study, the results are reported as mean BMI scores in four cells representing four groups formed by the independent factors: nutrition and exercise intervention, nutrition only intervention, exercise only intervention, neither intervention–control groups.

sum of the cases in the inner cells for women, such that A and B equal all women in this study, the number of cases in the first column (=E) equals the sum of the cases in the inner cells for diabetics, such that A and C equal all persons with diabetes in this study, and so forth. Finally, cell I refers to the table total, which is simply the sum of the frequencies in all inner cells, or the number of all study participants (=total sample size).

MEASURES OF ASSOCIATION FOR 2 × 2 TABLES

The Odds Ratio

The **odds ratio (OR)** is a very common measure of association in the biomedical and epidemiological literature. As the name "odds ratio" implies, the OR is a ratio of two odds.

Thus, we first begin by defining the odds themselves. In a 2 × 2 table, there are two row odds and two column odds. The row odds for the first row are defined as A/B and for the second row, they are defined as C/D. In the case of Table 16.2, A/B refers to the odds of having diabetes versus not having diabetes among female subjects (first row) and C/D refers to the odds of having diabetes versus not having diabetes among male subjects (second row). The column odds are, respectively, defined as A/C (first column) and B/D (second column). In Table 16.2, they represent the odds of being female versus male among diabetics (first column) and the odds of being female versus male among subjects who are not diabetic (second column).

Now we can define the odds *ratio*. The OR is a *symmetric* measure, which means it does not matter whether we use the column odds or the row odds in defining it; the result will be the same either way:

$$OR = \frac{\dfrac{A}{B}}{\dfrac{C}{D}} = \frac{\dfrac{A}{C}}{\dfrac{B}{D}} = \frac{AD}{CB}$$

Before we continue, let us use the numerical example in Table 16.3, substituting frequencies for the capital letters.

From Table 16.3 we get:

Odds of having diabetes among females: A/B = 100/300 = 0.333

Odds of having diabetes among males: C/D = 120/180 = 0.667

Odds ratio (male/female): OR = (120/180)/(100/300) = 2.0; according to the sample data in this table, the odds of having diabetes are 2.0 times greater (or twice as large) among men

TABLE 16.3 2 × 2 Table Showing Joint Distribution of Study Subjects Across Two Variables: Gender and Diabetes Status (Numerical Example)

		DIABETES STATUS		ROW MARGINAL FREQUENCIES
		HAS DIABETES	NO DIABETES	
Gender	Women	100	300	400
	Men	120	180	300
Column marginal frequencies		220	480	700

compared to women. (We can also take the inverse: $1/OR = (100/300)/(120/180) = 0.5$, which means the odds of having diabetes are only half as large among women than men, but it is easier to say it the other way around.)

Earlier we mentioned that the OR is a symmetric measure.[4] This means it does not matter whether we compute the OR as a ratio of the row odds (as above) or the ratio of the column odds. For the example in Table 16.3, we would get the following result with column odds:

$$OR = (B/D)/(A/C) = (300/180)/(100/120) = 2.0,$$

or using the inverse: $1/OR = (A/C)/(B/D) = (100/120)/(300/180) = 0.5$

Thus, the OR behaves like a correlation coefficient: It does not change, regardless of which variable we consider the dependent or independent variable.

There is an alternative way of writing odds and ORs that is also common in the literature. Odds are often defined as the *ratio of the probability of an event occurring over the probability of the event not occurring: odds = p/(1 − p)*. As a probability can be viewed as the proportion of an event occurring in the relevant universe, this alternative formulation of the odds is nothing new. For instance, in Table 16.3, we have 400 women, 100 of whom have been diagnosed with diabetes. Thus, the probability of diabetes among these women is $p = 100/400 = .25$. It follows, the probability of not having diabetes is .75, and the odds of having diabetes are: odds $= .25/.75 = .333$. As the probability of having diabetes among men is $p = .4$ (=120/300), it follows that the probability of *not* having diabetes among men is $1 − p = .6$; thus, the odds are again $p/(1 − p) = .4/.6 = .667$. Forming the ratio of the two odds among men and women, we again obtain:

$$OR = [p_m/(1 − p_m)]/[p_w/(1 − p_w)] = [0.4/0.6]/[0.25/0.75] = 2.0$$

Thus, whether we use the original cell frequencies or the probabilities, we get the same results. We mentioned earlier that ORs can be thought of as measures of association, just like a correlation coefficient. However, the neutral value of "no relationship" for correlation coefficients is zero; *for the OR, the neutral value is one*. To see why, consider the following example. Suppose the data in Table 16.3 had shown that 160 of the 400 women had been diagnosed with diabetes. In that case $p_w = p_m = .4$ or the probability of diabetes would be 40% among members of both genders. Given the formula for the OR, we would get the following results: $OR = (0.4/0.6)/(0.4/0.6) = 1$. If the odds of having diabetes are the same among men and women (which implies that $OR = 1$), then there is *no* relationship between diabetes and gender, as gender would not account for any variation in diabetes.

Another feature of the OR is that it can only be positive[5] and its distribution is *asymmetric* around the neutral value of 1. For instance, the inverse of 5 is 1/5; consequently, the following statements are perfectly equivalent: (a) "the odds of leukemia in population A are

---

[4]The symmetry of the OR is the reason why this measure of association is used in case-control studies, in which cases with a disease are compared to controls without the disease with respect to their odds of having been exposed to a suspected risk factor. As the OR is symmetric, we get the same estimate, whether we are looking for the odds of contracting the disease given exposure status or the odds of exposure given the disease state. For more detailed discussion of case-control studies, see Stommel and Wills (2004).

[5]Recall that ORs are based on frequency counts in cells, with zero being the lowest possible number of cases in a cell; however, a ratio with zero in the denominator ($N/0$) is not defined.

5 times larger than in population B," or (b) "the odds of leukemia in population B are only one-fifth of the odds in population A." We can, however, convert ORs using the natural logarithm transformation [ln(OR)], which results in a symmetric distribution around the value of zero.[6] As we will see in the following section, this transformation allows us to construct fairly easily the confidence intervals (CIs) for the OR.

CONFIDENCE INTERVALS FOR ODDS RATIOS

So far, we have only considered the sample OR, but as always, we must be able to draw inferences about the population OR. Given the asymmetry of OR values around one, it is no surprise that the sampling distribution of the original OR is positively skewed; however, the sampling distribution of the log-transformed OR is approximately normal. Thus, we can use the same procedure as for the t-test to construct 95% CIs of the OR. Recall from Chapter 8, that we obtain the 95% CI for a *mean* as follows: We calculate the point estimate of the mean from the sample data and add or subtract the t-value$_{.95}$ multiplied by the standard error of the mean (SEM):

$$\bar{x} - t \times \text{SEM} < \mu < \bar{x} + t \times \text{SEM}$$

Likewise, we can construct the 95% CI for the *log-transformed OR* as follows:

$$\ln(\text{sample-OR}) \pm t\text{-value} \times \text{SE}(\ln(OR)), \text{ or}$$

$$\ln(\text{sample-OR}) - t \times \text{SE}(\ln(OR)) < \ln(\text{population-OR}) < \ln(\text{sample-OR}) + t \times \text{SE}(\ln(OR))$$

All we need now to construct the 95% CI is an estimate of the standard error of the log-transformed OR and the appropriate t-value. The formula for the standard error of ln(OR) is:

$$\text{SE of } \ln(OR) = \sqrt{\frac{1}{A} + \frac{1}{B} + \frac{1}{C} + \frac{1}{D}}$$

where A, B, C, and D are the frequencies of the inner cells of the 2 × 2 table. With a sample of $n = 700$, the t-distribution is virtually identical to the normal distribution (see Appendix C) and the cut-off points for a 95% CI on the normal distribution equal ±1.96 standard errors. With this information, we can use the data in Table 16.3 to estimate the 95% CI for log-transformed OR as follows:

$$\ln(0.5) \pm 1.96 \times \sqrt{\frac{1}{100} + \frac{1}{300} + \frac{1}{120} + \frac{1}{180}}$$

$$-0.693 \pm 1.96 \times 0.165$$

$$-0.693 \pm 0.3234$$

$$-1.0164, -0.3696$$

Taking the antilog (exponentiating using the base e) of −1.0164 and −0.3696, we get the following estimate of the 95% CI of the *original* OR: 0.362 < pop(OR) < 0.691. Notice that this CI is not symmetric around the point estimate: 0.5 − 0.362 = 0.138 and 0.691 − 0.5 = 0.191. Also note that this CI does not contain the neutral value of one. Thus, we would reject the null

---

[6]For an informal refresher on how to use exponentiation and logarithms, see Appendix H.

TABLE 16.4 Cross-Tabulation of Gender and Diabetes Diagnosis

```
              |            diabetes:
              |
   gender     |   has diabetes   no diabetes   |   Total
--------------+-----------------------------------------
   female     |       100            300        |    400
   male       |       120            180        |    300
--------------+-----------------------------------------
   Total      |       220            480        |    700

              Pearson chi2(1)   =  17.8977   Pr = 0.000
              Fisher's exact    =            0.000
       1-sided Fisher's exact   =            0.000
```

```
-----------------------------------------------------------------------------------
   diabetes   |  OR(female/male)        z       P|z|     [95% Conf.    Interval]
-------------+---------------------------------------------------------------------
   gender     |       0.5             -4.20    0.000      .361850      .690894
-----------------------------------------------------------------------------------
```

```
-----------------------------------------------------------------------------------
   diabetes   |  OR(female/male)        z       P|z|     [95% Conf.    Interval]
-------------+---------------------------------------------------------------------
   gender     |       0.2             -4.20    0.000     1.447401     2.763574
-----------------------------------------------------------------------------------
```

```
-----------------------------------------------------------------------------------
   diabetes   |  OR(female/male)        z       P|z|     [95% Conf.    Interval]
-------------+---------------------------------------------------------------------
   gender     |       0.625           -4.20    0.00       .502008     0.778124
-----------------------------------------------------------------------------------
```

```
-----------------------------------------------------------------------------------
   diabetes   |  OR(female/male)        z       P|z|     [95% Conf.    Interval]
-------------+---------------------------------------------------------------------
   gender     |       1.6             -4.20    0.00      1.285142     1.991998
-----------------------------------------------------------------------------------
```

pwcorr gender diabetes, sig

```
              |    gender     diabetes
--------------+-------------------------
   gender     |   1.0000
              |
   diabetes   |  -0.1599     1.0000
              |   0.0000
```

hypothesis that the OR = 1 in the population, or that gender is not related to the odds of having a diabetes diagnosis. Table 16.4 shows the 2 × 2 table from Table 16.3, the OR and its inverse, the 95% confidence limits associated with the OR, and the p-value associated with a z-value of 4.2 on the normal distribution. Recall that our point estimate for the log-transformed OR was −0.693 and our standard error estimate was 0.165. The z-value of −0.693/0.165 = 4.2 indicates that the observed log-transformed OR is 4.2 standard errors away from the null hypothesis value of zero.[7] The associated p-value is smaller than .0005, making it very unlikely that the observed sample OR is just the result of random fluctuations.

---

[7]Remember: The neutral value for OR equals one, but the neutral value for the log-transformed OR equals zero.

THE RELATIVE RISK RATIO

The **relative-risk ratio (RRR)** is (sometimes) defined as the ratio of two probabilities. If the individuals in a study group are followed for the same period of time, the *risk* or *probability* of an adverse outcome is simply the proportion of people in any given group of interest that experiences the outcome (disease) in question.[8] The *relative risk* (RR) is the *ratio* comparing the risk in one group to that in another: $RR = p_1/p_2$.

Going back to Table 16.1, there are two rows indicating the gender of a person. In the second row, we have a total of H women; of these C men have been diagnosed with diabetes. Thus the proportion of diabetics among these men equals $C/H = p_m$. The first row shows the proportion of diabetics among women: $A/G = p_w$. The ratio of these two proportions or probabilities is the *relative risk* of having diabetes, with gender being the "risk factor":

$$RR = \frac{p_m}{p_w} = \frac{\frac{C}{H}}{\frac{A}{G}} = \frac{CG}{HA}$$

Even though it does not make much sense from a causal point of view, we could ask what is the "relative risk" of being a man, comparing diabetics and those not diagnosed with diabetes. This "RR" would be:

$$RR = \frac{\frac{C}{E}}{\frac{D}{F}} = \frac{CF}{ED}$$

Notice the important difference to the OR: While the OR is symmetric (it does not matter whether we start with the column odds or the row odds), the RRR is *not* symmetric:

$$\frac{CG}{HA} \neq \frac{CF}{ED}$$

As with the OR, the "neutral" value (indicating an absence of any association) is equal to one. If two groups, such as men and women, face the same risk of diabetes, then group membership (gender) is not related to the risk of diabetes; but if $p_1 = p_2$, RR = 1.

From the data in Table 16.3 we get:

Risk/probability of having diabetes among males: C/H = 120/300 = 0.4

Risk/probability of having diabetes among females: A/G = 100/400 = 0.25

Relative risk (male/female): RR = (120/300)/(100/400) = 0.4/0.25 = 1.6

In words: According to the sample data in this table, the risk of having diabetes is 1.6 times greater among men than among women.

(We can also take the inverse: 1/RR = (100/400)/(120/300) = 0.25/0.4 = 0.625, which means the risk of diabetes among women is only 62.5% as large as the risk among men.)

---

[8]*Note*: In Chapter 19, we encounter a more precise definition of RR as the ratio of two *incidence* rates. As mentioned, if individuals in the two comparison groups are observed for the same time, the two definitions are identical. Both definitions are used in the literature.

CONFIDENCE INTERVALS FOR RELATIVE-RISK RATIOS

Again, we have only considered the sample RR, but we need to be able to draw inferences about the population RR. Like the OR, RR values are always positive with no upper limit; it follows that they have a sampling distribution skewed to the right. Again, we can normalize this distribution through logarithmic transformation: ln(RR) is approximately normally distributed. Thus, in order to construct CIs, we only need an estimate for the standard error of ln(RR). It is given by the following formula:

$$\text{SE of } \ln(RR) = \sqrt{\frac{B}{A(A+B)} + \frac{D}{C(C+D)}}$$

With this information, we can use the data in Table 16.3 to estimate the 95% CI for the log-transformed RR as follows: ln(sample-RR) $\pm$ t-value $\times$ SE(ln(RR)), which yields the following estimates:

$$\ln(1.6) \pm 1.96 = \sqrt{\frac{300}{100(100+300)} + \frac{180}{120(120+180)}}$$

$$= 0.47 \pm 1.96 \times 0.1118 = 0.47 \pm 0.2191.$$

Consequently, the lower CI limit equals $0.47 - 0.2191 = 0.2509$ and the upper CI limit equals $0.47 + 0.2191 = 0.6819$. Taking the antilog of 0.2509, $e^{0.2509}$, yields an estimate of 1.2852 for the lower limit of the 95% CI of the *original* RR; the antilog of the upper limit, $e^{0.6891}$, yields 1.9919. Thus the 95% CI for this RR is: $1.2852 < \text{pop(RR)} < 1.9919$. Notice again, this CI is not symmetric around the point estimate of RR = 1.6: $1.6 - 1.2852 = 0.3148$ and $1.9919 - 1.6 = 0.3919$, but it is symmetric around the point estimate of ln(RR).

SIMILARITIES AND DIFFERENCES IN THE MAGNITUDES OF OR AND RR

In general, the point estimates of the OR and RR, when using the same data, are *not* identical or even of the same magnitude. In our numerical example, we computed an OR of 2.0 and an RR of 1.6. Their inverses are obviously also different from each other: 1/OR = 0.5, 1/RR = 0.625. However, epidemiologists sometimes invoke the *rare disease assumption* as an *exception* to this rule. If a disease is quite rare, say its overall prevalence in the population is 2 in 2,000, then the risk or probability of its occurrence is 2/2,000 and the odds of its occurrence is 2/1,998. Suppose further that we have collected case-control data from a large-scale registry. We find that the odds of exposure to a suspected risk factor among individuals with the disease are 5/1,995, while the odds of exposure among individuals without the disease are 1/1,999. Computing the OR, we get (5/1,995)/(1/1,999) = 5.01. In other words, the odds of exposure to the risk factor are approximately 5 times larger among people with the disease than among those without it. As we know that the OR is a symmetric measure, we might just as well say that the odds of contracting the disease among individuals exposed to the risk factor are 5 times larger than among people not exposed to the risk factor. However, with prospective data we could have computed an RR of (5/2,000)/(1/2,000) = 5. Thus, if the data involve rare diseases, the OR and RRR yield approximately the same values: OR $\approx$ RR.

THE CORRELATION COEFFICIENT PHI (Φ)

Another commonly used measure of association for a 2 × 2 table is the correlation coefficient **Phi (Φ)**. As shown in Appendix F, this measure is identical to Pearson's r correlation coefficient, but it can be computed in a simple way from the frequency counts in the 2 × 2 table:

$$Phi\,(\Phi) = \frac{(AD - BC)}{\sqrt{EFGH}}$$

In words, the Phi coefficient can be computed (using a calculator) by dividing the difference between the cross-products of the inner cells by the square root of the product of all marginal cells. Like the Pearson's r (and unlike the OR), this correlation coefficient is bounded by ±1, with *zero* (not one) indicating "no relationship." However, in most cases, the sign of this coefficient should be ignored. Recall that the two variables involved are often nominal or categorical variables with arbitrary numerical labels. Thus, recoding gender from "1 = women, 0 = men" to "0 = women, 1 = men" would reverse the sign of the coefficient, but leave the magnitude of the estimate unchanged. Only the latter, that is, the magnitude, is of interest in such a situation.

For a numerical example, we go back to Table 16.3:

$$Phi\,(\Phi) = \frac{(100 \times 180 - 300 \times 120)}{\sqrt{220 \times 480 \times 400 \times 300}} = \frac{(18000 - 36000)}{\sqrt{12672000000}} = \frac{-18000}{112569.9782} = -0.1599$$

Ignoring the sign, we can say that the observed sample correlation between gender and diabetes status is moderately small at 0.16. However, as the results in Table 16.4 show, the correlation is statistically significant at $p < .00005$. Thus again, we would reject the null hypothesis of no relationship between the two variables.

THE PEARSON CHI-SQUARED (χ^2) STATISTIC

So far, we have considered three measures of association commonly applied to data from 2 × 2 tables. The three measures of association we just introduced (the OR, the RRR, and Phi) were estimated from the available sample data. We reported p-values, based on the normal distribution test, for the null hypotheses that OR = 1 and RR = 1 and Phi = 0. There is another significance test frequently applied to categorical data, the **Pearson Chi-squared (χ^2) test**. It is easily one of the most frequently used statistical tests to determine whether two variables can be considered related "beyond a reasonable doubt." This is an *inferential* question rather than a descriptive one. As we have emphasized before, any study sample data are subject to numerous sources of measurement and sampling error; thus we can expect that another data set from the same target population would show somewhat different results. Consequently, we must ask: Is the observed sample pattern substantial enough, so that it cannot be easily "explained away" as the result of mere sampling fluctuations?

To answer such a question, we need (a) to construct an appropriate test statistic, and (b) to employ an appropriate probability model that tells us how likely or unlikely a particular sample result is under the conditions assumed in the null hypothesis.

In order to construct the χ^2-statistic, we first state a null hypothesis. The most common one would be to assume that the two variables (in Table 16.2, it is gender and diabetes status) are not related. If they are not related, what result should we expect to observe in the sample data? As stated before, we should expect the same prevalence of diabetes among both men and women. (Again, that is the same as saying: Knowing that someone is male or female does not help in improving the prediction of his or her diabetes status.)

For Table 16.2, the *expected* values in the inner cells, *if* gender and diabetes are not related, are as follows:

$$\text{for cell A:}\ \frac{E \times G}{I}, \quad \text{for cell B:}\ \frac{F \times G}{I}, \quad \text{for cell C:}\ \frac{E \times H}{I}, \quad \text{for cell D:}\ \frac{F \times H}{I}$$

(For instance, the overall proportion of individuals diagnosed with diabetes is E/I. If we multiply both the number of females [G] and the number of males [H] by E/I, we get the expected number of female and male sample subjects with diabetes, as we assume under the null hypothesis that male and female individuals do not differ with respect to their probability of having diabetes. Thus, the formula guarantees that the "expected" percentage of males or females with diabetes is the same. By the same token, the formula also guarantees that the percentage of males or females without diabetes is the same.)

In the final step, we can construct the Pearson χ^2-statistic. For each of the four inner cells, we subtract the expected cell frequency (Ex) from the observed cell frequency (Ob), square the difference, and divide it by the expected cell frequency number. This is our test statistic: $\chi^2 = \frac{\sum(Ob - Ex)^2}{Ex}$. Using the letters from Table 16.2, we can write out the χ^2-statistic as follows:

$$\chi^2 = \frac{\left(A - \dfrac{E \times G}{I}\right)^2}{\dfrac{E \times G}{I}} + \frac{\left(B - \dfrac{F \times G}{I}\right)^2}{\dfrac{F \times G}{I}} + \frac{\left(C - \dfrac{E \times H}{I}\right)^2}{\dfrac{E \times H}{I}} + \frac{\left(D - \dfrac{F \times H}{I}\right)^2}{\dfrac{F \times H}{I}}$$

Substituting the numbers from Table 16.3, we get:

$$\chi^2 = \frac{\left(100 - \dfrac{220 \times 400}{700}\right)^2}{\dfrac{220 \times 400}{700}} + \frac{\left(300 - \dfrac{480 \times 400}{700}\right)^2}{\dfrac{480 \times 400}{700}} + \frac{\left(120 - \dfrac{220 \times 300}{700}\right)^2}{\dfrac{220 \times 300}{700}} + \frac{\left(180 - \dfrac{480 \times 300}{700}\right)^2}{\dfrac{480 \times 300}{700}}$$

$$= \frac{(100 - 125.71)^2}{125.71} + \frac{(300 - 274.29)^2}{274.29} + \frac{(120 - 94.29)^2}{94.29} + \frac{(180 - 205.71)^2}{205.71}$$

$$= \frac{(-25.71)^2}{125.71} + \frac{(+25.71)^2}{274.29} + \frac{(+25.71)^2}{94.29} + \frac{(-25.71)^2}{205.71} = \frac{661.00}{125.71} + \frac{661.00}{274.29} + \frac{661.00}{94.29} + \frac{661.00}{205.71}$$

$$= 5.258 + 2.410 + 7.010 + 3.213 = 17.891$$

Except for small rounding errors, this is the χ^2-value reported in Table 16.4. To understand the use of this statistic, we need to look at its behavior under different assumptions. Suppose the null hypothesis is literally true. That means the observed frequency values in the inner cells do not deviate from the values expected on the basis of the null hypothesis. In that case, numerators associated with each cell must be equal to zero, as each cell difference, such as $(A - EG/I)$ or $(B - FG/I)$ must be zero. Now suppose the observed sample cell frequency A differs from the expected frequency EG/I. As the difference is squared, it does not matter, whether the difference is positive or negative. What we can say for sure though is that larger deviations lead to larger χ^2-values. Now, suppose the null hypothesis is true. It states that, in the population from which the study sample is drawn, gender and diabetes are *not* related. Because of the usual sampling fluctuations, we do not expect that any sample drawn from such a population would return an observed χ^2-value that is *exactly* equal to zero. Given the sampling fluctuations, we would be quite prepared to observe some deviations from zero. However, the larger the observed χ^2-statistic becomes, the less compatible it is with the null hypothesis, as it is unlikely that mere random sampling fluctuations would produce very large deviations of observed frequencies from expected frequencies. If the observed value is quite unlikely, say it occurs in less than 5% of all samples by chance, then we would reject the null hypothesis and would claim that the evidence is *inconsistent* with the null hypothesis.

In the numerical example of Tables 16.3 and 16.4, the observed sample χ^2-statistic is equal to 17.8977. Under the assumption that the null hypothesis is true, we ask: Could mere sampling fluctuations have produced a χ^2-value this large? In order to answer this question, we compare the observed sample value of the test statistic to the theoretical χ^2-distribution with 1 degree of freedom. Tabled values of this distribution (see Appendix G) show that a χ^2-value larger than 3.841 occurs in only 5% of all samples as a result of random chance alone.[9] In fact, χ^2-values larger than 7.879 would occur as a result of random fluctuations in fewer than 5 out of 1,000 samples. Thus, an observed χ^2-value of 17.9 is "almost certain" evidence that the sample observations are not the result of a mere random fluke. We conclude with a high degree of confidence that gender and diabetes status are related, or that this relationship is "statistically significant."

FISHER'S EXACT TEST

The Pearson chi-squared test is one of the most frequently used statistical tests for categorical data; however, it is inexact and produces misleading probabilities if the sample sizes are small. In particular, if any cell of an *m*-by-*n* frequency table has fewer than five cases and the total sample size is less than $n = 30$, we should use **Fisher's exact test** as an alternative. This test follows the so-called hypergeometric sampling distribution (we skip the details here) and is computationally demanding. Most statistical software programs print out the probabilities associated with Fisher's exact test. These *p*-values, computed under the null-hypothesis assumption of no relationship between the two variables examined, are interpreted the same way as the probabilities associated with the χ^2-test.

SUMMARY

In this chapter, we discussed the analysis of 2 × 2 frequency tables. Pearson's χ^2-test can easily be extended to frequency tables of variables with multiple categories (*m* × *n* tables). The Phi correlation coefficient is limited to the comparison of two variables with two categories, while the OR and RRR are indices that are used to compare binary outcomes in two groups at a time. What all the statistical methods introduced in this chapter have in common is that they are based on the assumption that the variables involved are categorical, which means that the basic mathematical "building material" for statistical indices is the frequency counts in all the cells defined by the cross-classifications of the categorical variables.

As we will see in the following chapters, both the OR and the RR are also basic building blocks of multivariate regression models with categorical outcomes. As such, a thorough understanding of these statistics is imperative for further discussion of such models as logistic and hazard regressions.

---

[9]In practice, we do not even have to look up the *p*-value associated with a χ^2-value of 17.9, as the computer printout usually provides it as shown in Table 16.4.

LITERATURE APPLICATION

Read: Baratin, D., Del Signore, C., Thierry, J., Caulin, E., & Vanhems, P. (2012). Evaluation of adult dTPaP vaccination coverage in France: Experience in Lyon city, 2010–2011. *BMC Public Health, 12*, 940.

(a) Provide a very brief (three to four sentences) summary of what this study is about.

(b) Define the target population to which the statistical analysis can be generalized. What were the eligibility and exclusion criteria for study participants? Is the study sample a random sample of the target population?

(c) Provide a clear definition of the outcome/dependent variables and a short description of the instrument used to measure them.

(d) Provide a clear definition of all independent/predictor variables and a short description of the instruments used to measure them.

(e) Describe the study design: How many comparison groups? Is the study cross-sectional or longitudinal?

(f) Table 3 on page 4 contains a column of *p*-values. For each of these *p*-values, formulate the null hypothesis and specify the statistical test that was used to test it. What do we learn from these *p*-values?

(g) Table 4 also contains a column of *p*-values. Again, for each of these *p*-values, formulate the null hypothesis and specify the statistical test that was used to test it. What do we learn from these *p*-values?

(h) Use ORs to test the *strength* of the relationship between age groups and vaccination coverage.

(i) Table 5 shows, for four types of vaccination, the number of study respondents who reported the vaccination and the number whose vaccination was confirmed. Create a 4 × 2 table to test the null hypothesis that there is no difference in the rate of confirmation among the four types of vaccinations, using the chi-squared test.

(j) Summarize the main findings in your own words. Are the conclusions of the authors consistent with the evidence presented?

EXERCISES

1. The following 2 × 2 table shows the distribution of smokers among juniors and seniors in a suburban high school:

	SMOKERS	NONSMOKERS
Seniors	100	350
Juniors	80	520

(a) Compute the ORs and RRs and compare their magnitudes.
(b) Compute 95% CI for ORs and RRs.
(c) Formulate the null hypotheses and compute the chi-squared test.
(d) Compute the Phi correlation.
(e) Write a short narrative conclusion about your findings concerning the relationship between class level and smoking.

2. If the OR for a particular 2 × 2 table equals 1, the RRR must also be equal to 1. True or false? Demonstrate why your conclusion is correct.

3. If RR > 1, it follows that OR > RR; if RR < 1, it follows that OR < RR. True or false? Demonstrate why your conclusion is correct.

4. Suppose that the RR of falling in two nursing home populations is 3 times larger in home A than home B. In addition, we also know that the absolute risk of falling is 0.1 (or 10%) in home B. Is it true that the odds of falling in home A are more than 4 times larger than in home B?

5. You are given the following information: Two shipments of blood tests are tested for contamination. You randomly select 60 tests from Shipment A and 40 tests from Shipment B. Your test samples from A show that 10 are contaminated, and your test samples from B show that 30 are contaminated. Can we conclude with high certainty that Shipment B is more contaminated than Shipment A? Calculate the Pearson chi-squared test statistic and use the table in Appendix G to make a decision.

6. You are given the following data: In nursing home A, out of 100 residents, 10 develop pneumonia during the winter quarter (January–March). In nursing home B, 30 out of 120 residents develop pneumonia during the same period.
   (a) What is the RR of developing pneumonia in B over A?
   (b) What is the OR comparing the odds of pneumonia in the two nursing homes?
   (c) Why is OR > RR?
   (d) True or false? If Phi = 0.23 in a study sample, then the OR for the same two variables must be different from 1.

REFERENCES

Hjermstad, M. J., Fayers, P. M., Haugen, D. F., Augusto Caraceni, A., Hanks, G. W., Loge, J. H., . . . Kaasa, S. (2011). Studies comparing numerical rating scales, verbal rating scales, and visual analogue scales for assessment of pain intensity in adults: A systematic literature review. *Journal of Pain and Symptom Management, 41*(6), 1073–1093.

Stommel, M., & Wills, C. E. (2004). *Clinical research.* Philadelphia, PA: Lippincott Williams & Wilkins.

CHAPTER 17

Logistic Regression With One Independent Variable

ODDS, ODDS RATIOS, AND PROBABILITIES

In the last chapter, we discussed the odds ratio (OR) as a measure of association for 2×2 frequency tables. As it turns out, the OR is also a major component of the logistic regression model. The methods we used in the last chapter to predict binary outcomes such as dead or alive, diagnosed with heart disease or not, rehospitalized or not, are limited as they can at best accommodate a few categorical predictor variables. **Logistic regression** on the other hand allows us to employ information from multiple, categorical as well as continuous independent variables to predict a binary outcome.

As we discussed in the last chapter, an OR is a ratio of two odds, which themselves are ratios of two probabilities. More precisely, the odds are a ratio of the probability of an event occurring over the probability of the event not occurring, where $p + (1 - p)$ always equals 1. Thus we have:

$$odds = \frac{p}{1-p}$$

One can always convert the odds back into a probability, if we only know the odds:

$$p = \frac{odds}{1 + odds}$$

From this it follows that, as a general rule, $p \neq odds$. If we compare the odds of an event occurring in two different population groups, where p_1 is the probability of the event in one group and p_2 the probability of the same event in another group, we get the OR:

$$OR = \frac{odds_1}{odds_2} = \frac{\dfrac{p_1}{(1-p_1)}}{\dfrac{p_2}{(1-p_2)}} = \frac{p_1(1-p_2)}{p_2(1-p_1)}$$

Suppose the probability of developing arthritis among persons older than 70 years of age is .25 ($=p_1$) and the probability of developing arthritis among persons between the ages 50 and 70 is .1 ($=p_2$); then the *odds$_1$* of developing arthritis among 70+ old persons are equal to:

$$odds_1 = \frac{p_1}{(1-p_1)} = \frac{.25}{(1-.25)} = \frac{.25}{.75} = \frac{1}{3} = .333$$

The *odds$_2$* of developing arthritis during the younger age of 50 to 70 are equal to:

$$odds_2 = \frac{p_2}{(1-p_2)} = \frac{.1}{(1-.1)} = \frac{.1}{.9} = \frac{1}{9} = .111$$

This yields the following OR:

$$OR = \frac{odds_1}{odds_2} = \frac{\frac{.25}{.75}}{\frac{.1}{.9}} = \frac{.333}{.111} = 3$$

In words, the odds of developing arthritis in the older population (70+ years of age) are three times larger than in the younger population (50–70 years of age). Note again that, as a general rule, the OR $\neq$ RR. The relative risk (RR) in this example would be: RR $= p_1/p_2 =$ .25/.1 = 2.5. While it would be correct to say in this instance that older persons (70+) are *2.5 times more likely* to develop arthritis than younger persons (50–70), it would be *incorrect* to say, based on the OR being equal to 3, that older persons (70+) are *three times more likely* to develop arthritis than younger persons (50–70). Instead, we should say something like this: The odds of developing arthritis are three times larger in the older age group.[1]

There are several important observations about ORs that we need to keep in mind when using and interpreting them:

1. We use ORs to compare the odds of an event occurring in two different groups. Often it is arbitrary which group is in the numerator and which is in the denominator. For instance, we could have expressed the above relationship between the age groups and the odds of arthritis as follows: The odds of developing arthritis in the *younger* population (50–70 years of age) are only *one third the odds* in the *older* population (70+ years of age). The strength of the relationship between age and arthritis is the same, whether we express it as 3 times larger in group A compared to group B, or as 1/3 as large in group B compared to group A. Thus, which group is in the numerator or the denominator can be changed through recoding, which may take into account which description is easier to verbalize.

2. Odds ratios are *multiplicative*: As $OR = odds_1/odds_2$, it follows that $odds_2 = odds_1 \times OR$. For example, if the odds of a specific disease are 3 times

---

[1]Comment: The (mistaken) interpretation of ORs as ratios of probabilities is unfortunately all too common in the clinical research literature. As mentioned in Chapter 16, in the case of a rare disease/event, the OR does *approximate* the RR ratio. Still, it is important not to confuse OR and RR, because sometimes they can be quite different in magnitude.

larger among low-income people (say, family income <$20,000) than among middle-income people ($40,000–$80,000), $OR_1 = 3$, and the odds of the same disease are 2 times larger among middle-income than among high-income people (>$80,000): $OR_2 = 2$, then the odds among low-income people are 6 times larger than among high-income people: $OR_1 \times OR_2 = 3 \times 2 = 6$.

3. Odds ratios produce highly skewed distributions, which is a direct result of their mathematical properties: From the discussion in Chapter 16, we know that the "neutral value" for an OR, indicating no relationship between two variables, is equal to 1. At the upper end, the OR is unrestricted in size, but at the lower end, the OR is greater than zero. For instance, the odds of an event occurring in one group could be 10,000 times larger than in the comparison group, but the inverse of that ratio is 1/10,000. In short: $0 < OR < \infty$ (infinity).

THE LOGISTIC REGRESSION MODEL

Suppose we are interested in predicting a binary outcome like a low birth weight (LBW = <2500 g) baby versus a normal birth weight (2500+ g) baby among 400 live births drawn randomly from the rosters of several hospitals in a large city. One of the predictor variables we have information on is gestational age at birth. For the time being, we divide the gestational age into a simple binary predictor variable: Babies are either premature, that is, born before the 37th week ($X = 1$) or not premature ($X = 0$). Table 17.1 shows the distribution of cases displayed in a 2×2 frequency table.

From the discussion in Chapter 16, we already know how to analyze a table like this. Among the term babies we have 12 low-weight births and 215 normal-weight births; thus the *odds* of a low-weight birth among term babies are $12/215 = 0.0558$. Among premature babies, these *odds* are $71/102 = 0.6961$. The *OR* comparing premature to term babies thus is $OR = 0.6961/0.0558 = 12.475$. In words: The odds of a low-birth-weight baby are approximately 12.5 times larger among premature than among term babies.

Given these facts, we can now construct a *multiplicative* model, in which the odds of a low-weight birth among *premature* babies are expressed as the *odds of a low-weight birth among term babies* (=0.0558) *times the OR* (=12.475), which shows the difference in the odds between premature and term babies: $0.0558 \times 12.475 = 0.6961$. If we refer to the odds of a low-weight birth among the term babies as $odds_0$, as X is coded 0 for this group, and the odds of a low-weight birth among premature babies as $odds_1$, as $X = 1$ for this group, we can express the latter odds as follows: $odds_1 = odds_0 \times odds_1/odds_0 = odds_0 \times OR$. In short, we have expressed the odds of an event occurring in one group (here: the premature babies) as a function of some *base-odds* (here: the odds of the event among term babies) *times the OR* that compares the two groups.

TABLE 17.1 2 × 2 Table of Joint Distribution of Prematurity and Low Birth Weight

		BIRTH WEIGHT STATUS		ROW MARGINAL FREQUENCIES
		NORMAL (2500+ g)	LBW (<2500 g)	
Premature birth (<37 weeks)	No	215	12	227
	Yes	102	71	173
Column marginal frequencies		317	83	400

If we now take the natural logarithm of both sides of this equation and multiply the OR by X, which is the binary independent variable, coded 0 (term baby) or 1 (premature baby),[2] we get the basic logistic regression model:

$$Y = \ln(odds_1) = \ln(odds_0 \times OR) = \ln(odds_0) + \ln(OR)X$$

In the final step, we rewrite this equation, setting $\ln(odds_0) = b_0$ and $\ln(OR) = b_1$, and we get:

$$Y = \ln(odds) = \ln\left(\frac{p}{1-p}\right) = b_0 + b_1 X$$

On the left side of the logistic regression equation we have the dependent variable Y, which is further specified as the *log-odds* or the *natural logarithm of the odds*; on the right side we have the familiar linear regression model with one intercept/constant (b_0) term and one independent variable (X) and its associated regression coefficient (b_1). Compared to the linear regression model, the only new part in the logistic regression model is the *logit link function* $\ln(p/1-p)$.[3]

In order to see how we can use this model to predict a binary outcome, we will go back to the analysis of the 2×2 frequency table in Table 17.1. We already established that the odds of having an low birth weight baby among term births are: $odds_0 = 0.0558$; and as $b_0 = \ln(odds_0)$, it follows that $b_0 = \ln(0.0558) = -2.8860$. Furthermore, $b_1 = \ln(OR) = \ln(12.475) = 2.5237$. Substituting these values into the logistic regression equation, we get:

$$Y = \ln(odds) = \ln\left(\frac{p}{1-p}\right) = b_0 + b_1 X = -2.8860 + 2.5237X$$

As the independent variable X is binary, coded 1 for premature babies and 0 for term babies, the logistic regression equation for term babies ($X = 0$) simplifies to:

$$Y_0 = -2.8860 + 2.5237(0) = -2.8860$$

For premature babies, the equation becomes:

$$Y_1 = -2.8860 + 2.5237(1) = -0.3623$$

We stated earlier that the dependent variable Y in the logistic regression model refers to the *log-odds* of an event occurring, $\ln(odds) = \ln(p/1-p)$. To get back to the odds, $(p/1-p)$, we take the antilog, that is, we exponentiate both sides of the equation, and get the following equation:

$$e^Y = odds = \frac{p}{1-p} = e^{b_0 + b_1 X}$$

---

[2]For the following, some familiarity with logarithms is required to follow the argument. Appendix H contains an informal discussion of exponentiation and logarithms, which is enough to follow the discussion here.

[3]A link function specifies the mathematical transformation that links the linear predictor model to the outcome variable. So far we have encountered the *identity* link, in which the linear predictor model predicts the actual values of Y. Here we have the *logit* link, which means the linear equation predicts the log-odds of an event occurring: $\ln(p/(1-p))$. Both models belong to a large class of statistical models known as the *General Linear Model*.

In the example, the specific results for the term babies ($X = 0$) are:

$$e^{Y_0} = e^{-2.8860+2.5237(0)} = e^{-2.8860} \times e^{2.5237(0)} = e^{-2.8860} \times e^0 = e^{-2.8860} = 0.0558$$

For the premature babies ($X = 1$), we get the following results:

$$e^{Y_1} = e^{-2.8860+2.5237(1)} = e^{-2.8860} \times e^{2.5237(1)} = 0.0558 \times 12.475 = e^{-0.3623} = 0.6961$$

Now we can see that the logistic regression model can reproduce the odds and ORs in a 2×2 table. It is a *linear* regression model predicting the *log-odds* of an outcome event; it is a *multiplicative* model predicting the *odds* of an outcome event. The regression coefficient representing the intercept (b_0) gives us the value of the dependent variable $Y = \ln(odds)$, if all independent variables are set to zero. For the data in Table 17.1, the term b_0 represents the value of Y, if the birth is not premature, that is, $X_1 = 0$. (To recover the base-odds, we take the antilog of b_0: $e^{b0} = e^{-2.8860} = 0.0558$.) The regression coefficient associated with the independent variable (b_1) gives us the *change* in the dependent variable Y, which is the change in the *log-odds*, for each one-unit change in the independent variable X. In the current example with a binary independent variable, a change in X from 0 to 1 represents the difference between a term and a premature baby. That means it represents the *logarithm* of the OR associated with that change. Taking the antilog, we get the OR again: $e^{b1} = e^{2.5237} = 12.475$. In words: The odds of a low-birth-weight baby are approximately 12.5 times larger among premature than among term babies.

ESTIMATING THE LOGISTIC REGRESSION MODEL

Table 17.2 shows the results from fitting the logistic regression model to the data in Table 17.1. In many ways, this output looks very much like the output from a linear regression model with an identity link function.[4] We already know the point estimates of the regression coefficients, as we calculated the log-odds directly from the 2×2 frequency table. However, Table 17.2 also provides the standard errors of the estimates of the regression coefficients, the associated OR estimates, and other information concerning statistical inference from the study sample to the target population.

TABLE 17.2 Logistic Regression Model Predicting Low Birth Weight From Prematurity Status

```
Iteration 0:     log likelihood  =  -204.25019
Iteration 5:     log likelihood  =  -164.07955


Logistic regression                            Number of obs   =       400
                                               LR chi2(1)      =     80.34
                                               Prob > chi2     =    0.0000
Log likelihood = -164.07955                    Pseudo R2       =    0.1967
```

Birth weight	Coef.	Std. Err.	z	P>|z|	Odds Ratio	[95% Conf.Interv. of OR]	
premature	2.52344	0.33447	7.54	0.000	12.4747	6.47457	24.02262
_cons	-2.88573	0.29662	-9.73	0.000	0.0558	0.31207	0.99822

---

[4]With an identity link function, the dependent variable is simply the measured variable rather than transformation of it, as is the case with the logit link function.

Analogous to the simple linear regression model discussed in Chapter 10, we can use the information in Table 17.2 and write out the regression equation as follows:

$$\hat{Y} = -2.886 + 2.523X$$

$$(0.297) \quad (0.334)$$

As we did for the linear regression with the identity link function, we test the null hypotheses that the intercept term and the regression coefficient associated with the independent variable are equal to zero in the population from which the sample is drawn. Our test statistic, known as the Wald statistic, is also similar: We divide the estimated coefficient by its standard error, which, for larger samples, follows the normal distribution. In Table 17.2, the test statistic for the intercept is $z = -2.886/0.297 = -9.73$; for the regression coefficient associated with the independent variable (X), we have $z = 2.523/0.334 = 7.54$. For both coefficients, the null hypothesis asserts that the population parameter is equal to zero. As the z-values exceed the critical value of ±1.96 (for an α-level of 0.05) by a substantial margin, the coefficients are highly significant ($p < .0005$). We conclude that prematurity is a significant predictor of low birth weight.

As already mentioned, the regression coefficients estimate the changes in *log-odds* as a result of a one-unit change in the independent variable, but we can take the antilog to obtain the base-odds, $e^{b0} = e^{-2.88573} = 0.0558$, and the OR, $e^{b1} = e^{2.52344} = 12.471$. Through exponentiation, we also obtain the confidence limits associated with the odds and OR. For example, the confidence limits for the original regression coefficient associated with prematurity are: $2.52344 \pm 1.96 \times 0.33447$, with the lower limit being $2.52344 - 1.96 \times 0.33447 = 1.86788$ and the upper limit $2.52344 + 1.96 \times 0.33447 = 3.179$. Taking the antilog of both values yields the OR confidence limits of $e^{1.86788} = 6.47456$ and $e^{3.179} = 24.02275$, allowing for some rounding errors.

MAXIMUM LIKELIHOOD ESTIMATION

We presented the estimation results from the logistic regression model without commenting on how we arrive at these estimates. When we use the logistic regression model to estimate particular regression coefficients on the basis of sample data, we need a *criterion* to fit the model to the data. Recall that, for the linear regression model, we employed the least squares criterion to estimate the regression coefficients. That means, we choose the linear regression coefficients so as to minimize the squared deviations of the observed Y variable from the predicted $\hat{Y}$ values based on the regression model. With logistic regression models, we cannot use the least squares criterion, because it requires a continuous outcome variable to compute the necessary sums of squares (SSs) and variances. Instead, our new criterion is the **maximum likelihood** criterion. That is, we choose estimates for the regression coefficients b_0 and b_1 in such a way that we maximize the likelihood of the observed outcome. We will go back to the example of Table 17.1 to clarify this point.

Among the 400 babies, 83 were low birth weight babies. If these 400 babies are a random sample of a much larger target population of all births in a city's hospitals over the last 5 years, we may want to know the probability that a baby in this target population is a low birth weight baby. To answer this question, we need to be able to predict the likelihood of the observed sample outcome based on different assumptions about the true population parameters. A function that connects the sample outcome to the assumed population values or parameters is called a **likelihood function (L)**. As the outcome variable is binary and as it is reasonable to assume that the events producing a low birth weight baby in one case are independent of those in another case, we can use the binomial probability distribution to predict the probability that a birth is low weight versus normal weight. The general form of the **binomial likelihood distribution** is as follows:

$$L(\pi|p) = \Pi \frac{n!}{k!(n-k)!} \pi^k (1-\pi)^{n-k}$$

This expression looks complicated, but when broken down into its components, it is not that difficult to follow. Let us start with the left side of the equation: $L(\pi/p)$. This shorthand expression simply indicates that the equation is used to compute the likelihood L (or probability) of observing a given *sample* proportion p of the binary variable for different (assumed) values of the population parameters, which in this case are the population proportions or probabilities π. On the right side of the equation we have the product operator Π ("pi"),[5] the symbol for the sample size, n, and for the number of cases in the sample that show the outcome in question, k. For the data in Table 17.1, we have: a sample size of $n = 400$, of which $k = 83$ births resulted in low birth weight babies. Thus, the sample proportion of low birth weight babies is: $p = k/n = 83/400 = 0.2075$. Now we use the binomial likelihood function to establish for which population values (π) the observed sample outcome of $p = k/n$ is most likely to occur:[6]

$$L(\pi|p) = \Pi \frac{400!}{83!317!} \pi^{83} (1-\pi)^{317}$$

As it turns out, if the population value π is equal to the sample proportion $p = k/n = 83/400 = .2075$, then we are most likely to observe the sample outcome of 83 low birth weight babies among 400 births. Put differently, for no other assumed π-value would a sample fraction of $83/400 = 0.2075$ be as likely to occur. Figure 17.1 shows a graph that depicts the likelihood function for different π-values in the range of $0.1 \le \pi \le 0.35$. If the true population proportion (π) is smaller than 0.1 or larger than 0.35, the likelihood of observing 83 low birth weight babies in a sample of 400 babies is essentially equal to zero; that is the reason why the graph has been cut off beyond those points on the horizontal axis. If we substitute 0.2075 for π in the equation, we see that, at its peak, $L = 400!/83!317! \, 0.2075^{83}(1 - 0.2075)^{317} = 0.049$, meaning for an assumed population value of $p = 0.2075$, there is a 4.9% probability of observing *exactly* 83 out of 400 low birth weight babies.

This same maximum likelihood estimation principle can be applied to the logistic regression model, except that we seek to maximize the likelihood function for the logistic model based on different values for b_0 and b_1: $L(\pi| b_0, b_1)$. In short, if we select our population parameters according to this principle, we get *maximum likelihood estimates* for these parameters.

The results in Table 17.2 already show the maximum likelihood estimates for the intercept: $b_0 = -2.88573$, and the regression coefficient: $b_1 = 2.52344$. Based on this, we can calculate the likelihoods for all four cells in Table 17.1:

1. First we can ask: What is the likelihood/probability of a low birth weight baby ($Y = 1$), if the baby is premature ($X = 1$)?

---

[5] Instead of summing terms, as does the summation operator Σx_k, Πx_k refers to the product of x_1 times x_2 times... x_k.
[6] Using a bit of calculus, we first convert the likelihood function into a log-likelihood: $\ln(L) = \ln((400!)/(83!317!)) + 83 \times \ln(p) + 317 \times \ln(1 - p)$ and take the derivative of that expression with respect to p: $\partial L/\partial p = 83/p - 317/1 - p$. Setting this derivative to zero yields the resulting estimate for which L is at a maximum: $\hat{p} = 83/400$.

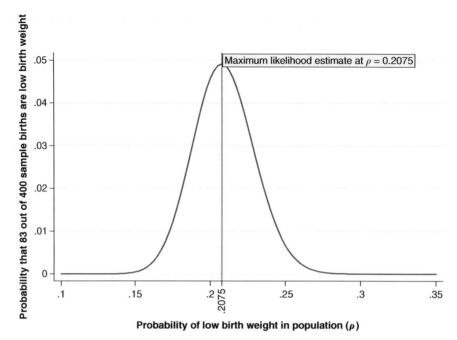

FIGURE 17.1 Likelihood Function Based on Binomial Distribution.

As, in general, $p = odds/(1 + odds)$ and the odds are estimated in the logistic model as $odds = e^{b_0 + b_1 X}$ we get:

$$\pi(X = 1) = \frac{e^{-2.88573 + 2.52344}}{1 + e^{-2.88573 + 2.52344}} = \frac{e^{-0.36229}}{1 + e^{-0.36229}} = \frac{0.69608}{1.69608} = 0.4104$$

2. For the second cell, we ask: What is the likelihood/probability of a low birth weight baby ($Y = 1$), if the baby is not premature ($X = 0$)?

$$\pi(X = 0) = \frac{e^{-2.88573}}{1 + e^{-2.88573}} = \frac{0.05581}{1.05581} = 0.05286$$

3. For the third cell, we ask: What is the likelihood/probability of a normal weight baby ($Y = 0$), if the baby is premature ($X = 1$)?

$$1 - \pi(X = 1) = 1 - \frac{e^{-2.88573 + 2.52344}}{1 + e^{-2.88573 + 2.52344}} = 1 - \frac{e^{-0.36229}}{1 + e^{-0.36229}} = 1 - \frac{0.69608}{1.69608} = 0.5896$$

4. For the fourth and last cell, we ask: What is the likelihood/probability of a normal weight baby ($Y = 0$), if the baby is not premature ($X = 0$)?

$$1 - \pi(X = 0) = 1 - \frac{e^{-2.88573}}{1 + e^{-2.88573}} = 1 - \frac{0.05581}{1.05581} = 0.94714$$

Now we have all the information to calculate the overall likelihood. For the 2×2 table we have four cells with different numbers of cases, n_i, but, within each cell, each case has the same estimated likelihood π_i or $1 - \pi_i$. Thus we have

n_1 = 71 cases in cell 1 (Y = 1, X = 1), each of which has the same probability of being a low birth weight baby (0.4104);

n_2 = 102 in cell 2 (Y = 0, X = 1), each of which has the same probability $(1 - \pi)$ of not being a low birth weight baby (0.5896);

n_3 = 12 in cell 3 (Y = 1, X = 0), each of which has the same probability of being a low birth weight baby (0.05286); and

n_4 = 215 in cell 4 (Y = 0, X = 0), each of which has the same probability $(1 - \pi)$ of not being a low birth weight baby (0.94714).

As the individual birth outcomes are assumed to be independent of each other, we can multiply the individual probabilities for each birth outcome and obtain the model likelihood based on the maximum likelihood estimates of the regression coefficients:

$$L_M = 0.4104^{71} \times 0.5896^{102} \times 0.05286^{12} \times 0.94714^{215}$$

This number is usually very small, close to zero. For that reason, and ease of mathematical manipulation, we usually compute the **log-likelihood**:

$$\ln(L_M) = 71 \times \ln(0.4104) + 102 \times \ln(0.5896) + 12 \times \ln(0.05286) + 215 \times \ln(0.94714)$$
$$= -164.07955$$

This log-likelihood estimate of -164.07955 is shown as part of the output in Table 17.2. In and of itself, it is not all that interesting, but it obtains meaning in the comparison to another log-likelihood. Table 17.2 also shows a log-likelihood value listed under "iteration zero." This is the *initial* likelihood for the so-called *null model*, in which all logistic regression coefficients are assumed to be zero (null hypothesis). If the logistic regression coefficient is equal to zero, the OR comparing premature to term babies is equal to one, which implies that both the odds and the probabilities of a low birth weight baby are the same for premature and term babies. If that null-hypothesis assumption is true, then the log-likelihood function would be based just on the fact that all babies share the same low birth weight risk π = 0.2075 and its complement, the probability of not being low birth weight, $1 - \pi$ = 0.7925. Overall there were 83 low birth weight babies and 317 normal weight babies; thus we can compute a simplified log-likelihood:

$$\ln(L_0) = 83 \times \ln(0.2075) + 317 \times \ln(0.7925) = -204.25019$$

In Table 17.2, this log-likelihood value is listed under "iteration zero." If we subtract the log-likelihood of the regression model (L_M) from the log-likelihood of the null model (L_0) and multiply the difference by (-2), we get a test statistic that is distributed like a chi-square distribution with degrees of freedom (df) equal to the difference in the number of parameters estimated in the null model and the regression model:

$$(-2) \times \ln(LR) = [\ln(L_0) - \ln(L_M)] \times (-2)$$

For the data in Table 17.1, we get: $-2 \times \ln(LR) = [-204.25019 - (-164.07955)] \times (-2) = 80.34$. The associated df equal $2 - 1 = 1$. The reason is that, in the null model, we set b_1 = 0, so that the constant b_0 remains as the only parameter to be estimated; in the regression model, we estimate both b_0 and b_1, and thus two parameters are estimated.

Table 17.2 shows the estimate for the *difference* between the two log-likelihoods times (−2) under the label "LR" or "likelihood ratio." As this ratio (or its log-transformation, which is also known as the *deviance*) compares the likelihood under the null hypothesis with no explanatory independent variables to the likelihood under the regression model with the maximum likelihood estimates for the regression coefficients, a statistically significant ($\alpha < 0.05$) difference would tell us that the independent variable or variables in the model *do* contribute to explaining variation in the outcome. Thus, in the output from the software shown in Table 17.2, you see an overall *p*-value associated with the deviance or LR test of $p < .0005$. Based on this test, we reject the null hypothesis that the independent variable does not contribute to explaining variance in the outcome. This multivariate LR test functions like the *f*-test in linear regression or analysis of variance: It tests whether at least one of the independent predictor variables improves the prediction compared to the null model.

Finally, Table 17.2 also displays a statistic by McFadden, called the Pseudo R-squared.[7] This statistic can be easily computed from the results in the table:

$$\text{Pseudo R}^2 = 1 - \frac{\ln(L_M)}{\ln(L_0)}$$

The fraction $\ln(L_M)/\ln(L_0)$ is simply a ratio of the log-likelihood for the regression model L_M over the null model L_0. The log-likelihood of the null model is based on a model that does not explain any variation in the outcome probabilities; it can be thought of as *conceptually* similar to the total (unexplained) SS in linear regression. If the regression model with the maximum likelihood estimates for the regression coefficients explains some of the variation in the outcome probabilities among different groups defined by the independent variable, then its likelihood must be larger than the likelihood of the null model: $L_M > L_0$. This implies that $\ln(L_M) < \ln(L_0)$ and that the ratio of $\ln(L_M)/\ln(L_0) < 1$, if $L_M > L_0$. In other words the McFadden statistic can be thought of as being similar to a proportional reduction in error variance: if more variation in outcome probabilities is explained by the model, $\ln(L_M)$ becomes smaller and the value of the Pseudo R² becomes larger. For the logistic regression model in Table 17.2, we have:

$$\text{Pseudo R}^2 = 1 - \frac{\ln(L_M)}{\ln(L_0)} = 1 - \frac{-164.07955}{-204.25019} = 0.1967$$

Using the language borrowed from linear models with continuous outcome variables, we may say, somewhat loosely, that this logistic regression model accounts for almost 20% in unexplained variation of the outcome variable.

LOGISTIC REGRESSION MODEL WITH A CONTINUOUS INDEPENDENT VARIABLE

The reader may wonder why we used a complicated model like the logistic regression model to compare just the odds or probabilities of a binary outcome in two groups. The analysis of a 2 × 2 frequency table is clearly easier using the straightforward methods of the last chapter. However, the great value of the logistic regression model is that it can be used for estimating the relationship between a binary outcome and any combination of continuous and categorical

---

[7]There are several different Pseudo R-squared statistics, but we will confine the discussion to this commonly encountered statistic.

TABLE 17.3 Logistic Regression Model Predicting Low Birth Weight From Weeks of Gestation

```
Iteration 0:     log likelihood  =  -204.25019
Iteration 5:     log likelihood  =  -110.63846


Logistic regression                        Number of obs =      400
                                           LR chi2(1)    =   187.22
                                           Prob > chi2   =   0.0000
Log likelihood = -110.63846                Pseudo R2     =   0.4583
```

Birth weight	Coef.	Std. Err.	z	P>|z|	Odds Ratio	[95% Conf.Interv. of OR]	
gestation(t)	-0.32740	0.03403	-9.62	0.000	0.72080	0.67428	0.77052
_cons	2.01365	0.31848	6.32	0.000	7.49061	4.01246	13.98319

predictor variables, just as the linear regression model extends beyond the two-group comparison of the *t*-test. For the remainder of this chapter, we expand the logistic regression model to include just a single *continuous* independent variable. In Table 17.2, we applied the logistic regression model to the data in Table 17.1, which divided the predictor variable into a single dichotomy: premature versus term babies. However, if we have actual data on gestational weeks, we can ask how the odds of having a low birth weight baby change *for each additional week* of gestation. Table 17.3 shows the results from a regression model, in which X = weeks of gestation minus 21. The actual range of gestation is 21 to 44 weeks, but using the original variable would result in an intercept term that estimates the log-odds of a low birth weight baby, if gestation equals zero weeks.

That is obviously a meaningless estimate. By subtracting 21 weeks from the actual gestation variable, the value zero on the transformed gestation variable is equivalent to the lowest observed gestational week of 21. Thus, the intercept term becomes interpretable: Its antilog estimates the odds of a low birth weight baby, if a baby is born after 21 weeks of gestation.

The output in Table 17.3 is formally similar to that in Table 17.2, but the interpretation of the regression coefficient differs slightly, as the predictor variable is continuous (measured in weeks). As before, we can write the regression equation based on the information in Table 17.3 as follows:

$$\hat{Y} = 2.014 - 0.3274X$$

$$(0.318)\ (0.034)$$

Again we divide the coefficients by their respective standard errors to obtain the z-scores, which are the basis for the tests of the null hypotheses that a coefficient does not differ from zero in the population from which the sample is drawn.[8] Thus we have the test for the intercept coefficient, 2.01365/0.31848 = 6.32, and the regression coefficient associated with the independent variable, -0.32740/0.03403= -9.62. Both far exceed the critical value of ±1.96, at which the α-level = 0.05, leading us to conclude that both coefficients differ from zero. To interpret the results, it is easier to exponentiate the whole equation, which shows us how the *odds* of having a low birth weight baby *change* based on different levels of the independent predictor variable, here indicating weeks of gestation after week 21.

---

[8]The Wald Test is analogous to the *t*-test of regression coefficients in linear models.

Here is the antilog form of the regression equation, using the information in Table 17.3:

$$e^{\hat{Y}} = \frac{p}{1-p} = e^{b_0 + b_1 X} = e^{b_0} \times e^{b_1 X} = baseodds \times OR^X = 7.4906 \times 0.7208^X$$

We already showed that the original regression coefficients, predicting the log-odds of the outcome variable, differ significantly from zero. This implies that, in the antilog form of the equation, the base-odds and the OR differ significantly from one. This is also confirmed by the 95% confidence intervals (CIs) for e^{b_0} and e^{b_1}, neither of which contains the value of one. The interpretation of the equation is straightforward: If we substitute the value zero for X, the equation simplifies to $p/(1-p) = 7.4906 \times 0.7208^0 = 7.4906 \times 1 = 7.4906$.[9] As we employed a transformed gestation variable, subtracting 21 weeks from the original gestation variable, setting $X = 0$ is equivalent to looking at babies born after 21 weeks of pregnancy. Our equation predicts that the odds of having a low birth weight baby in that gestation group are almost 7.5 to 1. Now we assign $X = 1$, which refers to babies who have been born after 22 weeks of gestation. that is, one week after the baseline week. It follows that the predicted odds of having a low birth weight baby fall to $7.4906 \times 0.7208 = 5.3992$; for babies born after 23 weeks of gestation, we have $7.4906 \times 0.7208^2 = 3.8918$, and so forth. Consequently, the interpretation of the OR = 0.7208 is that, *for each additional week of gestation, the odds of having a low birth weight baby fall by about 28%* $(1 - 0.7208 = 0.2792)$.[10]

This logistic regression model with a continuous gestation variable as predictor is superior to the previous binary predictor of premature versus term babies, as it can explain more variation in the odds of low birth weight births. This is indicated both by the larger value of McFadden's Pseudo R^2 statistic (0.4583 in Table 17.3 versus 0.1967 in Table 17.2) and the larger value of the deviance statistic, which is a measure of the difference between the two log-likelihoods: 187.22 in Table 17.3 versus 80.34 in Table 17.2.

JUDGING THE ASSUMPTIONS OF THE LOGISTIC REGRESSION MODEL

As with all statistical models, we need to assess how well the model fits the data. In the discussion of linear regression models, we examined the behavior of individual error terms, which represent the deviations of observed values from predicted values, to obtain clues about the fit of the model. Error terms of the logistic model do not follow a normal distribution, but they follow the binomial distribution. The reason is obvious: The dependent outcome variable either takes on the value 1 (presence of the event or condition to be predicted) or the value 0 (absence of the event or condition to be predicted). However, if we group the data based on categories of the continuous independent variable in question, we can examine whether certain assumptions of the model are borne out by the data or whether we need to modify the model for a better fit. For instance, the logistic regression model is a *linear* model in the log-odds:

$$Y = \ln\left(odds\right) = \ln\left(\frac{p}{1-p}\right) = b_0 + b_1 X$$

It is important to realize that, just like the linear regression model assumes a linear relationship between the outcome variable Y and the continuous predictor variables (Xs), so does the logistic regression model, except that the dependent variable takes on the form of the logit

---

[9]Recall that any number raised to the power of zero equals one; see Appendix H.
[10]Alternatively, you could say that for each additional week of gestation the odds of having a low birth weight baby are only 72% as large as for babies born a week earlier, but that is a cumbersome way of putting it.

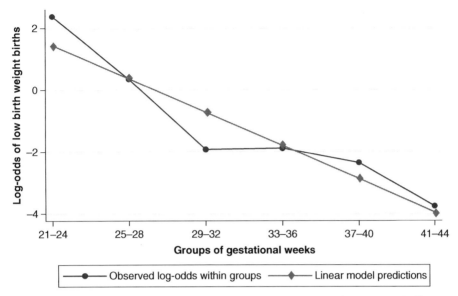

FIGURE 17.2 Linear Predictions of Log-Odds Versus Observed Log-Odds: Logistic Regression Models With Linear Versus Categorical Predictors.

link function, which *assumes* that the log-odds change by a constant amount (b_1) for each unit increase in the independent variable X. We can test this assumption by comparing the log-odds predicted in the linear model to the log-odds observed within the categories of the independent variable without imposing the linear constraint (Figure 17.2).

Figure 17.2 compares the results from two logistic regression models: a simple logistic regression model assuming a linear relationship between gestational weeks (X) and the log-odds of low birth weight births: $Y = \ln(odds) = \ln(p/1 - p) = b_0 + b_1X$. However, compared to the earlier model, the independent variable "gestational weeks" has been combined into 6 groups, 21 to 14 weeks, 25 to 28 weeks, and so forth, because we need sufficient numbers of cases within each category of the independent variable in order to compute odds and log-odds. In the graph of Figure 17.1, the linear model is represented by the gray line. The second logistic regression model employed five dummy-coded independent variables,[11] so that the log-odds within each of the six categories were not constrained to lie on a straight line. The unconstrained log-odds are connected by black lines in Figure 17.2. On the face of it, there seems to be some nonlinearity in the log-odds of low birth weight births. In fact, we can test whether the unconstrained model with the independent, dummy-coded, categorical variables is a better predictor than the linearly constrained model. For this test, we can use the LR test: If we compare the deviance of the categorical, that is, linearly unconstrained model (182.12) to the deviance of the linearly constrained model (165.26), we obtain a new deviance (or log-LR) statistic (16.86) with 4 df. (The first model contains five categorical predictors plus the intercept requiring the prediction of six parameters; the second model contains the intercept term and one linear regression coefficient; thus df $= 6 - 2 = 4$.) The p-value associated with the chi-squared statistic of 16.86 and 4 df is $p < .002$. Thus we conclude that the logistic regression model with linear predictors of the log-odds is not fully consistent with the data.[12]

---

[11]See Chapter 10 for a more detailed discussion of dummy codes.
[12]Similar to the problem in Chapter 10, a polynomial regression model of third degree, $Y = \ln(odds) = b_0 + b_1X + b_1X^2 + b_1X^3$, does provide a better model fit, as is indicated by a nonsignificant ($p > .146$) LR test comparing the polynomial model to the categorical predictor model.

As a reader of research reports that employ the logistic regression model, you may not be interested in all the technical details of fitting such models, but you should be aware that the problem of checking the assumptions of a model is part and parcel of good data analysis practice. Readers of research reports in professional journals should expect some assurance in the methods section of an article that the appropriate tests have been run. Box 17.1 provides a summary of the assumptions underlying the use of the logistic regression model.

BOX 17.1	ASSUMPTIONS OF LOGISTIC REGRESSION MODEL

- Binary outcome variable
- Linearity of relation between the logarithm of the dependent odds and independent (interval/ratio-level) variable(s)
- Independence of individual observations (uncorrelated error terms)
- Binomial distribution of error terms, that is, binomially distributed variables *within* the categories defined by the independent variable
- Randomly drawn study sample for population inferences

SUMMARY

In this chapter, we have introduced the logistic regression model, which has become a "popular" model for analyzing data with binary outcome variables (e.g., Forsman, Rudman, Gustavsson, Ehrenberg, & Wallin, 2012; Gaugler, Mittelman, Hepburn, & Newcomer, 2010; Shahin et al., 2010). Its strength lies in the fact that the antilog forms of the estimated logistic regression coefficients can be readily interpreted in terms of odds and ORs. The logistic model presents a straightforward extension of the analysis of 2 × 2 frequency tables, while the basic statistical measures of odds and ORs are also the basic building blocks for the analysis of case-control studies.

So far, we have dealt only with logistic models containing a single independent variable. In the next chapter, we turn to the multiple logistic regression model as well as a few other extensions, such as multinomial and ordinal logit regression models.

	LITERATURE APPLICATION

Read: Shahin, E. S. M., Meijers, .J. M. M., Schols, J. M. G. A., Tannen, A., Halfens, R. J., & Dassen, T. (2010). The relationship between malnutrition parameters and pressure ulcers in hospitals and nursing homes. *Nutrition, 26*(9), 886–889.

(a) Provide a very brief (three to four sentences) summary of what this study is about.

(b) Define the target population to which the statistical analysis can be generalized. What were the eligibility and exclusion criteria for study participants? Is the study sample a random sample of the target population?

(c) Provide a clear definition of the outcome/dependent variable and a short description of the instrument used to measure it.

(d) Provide a clear definition of all independent/predictor variables and a short description of the instruments used to measure them.

(e) In Tables 1 and 2 of the article, the authors compare the prevalence of "poor nutritional intake" among patients who experience pressure ulcers and those who did not. Using the figures provided in the tables, reconstruct the ORs predicting the odds of having a pressure ulcer based on poor nutritional intake or its absence. Is the relationship between nutritional intake and pressure ulcers greater or smaller among hospital or nursing home patients/residents?

(f) In Tables 3 and 4 of the article, the authors report the results from (multiple) logistic regression models. Show how the 95% CIs for the ORs are obtained from the logistic regression coefficients and the standard errors.

(g) Summarize the main findings in your own words. Are the conclusions of the authors consistent with the evidence presented?

EXERCISES

1. Researchers of a study conducted in several hundred hospitals report the results of a logistic regression model designed to predict the occurrence of urinary tract infections (UTIs), Y, based on the patient/nurse staffing ratio X:

$$\hat{Y} = -4.595 + 0.2864X$$

$$(0.238) \quad (0.031)$$

where $\hat{Y}$ refers to the predicted log-odds of UTI occurrence in a hospital and X equals the number of patients per RN, ranging from a minimum of 1.5 to 9.

(a) What are the odds of a UTI if the patient–nurse ratio equals 2?
(b) What are the odds of a UTI if the patient–nurse ratio equals 8?
(c) Are the intercept and slope coefficients statistically significant at the 0.05 level?
(d) What is the 95% CI for the OR predicting the change in UTI?
(e) In your own words: What is the meaning of the intercept term? Is it interpretable?

2. A survey of 320 adults finds that 120 respondents are smokers ($X = 1$) and 200 are nonsmokers ($X = 0$). The survey respondents were asked whether they experienced pneumonia during the 12 months prior to the interview. Using a logistic regression model, analysts obtain the following estimates for the equation predicting the log-odds of pneumonia:

$$\hat{Y} = -3.6889 + 1.6094X$$

$$(0.1993) \quad (0.0422)$$

(a) What are the odds of nonsmokers experiencing pneumonia?
(b) What are the odds of smokers experiencing pneumonia?
(c) How many nonsmokers experienced pneumonia?
(d) How many smokers experienced pneumonia?

3. In a study of over 2,000 primary care patients, researchers report on a logistic regression model, which contains estimates to predict the log-odds of coronary heart disease (CHD) as follows:

$$\hat{Y} = \ln(p/(1 - p)) = -2.3 + 0.47 \, (\text{HTN}) + 0.01 \, (\text{AGE}),$$

where HTN (hypertension) is coded 0 = person has no HTN, 1 = person has HTN, and AGE is coded in years.

What are the odds that a 50-year old adult with HTN has CHD (all regression coefficients are statistically significant)?

4. Suppose you have a sample of 100 obese and 100 normal weight adults. Among the normal weight adults, the odds of having diabetes are 4/96. The logistic regression equation that predicts the log-odds of diabetes (Y) equals: $Y = \ln(p/(1 - p)) = -3.178 + 1.792X$, where $X = 0$ if the adult has normal weight and $X = 1$ if the adult is obese. How many obese adults in this study sample have diabetes?

5. The following table shows how many men (among 1,000 men) and how many women (among 1,000 women) are involved in car accidents per year. Write out the logistic regression equation, including the estimates of the regression coefficients, which reflects these facts.

	INVOLVED IN CAR ACCIDENTS		
	YES = 1	NO = 0	
Male = 0	40	960	1000
Female =1	20	980	1000
Total	60	1940	2000

REFERENCES

Forsman, H., Rudman, A., Gustavsson, P., Ehrenberg, A., & Wallin, L. (2012). Nurses' research utilization two years after graduation—A national survey of associated individual, organizational, and educational factors. *Implementation Science*, 7, 46.

Gaugler, J. E., Mittelman, M. S., Hepburn, K., & Newcomer, R. (2010). Clinically significant changes in burden and depression among dementia caregivers following nursing home admission. *BMC Medicine*, 8, 85.

Shahin, E. S. M., Meijers, J. M. M., Schols, J. M. G. A., Tannen, A., Halfens, R. J., & Dassen, T. (2010). The relationship between malnutrition parameters and pressure ulcers in hospitals and nursing homes. *Nutrition*, 26(9), 886–889.

CHAPTER 18

Logistic Regression Models With Multiple Predictors

MULTIPLE LOGISTIC REGRESSION

In the last chapter, we introduced the logistic regression model to predict the odds of an event occurring based on either a binary or a single continuous predictor variable.

The general form of the multiple linear regression model looks very much like the general form of the linear regression model with the identity link function.[1] The only difference is that the link function for the logistic model is the logit or the log-odds of the event occurring:

$$Y = \ln(odds) = \ln\left(\frac{p}{1-p}\right) = b_0 + b_1 X_1 + b_2 X_2 + b_3 X_3 + \cdots + b_k X_k$$

where $Y = \ln(p/1-p)$ refers to the dependent variable, b_0 is the intercept (or "constant") in the equation, and the $b_k X_k$ terms refer to k independent variables, X_k, multiplied by their respective regression coefficients, b_k.

Compared to the simple logistic regression models with one independent variable, the multiple logistic regression model contains two or more predictor variables. As with all multiple regression models, this leads to the additional complications of confounding and interaction effects.[2]

Before we address the problems of confounding and interaction effects in the logistic model, we will first take a look at the output from a multiple logistic regression model and explain how to interpret its coefficients.

EMPIRICAL EXAMPLE OF A MULTIPLE LOGISTIC REGRESSION ANALYSIS

Table 18.1 shows the output from a logistic regression model that predicts low birth weight based on the marital status and formal education of the mother. The table contains the estimates of the logistic regression coefficients as well as the associated odds and odds ratios (ORs).

---

[1]With the identity link function, the dependent variable is equal to the measured scores; the logit link function represents a logarithmic transformation of the original scores.

[2]See the discussion in Chapter 12.

TABLE 18.1 Logistic Regression Model Predicting Low Birth Weight From Marital Status and Years of Formal Education

```
Logistic Regression model with maritalstat (1=married, 0=not married) and years of education
(8-17) as predictors

Iteration 0:   log likelihood = -204.25019

Logistic regression                                     Number of obs  =      400
                                                        LR chi2(2)     =    25.67
                                                        Prob > chi2    =   0.0000
Log likelihood = -191.41563                             Pseudo R2      =   0.0628

------------------------------------------------------------------------------------
Birth weight |   Coef.    Std. Err.    z     P>|z|   Odds Ratio   [95% Conf. Interv. of OR]
-------------+----------------------------------------------------------------------
  maritalstat |  -.58636   .28275    -2.07   0.038     .55635      .31964      .96834
    educatyrs |  -.34871   .07406    -4.71   0.000     .70560      .61026      .81582
        _cons |  3.16751   .92827     3.41   0.001   23.74828     3.85011    146.48297
------------------------------------------------------------------------------------
```

Employing this information, we can write the logistic regression equation with the standard errors as follows:

Estimated equation[3]: $\hat{Y} = 3.168 - 0.586X_1 - 0.349X_2$

Standard error of coefficients: (0.928) (0.283) (0.074)

p-values: $\leq.038$ $\leq.001$ $\leq.001$

Summary statistics: log-likelihood ratio (2 df): 25.67; $p < .00005$; Pseudo $R^2 = 0.628$

Antilog form of equation: $e^{\hat{Y}} = (23.748)\,(0.556)^{X_1}\,(0.706)^{X_2}$

In many research reports published in nursing and medical journals, only the ORs, their associated p-values, or the 95% confidence intervals (CIs) are reported. Often the information about the log-likelihood ratio (LR) is not provided to the reader, even though it is essential for judging whether the equation as a whole has any predictive power.[4] As is often the case in multiple regression models, the constant or intercept has no readily interpretable meaning, but that does not mean we should skip the base-odds, which are the antilog of the intercept term, in tables reporting the OR. As we will see, there is value in having this information for predictive purposes.

Before we interpret the estimates of the logistic regression coefficients, we begin by noticing that the log-LR, which equals *twice* the difference between the log-likelihood of the estimated regression model minus that of the null model, $2 \times [(-191.41563) - (-204.25019)] = 25.67$, is statistically significant: $p < .00005$. Thus we conclude that the model as a whole does predict to some extent which babies are born with a low birth weight, but the predictive power is moderate (Pseudo $R^2 = 0.063$). The intercept term, 3.168 for the log-odds, or 23.748 for the base-odds, is not interpretable, because it represents the estimate of $\hat{Y}$, or $e^{\hat{Y}}$, when the

---

[3] All coefficients in the book have been rounded to the third decimal.
[4] By contrast, f-tests for linear regression models are usually reported in applied journal articles.

two independent variables are set to zero. For the binary marital status variable, zero denotes unmarried subjects, but zero for the education variable would literally refer to persons with no formal education at all, even though the data set only includes subjects with exposure to formal education ranging from 8 to 17 years. As there are no unmarried subjects without any formal education in the data set, we cannot use these estimates to extrapolate to such persons, as they are not represented at all in the data. However, while the estimate of the base-odds (23.748) is suspect and should not be interpreted to mean that unmarried mothers with no education face a 96% probability of having a low birth weight baby,[5] we can make predictions for women with educational attainments within the observed range of 8 to 17 years. For instance, an unmarried woman with 8 years of formal education faces the following odds of giving birth to a low-weight baby: $e^{\hat{y}} = (23.748)(0.556)^0(0.706)^8 = (23.748)(0.0617) = 1.4657$, which translates into a 0.59 probability. By contrast, a married woman with 17 years of education would face a 3.4% probability: $e^{\hat{y}} = (23.748)(0.556)^1(0.706)^{17} = (23.748)(0.556)(0.00269) = .0355$; thus

$$p = \frac{0.0355}{1.0355} = .0343$$

CONFOUNDING IN MULTIPLE LOGISTIC REGRESSION MODELS

Just as with multiple linear regression models applied to observational data, confounding is also an issue in multiple logistic regression models. Only if all the independent variables are uncorrelated would confounding be absent, but that rarely happens in observational studies. For the current data, a comparison of the output in Tables 18.1 and 18.2 shows how the estimates of the logistic regression coefficients and their associated ORs are affected by confounding. Notice first (at the bottom of the table) that marital status and educational attainment are negatively correlated, meaning that in this data set, married mothers have a somewhat lower average educational attainment than single mothers, primarily because of relatively few married mothers with college degrees among these women. As a consequence, the association between marital status and the odds of giving birth to a low-weight baby is "suppressed." If you compare the magnitudes of the logistic regression coefficients and their associated ORs in Tables 18.1 and 18.2, you see that the coefficients for the years-of-education variable change little between the simple model with only the education variable as predictor ($b = -0.316$) and the model with both education and marital status as predictor ($b = -0.349$). On the other hand, the change in the regression coefficient for the marital status variable is substantial: In the bivariate model with only marital status as predictor (Table 18.2) we do not see any significant effect ($p > .314$) with an estimate of the OR of 0.77 and a CI including one. In the multiple regression model of Table 18.1, the OR estimate is 0.56 ($p \leq .038$) and the 95% CI ranges from 0.32 to 0.97. Thus, *after controlling for years of education*, we see that married women are less likely to have low-weight births.[6] This effect was obscured in the simple regression model, because married women in this study had less education than the unmarried women, and less education is associated with a greater risk of low-weight births.

---

[5] $p = \dfrac{odds}{1 + odds} = \dfrac{23.748}{1 + 23.748} = 0.9596.$

[6] The careful reader of the last chapter may wonder why we used the phrase "less likely" here after warning before that an OR should not be confused with an RRR. That still remains the case, but it is legitimate to say "less likely" as long as we do not put the specific OR figure to this statement, because it is the case that whenever OR < 1, RR also must be less than 1.

TABLE 18.2 Logistic Regression Model Predicting Low Birth Weight From Marital Status and Years of Formal Education Separately

Logistic Regression model with maritalstat (1=married, 0=not married) and years of education (8–17) as predictors

Logistic regression							
					Number of obs	=	400
					LR chi2(1)	=	1.00
					Prob > chi2	=	0.3179
Log likelihood = –203.75133					Pseudo R2	=	0.0024

bwt2	Coef.	Std. Err.	z	P>|z|	Odds Ratio	[95% Conf. Interv. of OR]	
maritalstat	–.26558	.26366	–1.01	0.314	.76676	.45733	1.28555
_cons	–1.15643	.21668	–5.34	0.000		–1.58112	–.73175

Iteration 0:   log likelihood = –204.25019

Logistic regression							
					Number of obs	=	400
					LR chi2(1)	=	21.45
					Prob > chi2	=	0.0000
Log likelihood = –193.52757					Pseudo R2	=	0.0525

bwt2	Coef.	Std. Err.	z	P>|z|	Odds Ratio	[95% Conf. Interv. of OR]	
educatyrs	–.31560	.07123	–4.43	0.000	.72935	.63431	.83863
_cons	2.37153	.82770	2.87	0.004	10.71377	2.11539	54.26188

. corr maritalstat educ3, sig

	marita~t	educat~s
maritalstat	1.0000	
educatyrs	–0.2111	1.0000
	(0.0000)	

In principle, confounding is always an issue, when independent predictor variables are correlated. If confounding exists, we need to "control for" the confounding effect, because it *obscures* the "true" effect of or "true" association involving the variable of interest. In our example, statistically controlling for the effect of mothers' education means that we must get an estimate of the strength of the relationship between the mother's marital status and the odds of a low-weight birth that is unaffected by the mother's education. This estimate is given by the OR in the multiple logistic regression model as OR = 0.556 (Table 18.1). Its meaning is straightforward: Suppose we computed the ORs within each of the subsamples formed by the years of educational achievement; for instance, there are mothers with 8, 9, … 16 years of schooling, and we compute the OR between marital status and low-weight births within each of these educational achievement groups. As mothers *within* these groups share the *same* educational attainment, these ORs are not affected by difference in educational attainment.

Thus, all we need in the end is to compute a *weighted average of these within-group ORs*, weighted that is by the number of cases within each group. This weighted average or pooled summary OR is the *adjusted* OR we seek: It reflects the average association of marital status with the odds of low-weight births, independent, or net of, educational attainment.

INTERACTIONS IN MULTIPLE LOGISTIC REGRESSION MODELS

Whenever we have more than one independent predictor in a regression model, we must also test for interaction effects.[7] In order to show how to interpret an interaction effect within the context of a multiple logistic regression model, we expand the model in Table 18.1 and add a binary variable for smoking status (1 = smoker, 0 = nonsmoker) as well as an interaction variable involving smoking status and years of educational attainment, as shown in Table 18.3.

TABLE 18.3 Logistic Regression Model Predicting Low Birth Weight From Marital Status, Years of Formal Education, Smoking Status, and the Interaction of Smoking × Formal Education

```
Logistic Regression model with maritalstat(1=married, 0=not married), years of education
(8-17), smoking status(1=smoker, 0=non-smoker) and the interaction of smoking status &
years of education as predictors

Log likelihood = -191.41563                          Pseudo R2  = 0.0628

Iteration 0:      log likelihood = -204.25019

Logistic regression                                  Number of obs  =    400
                                                     LR chi2(4)     =  33.73
                                                     Prob > chi2    = 0.0000
Log likelihood = -187.38479                          Pseudo R2      = 0.0826

------------------------------------------------------------------------------
Birth weight |   Coef.   Std. Err.    z    P>|z|  Odds Ratio  [95% Conf. Interv. of OR]
-------------+----------------------------------------------------------------
 maritalstat |  -.66527   .28716   -2.32  0.021    .51413     .29285      .90262
    educatyrs |  -.41334   .08522   -4.85  0.000    .66144     .55969      .78168
      smoker |  -3.62825  1.76174  -2.06  0.039    .02656     .00084      .83921
 I:smoker-edu |   .20617   .08773    2.35  0.019   1.22896    1.03481     1.45954
        _cons |  4.62006  1.19381    3.87  0.000  101.50012   9.77856   1053.55728
------------------------------------------------------------------------------

. lrtest Table 18.1 model vs. Table 18.3 model, stats

Likelihood-ratio test              LR chi2(2) = 8.0617
(Assumption: models are nested)    Prob > chi2 = 0.0178
----------------------------------------------------------
    Model |  Obs    ll(null)   ll(model)   df
----------+-----------------------------------------------
 basemodel |  400  -204.2502  -191.4156    3
  newmodel |  400  -204.2502  -187.3848    5
----------------------------------------------------------
```

[7]Other names for "interaction effects" in the health care literature are "effect modifiers" (epidemiology) or "moderator variables" (social science and nursing research).

First, we compare this expanded model to the simpler one in Table 18.1 and ask whether the addition of two new predictors (smoking status and its interaction with years of education) improves our ability to predict the odds of a mother having a low-weight baby. Comparing the new log-likelihood in Table 18.3 (-187.38479) to the one for the model in Table 18.1 (-191.41563) gives us the basic for the LR with 2 df,[8] which is our multivariate test statistic: $2 \times [(-187.38479) - (-191.41563)] = 8.06168$. The p-value associated with this test is $p \leq .0178$ leading us to reject the null hypothesis that the new variables do not add any predictive power. In addition, we see that McFadden's Pseudo R^2 is larger in the new model, increasing from 0.0628 to 0.0826.

In order to interpret the interaction effect depicted in the model correctly, we first go back to the logistic model with linear predictors of the log-odds of the outcome. The interaction in this model is interpreted in the same way as an interaction in a linear regression model with an identity link:

Estimated equation: $\hat{Y} = 4.620 - 0.665X_1 - 0.413X_2 - 3.628X_3 + 0.206X_4$

Standard error of coefficients: (1.194) (0.287)   (0.085)   (1.762)   (0.088)

p-values: $\leq.001$ $\leq.021$ $\leq.001$ $\leq.039$ $\leq.019$

Summary statistics: log-LR (4 df): 33.73; $p < .00005$; Pseudo $R^2 = 0.826$

Antilog form of equation: $e^{\hat{Y}} = (101.5)(0.514)^{X_1}(0.661)^{X_2}(0.027)^{X_3}(1.229)^{X_4}$

In this model, X_1 refers to the binary marital status variable, X_2 refers to the continuous years of education variable, X_3 refers to the binary smoking status variable, and X_4 is the multiplicative interaction term involving education and smoking: $X_4 = X_2 \times X_3$. As the interaction term involves the binary smoking status variable (X_3), it is easy to construct separate equations for smokers ($X_3 = 1$) and nonsmokers ($X_3 = 0$):

Nonsmokers: $\hat{Y} = 4.620 - 0.665X_1 - 0.413X_2 - 3.628(0) + 0.206(0)$

$\hat{Y} = 4.620 - 0.665X_1 - 0.413X_2$

Antilog version of nonsmoker equation: $e^{\hat{Y}} = (101.5)(0.514)^{X_1}(0.661)^{X_2}$

Smokers: $\hat{Y} = 4.620 - 0.665X_1 - 0.413X_2 - 3.628(1) + 0.206(X_2)$

$\hat{Y} = (4.620 - 3.628) - 0.665X_1 - (0.413 - 0.206)X_2$

$\hat{Y} = 0.992 - 0.665X_1 - 0.207X_2$

Antilog version of smoker equation: $e^{\hat{Y}} = (2.697)(0.514)^{X_1}(0.813)^{X_2}$

Figure 18.1 presents a graph depicting the interaction term between years of education and mothers' smoking status. The graph shows that the odds of having a low birth weight baby are quite low for all nonsmoking mothers, even though additional years of education is associated with a slight decline in these odds. By contrast, smoking mothers with 8 years of education have very high odds of giving birth to a low-weight baby, but these odds rapidly decline with additional years of education, until they almost come down to the levels experienced by nonsmoking mothers. While the effect is linear at the level of log-odds, the decline in odds is exponential. As always, the existence of such an interaction means that the effect of one

---

[8]The LR test has 2 degrees of freedom (df), as we added two parameter estimates to the model.

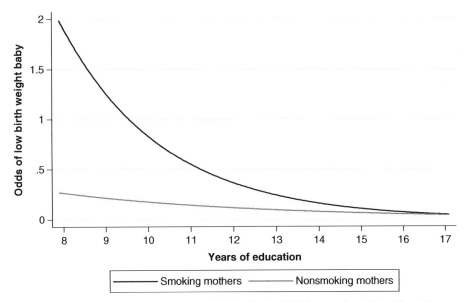

FIGURE 18.1 Changing Odds of Low Birth Weight Baby With Increasing Education: Comparison of Married Smokers and Married Nonsmokers.

variable (here: mothers' education) differs, that is, has differential effects, depending on the level of another variable (here: smoking status).[9]

MODEL FIT

As always, we must ask whether the statistical model we employed fits the data at hand. While the log-LR in Table 18.3 tells us that the model has some predictive power, and the Pseudo R^2 tells us that the predictive power is quite modest, we also need to consider whether the data show patterns that are inconsistent with the assumptions of the model employed. Recall from the discussion of the linear regression model with an identity link, that we use the difference between the actually observed outcome score and the score predicted on the basis of the linear model (the error term) as an index of how well, or not so well, the model matches the data. Thus, the sum of squares (SS) of the error terms or residuals and its complement, the regression SS, can be used as an index of the relative fit of the model. In principle, we can do the same thing with the logistic regression model. The outcome variable either takes on the value one, which means the event of interest occurred, or zero, that is, the event of interest did not occur. In addition to the observed outcome, the logistic model gives us estimates of the

---

[9]Here we are interested only in establishing a *pattern* of interaction between two independent variables. The *interpretation* of this pattern is less certain, as the smoking variable only indicates whether or not the mother is a smoker, but not how much she smokes. There may well be additional confounding between the smoking and education variable not captured in these measures. For instance, female smokers with higher education may be more likely to interrupt their smoking during pregnancy compared to female smokers with less education. This could explain at least in part, the precipitous decline in low birth weight babies among smoking mothers with higher education.

TABLE 18.4 Covariate Patterns for Logistic Regression Model in Table 18.3 With Predicted Probabilities of Low Birth Weight Babies

```
. list birthwt prob maritalstat educyrs smoker if pattern==1
     +-------------------------------------------------------- +
     |  birthwt     prob     maritalstat    educyrs    smoker  |
     |-------------------------------------------------------- |
287. |     0      .3494843   0. not married    13     1. smoker |
288. |     1      .3494843   0. not married    13     1. smoker |
289. |     1      .3494843   0. not married    13     1. smoker |
290. |     0      .3494843   0. not married    13     1. smoker |
291. |     0      .3494843   0. not married    13     1. smoker |
     |-------------------------------------------------------- |
292. |     1      .3494843   0. not married    13     1. smoker |
293. |     0      .3494843   0. not married    13     1. smoker |
294. |     1      .3494843   0. not married    13     1. smoker |
293. |     0      .3494843   0. not married    13     1. smoker |
294. |     0      .3494843   0. not married    13     1. smoker |
     +-------------------------------------------------------- +

. list birthwt prob maritalstat educyrs smoker if pattern==2
     +-------------------------------------------------------- +
     |  bwt2        prob     maritals~t     educ3     smoker   |
     |-------------------------------------------------------- |
247. |     0      .0246361   1. married       16   0. non-smoker |
248. |     0      .0246361   1. married       16   0. non-smoker |
249. |     0      .0246361   1. married       16   0. non-smoker |
250. |     0      .0246361   1. married       16   0. non-smoker |
251. |     0      .0246361   1. married       16   0. non-smoker |
     |-------------------------------------------------------- |
252. |     0      .0246361   1. married       16   0. non-smoker |
253. |     0      .0246361   1. married       16   0. non-smoker |
254. |     0      .0246361   1. married       16   0. non-smoker |
255. |     0      .0246361   1. married       16   0. non-smoker |
256. |     0      .0246361   1. married       16   0. non-smoker |
     |-------------------------------------------------------- |
257. |     0      .0246361   1. married       16   0. non-smoker |
258. |     0      .0246361   1. married       16   0. non-smoker |
259. |     0      .0246361   1. married       16   0. non-smoker |
260. |     0      .0246361   1. married       16   0. non-smoker |
261. |     0      .0246361   1. married       16   0. non-smoker |
     |-------------------------------------------------------- |
262. |     0      .0246361   1. married       16   0. non-smoker |
     +-------------------------------------------------------- +
```

probability of the event occurring for each unique covariate pattern.[10] Thus, we could apply a Pearson chi-squared test based on the differences between the observed number of outcomes and the expected number for each covariate pattern. Here is how this works.

Going back to the logistic regression model in Table 18.3, consider the independent variables. There are: a marital status variable with two categories (married or not), a smoking status variable with two categories (smoker or not), and a years-of-education variable with potentially 10 categories (each year forming a separate group). Thus, the different combinations of

---

[10]While the model predicts log-odds, they can be converted to odds and ORs, which in turn can be converted to probabilities.

the independent variables form $2 \times 2 \times 10 = 40$ *possible* covariate patterns. In this particular data set, there are actually only 20 unique covariate patterns, because not all combinations of covariates actually occur in the data. Table 18.4 shows just two such covariate patterns: Pattern 1 shows 10 study participants who are smokers, have 13 years of formal education, and are not married. The logistic model assigns a probability 0.349 that mothers with these characteristics would give birth to a low birth weight baby. We also see that, for the 10 births in question, 4 actually are low birth weight babies. Thus the observed proportion (0.4) and the predicted probability (0.35) are quite close. Similarly for the covariate pattern of nonsmoking mothers with 16 years of formal education, the logistic model assigns a probability of 0.025 to the occurrence of a low-weight birth, and we actually observe no case among the 21 births.

Not all of the covariate patterns produce similar closeness between the observed proportions of low birth weight babies and the predicted probabilities, but overall the Pearson chi-squared (df = 15) equals 14.99 with an associated *p*-value of .453. Thus, we would *not* reject the *null hypothesis* that the observed number of cases among all the covariate patterns equals the number predicted by the model.

A similar goodness-of-fit test for logistic regression models is the Hosmer–Lemeshow (2000) test. The Pearson chi-squared test would be difficult to apply, if the number of covariate patterns approaches the number of cases (*n*) in the sample—in the extreme, each covariate pattern would contain only one case and we could not observe *proportions* of cases within a covariate pattern experiencing the event of interest. For this reason, Hosmer and Lemeshow proposed a different grouping strategy. The proposed to rank-order all cases by their predicted probability from lowest to highest and to divide the sample into percentile groups, often between 8 and 12, depending in part on the size of the sample. For each of the percentile groups we have (a) the number of observed low birth weight babies and the number of normal weight babies, and (b) the number of expected low birth weight and normal babies based on the average probabilities predicted by the logistic model. Table 18.5 shows results after dividing the data into nine percentile groups. The groups are uneven in size because boundaries are

TABLE 18.5 Hosmer–Lemeshow Test: Observed and Expected Numbers of Low Birth Weight (L) and Normal Weight (N) Babies in Nine Percentile Groups Ranked by Average Probability of Low Birth Weight Babies

Group	Prob.	Obs_L	Exp_L	Obs_N	Exp_N	Total
1	0.0921	7	6.5	84	84.5	91
2	0.1388	9	9.4	59	58.6	68
3	0.1647	6	5.6	28	28.4	34
4	0.2164	4	4.5	18	17.5	22
5	0.2352	8	7.5	24	24.5	32
6	0.2759	18	14.3	38	41.7	56
7	0.2893	10	13.6	37	33.4	47
8	0.3495	5	4.4	8	8.6	13
9	0.6667	16	17.1	21	19.9	37

number of observations = 400
number of groups = 9
Hosmer-Lemeshow chi2(7) = 3.06
Prob > chi2 = 0.8789

determined by how many cases fall into adjacent covariate patterns, ordered by the size of the predicted probabilities associated with each covariate pattern. Based on these numbers, the Hosmer–Lemeshow chi-squared test (df = number of groups − 2 = 9 − 2 = 7) returns a value of 3.06 with $p > .878$. From this we conclude that the predictions of the model are consistent with the observed outcome events.

TESTING FOR INFLUENTIAL OUTLIER PATTERNS

As with linear regression models, in addition to examining the overall goodness-of-fit, we need to go beyond summary statistics and examine the data for outliers or influential observations before accepting the model as a good representation of the patterns in the data. As we saw in the last section, the predictor variables for the logistic model in Table 18.3 combine to produce 20 unique covariate patterns, for each of which we obtain a standardized residual comparing the observed number of events within the covariate pattern to the predicted number based on the model. While the standardization formula is a bit complicated,[11] for our purposes it suffices to inspect the results in Figure 18.2. First notice that the graph in Figure 18.2 depicts *squared* standardized Pearson residuals. As for a normal distribution, the 95% confidence limits (CIs) would be ±1.96, the limits for the squared values would be $1.96^2 = 3.8416$.

Assuming the Pearson residuals follow the normal distribution, we would expect only 5% of the covariate patterns to produce residuals that fall outside the 95% CIs. That means we expect not more than 1 out of the 20 covariate patterns to have standardized residuals larger than 3.84. That is the case with these data: Only one positive standardized residual exceeds 3.84; this covariate pattern involves 26 married smokers with 10 years of formal education. Among these, the model predicts the probability of a low birth weight baby to be .276, but the observed proportion is 11/26 = 0.423. The deviation also has the largest *influence statistic* ($\Delta\hat{b}_j$). This statistic measures by how much the estimated regression coefficients *change*, if cases with a particular covariate pattern were excluded from the analysis. The *relative*

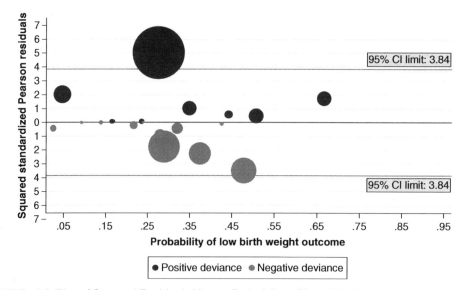

FIGURE 18.2 Plot of Squared Residuals Versus Probability of Low Birth Weight Outcome.

Note: Sizes of circles represent relative influence of covariate pattern on changes in estimates of logistic regression coefficients.

---

[11] Interested readers may consult Hosmer and Lemeshow (2000).

influence that a particular covariate pattern has on the magnitude of the estimated regression coefficients is indicated in the graph of Figure 18.2 by the diameter of the circles. In much of the published clinical literature, it is assumed that logistic (and other) regression models have been examined for their overall fit and sensitivity to outliers, but in many journals it is not a general practice to reassure the reader that such testing has actually occurred.

EXTENSIONS OF THE LOGISTIC REGRESSION MODEL

Logistic or logit regression models are not only confined to binary outcome measures. One important extension is the **multinomial logistic regression model**,[12] in which the outcome variable consists of three or more discrete categories without inherent ordering. For example, Intrator, Zinn, and Mor (2004) examined hospitalization patterns among nursing home residents. In particular, these researchers wanted to know whether the presence of a nurse practitioner and the nursing-staff-to-residents ratio have any effect on the rate of preventable hospitalizations, defined as hospitalizations for ambulatory-care-sensitive (ACS) conditions. In the study, the researchers considered four possible, mutually exclusive outcomes comprising: (a) any hospitalization(s) with a primary discharge ACS diagnosis, (b) any other hospitalization(s), (c) death of resident, (d) or remaining in facility without hospitalization (reference group). Another frequent use of multinomial logit regressions is the prediction of multiple, but mutually exclusive disease outcomes based on a variety of continuous and categorical independent variables (Arif & Delclos, 2012).

In order to discuss the multinomial logistic regression model, we turn to the example in Table 18.6. The goal of the analysis is to predict medication use among 400 mothers after birth depending on their formal education and age (measured in years), their weight (in pounds), current alcohol consumption (yes or no), and current smoking (yes or no). The dependent variable, medication use, comprises four mutually exclusive outcome categories: (a) taking neither headache nor antidepressant medications, (b) taking headache medications only, (c) taking antidepressants only, and (d) taking both types of medicines. The regression coefficients in the table have been converted to relative-risk ratios (RRRs) instead of ORs,[13] but other than that, there is not much change between the multinomial and the binary logistic regression model. Overall, the log-LR (41.69, df = 15) is statistically significant ($p \leq .0003$), suggesting that at least some of the independent variables contribute to explaining variation in medication use, but the Pseudo R^2 of 0.637 implies only modest predictive power. The output is organized into three sections containing the exponentiated regression coefficients and their associated p-values. The top section compares the risks of taking two types of medicines (only for headaches, only for depression, for both) to not taking either medicine types. For instance, compared to nonsmokers, smokers are 3.48 times ($p < .0005$) more likely to take depression medicines than nonsmokers; they are also three times (RRR = 3.05, $p \leq .017$) more likely to take both headache and depression medicines. However, we *cannot* reject the null hypothesis that smokers are not more likely than nonsmokers to use headache medicines without depression medicines (RRR = 1.233, $p \geq .624$). Similarly, mothers' weight also predicts the use of depression medicines (RRR = 1.01, $p < .005$) and the combination of depression and headache medicines (RRR = 1.01, $p \leq .006$): In both cases, each additional pound of weight increases the probability of taking these medicines by about 1%. Alcohol consumption may also contribute to the risk of taking both depression and headache medicines (RRR = 2.8, $p \leq .03$),

---

[12] Another name for this model is *polytomous logistic regression*.

[13] Recall that an RR is a ratio of two probabilities, which in turn can be estimated from the odds involved, as $p = odds/(1 + odds)$.

TABLE 18.6 Multinomial Logistic Regression Model With Four Categorical Outcomes

```
. mlogit medications education age weight alcohol smoker, rrr

Iteration 0:     log likelihood = –327.28534

Multinomial logistic regression                        Number of obs   =     400
                                                       LR chi2(15)     =   41.69
                                                       Prob > chi2     = 0.0003
Log likelihood = –306.43833                            Pseudo R2       = 0.0637
```

medications	RRR	P>|z|	RRR	P>|z|	RRR	P>|z|	LR(df=3)	P>chi2
base outcome:		comparison to base outcome:					LRs for models	
no meds	headache meds		depression meds		both meds		w/o predictor	
education	.941	0.567	1.013	0.889	1.125	0.339	1.35	0.717
age	.968	0.267	.997	0.884	1.006	0.851	1.49	0.684
weight	1.004	0.240	1.010	0.002	1.011	0.006	14.51	0.002
alcohol	1.252	0.631	1.608	0.222	2.821	0.030	5.35	0.148
smoker	1.233	0.624	3.480	0.000	3.051	0.017	15.93	0.001
base outcome:	comparison to base outcome:							
headache meds	depression meds		both meds					
education	1.078	0.580	1.196	0.251				
age	1.030	0.417	1.039	0.351				
weight	1.005	0.245	1.007	0.190				
alcohol	1.285	0.658	2.253	0.197				
smoker	2.823	0.044	2.474	0.131				
base outcome:	comparison to base outcome:							
depress meds	both		meds					
education	1.110	0.467						
age	1.009	0.800						
weight	1.002	0.734						
alcohol	1.754	0.319						
smoker	.877	0.807						

but does not predict the use of depression medicines alone. The two demographic variables (mother's age and education) do not predict any use of medications.

The two lower sections in Table 18.6 show additional risk comparisons, juxtaposing different combinations of medicine use: depression medicines versus headache medicines, depression and headache medicines versus headache medicines alone, and depression and headache medicines versus depression medicines alone. It is not difficult to see that these comparisons are *redundant* and can be derived from the previous risk comparisons. For instance, the (nonsignificant) *sample* estimate of the risk of taking headache medicines as opposed to no medicines is 1.233 times larger for smokers than nonsmokers. In the second section we see that, compared to nonsmokers, smokers are 2.823 times more likely to use depression medicines rather than headache medicines. It follows that, compared to nonsmokers, smokers are 3.48 times more likely to use depression medicines rather than no medicines, as $1.233 \times 2.823 = 3.48$.

As a general rule, if we have k outcome categories, labeled A, B, ... K, and if we choose K as the reference category, then we could, for instance, estimate the RRRs comparing the risks of the outcomes A versus K, B versus K, and A versus B. But if we have an estimate for A versus K and B versus K, we also have an implied estimate of A versus B. Let us assume the logistic regression model gives us the following RRR estimates: $RRR_{A-K} = 4/2$ and $RRR_{B-K} = 3/2$. It follows that $RRR_{A-B} = (4/2)/(3/2) = 4/3$.[14]

One additional advantage of employing the multinomial logistic regression model over separate binary logistic regression models, each comparing only two outcomes at a time, is that we can determine whether any of the predictor variables have significant associations across *all* comparison groups. Table 18.6 shows the log-LRs comparing the full model with all five predictor variables to five models with four predictor variables, after eliminating one predictor at a time from the full model. The results show that only the omission of weight and smoking status would appreciably reduce the predictive power of the multinomial model.

Multinomial logistic regression models make the same assumptions about the data as the binary logistic regression model, except for one addition: The model assumes that, if we eliminate one of the outcome categories, the estimates of the coefficients for the remaining binary outcome comparisons are not affected. For instance, in the example of Table 18.6, the RR probability of taking depression medicines associated with smoking should remain the same, whether or not the risk of taking headache medicines is considered in the model. This "independence of irrelevant alternatives" assumption can be tested using Hausman's specification test, but we leave this problem for the interested reader to explore (Kwak & Clayton-Matthews, 2002).

Another extension of the logistic regression model is the **ordinal logistic regression models**. In Chapter 15, we have already considered several statistical models for ordinal outcome variables, such as the Wilcoxon rank-sum tests or the Kruskal–Wallis test. However, these tests are limited to a single independent variable. Ordered logit regression models may be employed if the categories of the outcome variable can be ordered from least to most and the independent variables represent a mixture of continuous and categorical variables. There are several subtypes of this model, but the most common is the *proportional-odds model*. Suppose we want to predict self-rated responses to a survey question about a person's health, with the ratings ranging from "poor" to "fair" to "good" to "excellent." We could cut the responses in the following way: comparing poor to fair through excellent, poor and fair to good and excellent, and poor–good to excellent. Each time we estimate ORs comparing two groups. If the ORs are similar across all three splits of the outcome categories, then the data are consistent with the model assumption of proportional odds, and a single averaged OR would represent how the odds of higher self-rated health change at every cut-off point. As with all statistical models, the model assumptions need to be tested. For the *proportional-odds* model, the so-called Brant test and the score test can be used for this purpose; further reading on this topic is provided in Hosmer and Lemeshow (2000). Examples of the application of this model to clinical and nursing data can be found in Murray and colleagues (2007) and Wyatt, Sikorskii, Wills, and Su (2010).

SUMMARY

This chapter concludes our discussion of models for categorical outcome variables. Models for categorical outcome variables (both ordered and unordered) have become much more common in the clinical literature, because many outcomes of interest in nursing and medicine

---

[14]The argument holds for ORs as well.

are not measured at an interval or ratio level, which makes the application of linear models for continuous outcome variables suspect. By contrast, the logit regression models discussed in this chapter are capable of analyzing data containing outcome variables with few categories, which may or may not be ordered. Such qualitative variables are part and parcel of clinical judgments and a basic understanding of statistical models to analyze them is more and more required to read the clinical research literature.

In the next section of this book (Part IV), we turn to another class of statistical models that can be used to analyze yet another type of data that is relevant to clinical practice. Clinicians often evaluate the success or failure of treatments in terms of outcomes that lie in the future and may or may not occur. In such cases, we are not only interested in whether or not the event occurs (for that we could employ the logistic regression models discussed in this chapter), but also in when they occur. For example, we may want to be able to predict which patients discharged from a hospital will be rehospitalized for the same illness and at what time within the next 5 years. Or we may want to know for how long patients survive after a particular surgery or cancer treatment. Information about such events is often "censored" at a certain time, that is, we usually have incomplete follow-up information, as the observation periods are inevitably limited. This requires special kinds of analysis models, to which we will turn next.

LITERATURE APPLICATION

Read: Nojkov, B., Rubenstein, J. H., Chey, W. D., & Hoogerwerf, W. A. (2010). The impact of rotating shift work on the prevalence of irritable bowel syndrome in nurses. *American Journal of Gastroenterology, 105*(4), 842–847.

(a) Provide a very brief (three to four sentences) summary of what this study is about.

(b) Define the target population to which the statistical analysis can be generalized. What were the eligibility and exclusion criteria for study participants? Is the study sample a random sample of the target population?

(c) Provide a clear definition of the outcome/dependent variable and a short description of the instrument used to measure it.

(d) Provide a clear definition of all independent/predictor variables and a short description of the instruments used to measure them.

(e) From the data in Table 3, reconstruct the bivariate ORs for each of the sleep-quality measures and the presence or absence of irritable bowel syndrome. Compare these ORs to the estimates in Table 4. Why are they different?

(f) Do the data in Table 3 suggest a possible interaction effect between the sleep-quality measures and the different shifts? If no, why not; if yes, why?

(g) Should the authors have presented only evidence from a main-effects model in Tables 4 and 5? Defend your answer.

(h) In a sentence, how would you describe the OR for Age in Table 5?

(i) Do the authors provide enough information for the reader to judge the goodness-of-fit of the model?

(j) Summarize the main findings in your own words. Are the conclusions of the authors consistent with the evidence presented?

EXERCISES

1. A binary logistic regression equation estimates the log-odds of coronary heart disease (CHD) as follows: $Y = \ln(p/(1-p)) = -2.3 + 0.47$ (HTN) $+ 0.01$ (AGE), where HTN is coded $0 =$ person has no hypertension (HTN), $1 =$ person has HTN, and AGE is coded in years. What are the odds that a 50-year old adult with HTN has CHD (all regression coefficients are statistically significant)?

2. Suppose you have a sample of 100 obese and 100 normal weight adults. Among the normal weight adults, the odds of having diabetes are 4/96. The logistic regression equation that predicts the log-odds of diabetes (Y) equals: $Y = \ln(p/(1-p)) = -3.178 + 1.792X$, where $X = 0$ if the adult has normal weight and $X = 1$ if the adult is obese. How many obese adults have diabetes?

3. The following logistic regression model predicts the odds of incurring a myocardial infarction (MI) based on age (in years), education (years of formal education), and sex ($1 =$ female, $0 =$ male): $Y = \ln(p/(1-p)) = -2.996 + 0.0198$ (AGE) $- 0.0513$ (EDUC) $- 0.1054$ (SEX). All regression coefficients and the intercept are highly significant ($p < 0.001$). What is the OR that compares the odds of an MI among 60-year old men with a high school degree (12 years of education) compared to 45-year old women with a college degree (16 years of education)?

4. Observe the following output from a logistic regression, in which the outcome/dependent variable refers to the odds of having a major functional limitation (e.g., cannot walk independently, cannot dress oneself, cannot feed oneself), and age, education, sex, and marital status are all predictor/independent variables:

Variables in the Equation

	B	S.E.	WALD	DF.	SIG.	EXP(B)	95% C.I. FOR EXP(B)	
							LOWER	UPPER
Age (in years)	.041	.001	2732.53	1	.000	1.042	1.040	1.043
Education (years of formal education)	−.105	.004	694.57	1	.000	.900	.894	.906
Sex (female vs. male)	−.140	.024	34.49	1	.000	.869	,829	.911
Poverty (<100% vs. higher income)	.831	.034	602.97	1	.000	2.295	2.147	2.452
Marital status: (reference category: married)			189.51	5	.000			
(widowed vs. married)	.116	.039	8.76	1	.003	1.123	1.040	1.213
(divorced vs. married)	.462	.041	127.47	1	.000	1.587	1.465	1.720
(separated vs. married)	.466	.067	48.09	1	.000	1.594	1.397	1.819
(single/never mar. vs. married)	.283	.037	57.83	1	.000	1.328	1.234	1.428
Constant	2.494	.089	786.07	1	.000	.083		

(a) In a single sentence, state how age affects having a serious functional limitation.

(b) Suppose you are comparing a person with 10 years of formal education to one with 7 years of formal education; by how much do the odds of having a serious functional limitation differ between persons with 10 years, as opposed to 7 years, of formal education?

(c) Based on the information provided in the table, is it possible to say that, for separated persons, the odds of having functional limitations are significantly higher than for widowed persons?

REFERENCES

Arif, A. A., & Delclos, G. L. (2012). Association between cleaning-related chemicals and work-related asthma and asthma symptoms among healthcare professionals. *Occupational and Environmental Medicine, 69*(1), 35–40.

Hosmer, D. W., & Lemeshow, S. (2010). *Applied logistic regression* (2nd ed.). New York, NY: John Wiley & Sons.

Intrator, O., Zinn, J., & Mor, V. (2004). Nursing home characteristics and potentially preventable hospitalizations of long-stay residents. *Journal of the American Geriatrics Society, 52*(10), 1730–1736.

Kwak, C., & Clayton-Matthews, A. (2002). Multinomial logistic regression. *Nursing Research, 51*(6), 404–410.

Murray, G. D., Butcher, I., McHugh, G. S., Lu, J., Mushkudiani, N. A., Maas, A. I. R., . . . Steyerberg, E. W. (2007). Multivariable prognostic analysis in traumatic brain injury: Results from the IMPACT study. *Journal of Neurotrauma, 24*(2), 329–337.

Wyatt, G., Sikorskii, A., Wills, C. E., & Su, H. A. (2010). Complementary and alternative medicine use, spending, and quality of life in early stage breast cancer. *Nursing Research, 59*(1), 58–66.

PART IV. MODELS FOR TIME-TO-EVENT DATA/SURVIVAL ANALYSIS

CHAPTER	19

Incidence Rates, Life Tables, and Survival Function

CENSORING

So far, we have examined statistical models that predict outcomes without taking into account exactly when these outcomes or events occur. While repeated-measures analysis of variance (ANOVA) models can be used to analyze changes in outcome scores over selected time intervals, such as the predetermined time intervals of repeated measurements in a panel study, these models do not take into account individual variations in the timing of the outcome of interest. Yet, in prospective studies of patients,[1] we often follow a given set of individuals, defined by a common treatment or intervention or a common diagnosis, for a specified time to record adverse events or other outcomes of interest. These events, which include death, rehospitalizations after an initial discharge, or other critical endpoints such as a patient experiencing the onset of specified symptoms, occur at different times for different individuals. As individuals cannot be followed for an indefinite period of time or data collection may be cut short due to death or unwillingness to participate further in a study, eventually all prospective longitudinal studies share the common problem of **censoring**.

Suppose we want to know whether, and when, a patient who is discharged from a hospital after a triple bypass surgery will be hospitalized again. We may be able to follow patients for up to 1 year, during which we ascertain all rehospitalizations. However, hospitalizations occurring 12 months or later after the initial discharge would not be recorded. Thus, information about rehospitalization would be incomplete: We would know about hospitalizations during the 12-month observation period, but not after it. This incomplete information about rehospitalization is an example of censoring. Figure 19.1 presents a graphical illustration of censoring.

Suppose that some researchers follow newly diagnosed colon cancer patients for up to 18 months. Such a study may focus on several adverse events of interest: death, rehospitalization, immobility, adverse reactions to toxicity of chemotherapy, loss of hair or appetite, and so forth. Adverse events other than death and rehospitalization are recorded monthly at home visits of the patient/study participant. For each individual study participant, the researchers record the time he or she is enrolled in the study, counting from the day of diagnosis.

---

[1]A prospective longitudinal study may be experimental (clinical trials) or observational (cohort studies).

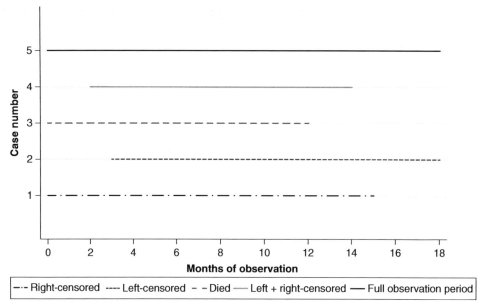

FIGURE 19.1 Observation Periods for Five Participants in a Cohort Study.

As Figure 19.1 shows, study participants 1, 3, and 5 are enrolled immediately after diagnosis, but participant no. 4 was enrolled in the second month and participant no. 2 in the third month after diagnosis. The observations on these two study participants are said to be "left-censored," as information about their health status at early home visits is missing.[2] In addition, there is also the problem of right-censoring. For instance, participant no. 1 may have refused to continue in the study after 15 months; thus, no information on this patient's morbidity and mortality status is available after this time. Likewise, participant no. 4 is lost to follow-up after the 14th month—perhaps the patient moved away without notifying the study personnel. Whatever the reason, these five individuals have been observed during time periods of different lengths. However, when we observe one individual for a longer time than another individual, the *opportunity* to observe an event or outcome of interest will be greater for the former than for the latter. From this it follows that simply comparing the incidences of an adverse event in different groups of individuals would lead to biases if the different observation times are not taken into account.

INCIDENCE RATES

Given the inherent time dimensions of the occurrences of adverse events, the way to get unbiased information is to employ *rates* rather than proportions of people experiencing specific event outcomes. The crucial part of the definition of an **incidence rate** (IR) is that it involves both counts of events (incident cases of diseases for instance or of persons experiencing an adverse event) and explicitly defined time periods of observation. Thus, a rate is not simply a proportion of persons newly diagnosed with a specific disease over the total number of persons in a particular population. The denominator of the "population at risk for the disease" is the *product of the number of persons exposed times their associated average exposure time.*

---

[2]Of course, if we were interested in death as the sole outcome, left-censoring would not be an issue, as the study participants must all be alive at the time of enrollment.

DEFINITION OF INCIDENCE RATE

An *incidence rate (IR)* is a ratio of two quantities: the number of new ("incident") cases diagnosed with a particular disease, or experiencing an adverse event for the first time, within a given time period over the *population at risk* for the disease or adverse event in that time period.

$$IR = \frac{Number\ of\ persons\ experiencing\ incident\ events}{Total\ person\text{-}time\ of\ observation}$$

An example will illustrate this definition: Suppose a researcher follows 10 smokers and 10 nonsmokers, initially all 55 years old, for 10 years with the objective of documenting their first incidence of an acute myocardial infarction (AMI), should there be any. Given an observation period of 10 years, some of the study participants are quite likely to be lost to follow-up: They may move away without leaving an address, refuse further participation, or die due to unrelated causes such as car accidents.

Table 19.1 shows some data for this hypothetical study.[3] The first and fifth columns indicate the years of exposure, that is, the year during which a person smoked or did not smoke. The second and sixth columns show the number of smokers or nonsmokers in each year, who were at risk for experiencing an AMI. The third and seventh columns incorporate a simplifying assumption about death or follow-up: We assume here that, if a person dies or is lost to follow-up, this event always occurred exactly on the last day of the observation year, so that the person was at risk for an AMI during the entire year of observation.[4] Finally, the fourth and eighth columns show the disease outcome of interest: the first occurrence (incidence) of an AMI for a given person. Note that we defined the event of interest as the *first* occurrence of an AMI. That means, once a person has had an AMI, he or she no longer is at risk for another first AMI.

TABLE 19.1 10-Year Follow-Up Data for 10 Smokers and 10 Nonsmokers to Record Incidences of a First Acute Myocardial Infarction

	Non-Smokers:				Smokers:		
Year	Persons At Risk for AMI	Loss to Follow-up	New AMI		Year	Persons At Risk for AMI	Loss to Follow-up	New AMI
0–1	10	0	0		0–1	10	1	0
1–2	10	1	0		1–2	9	0	0
2–3	9	0	0		2–3	9	0	1
3–4	9	0	1		3–4	8	0	1
4–5	8	0	0		4–5	8	1	0
5–6	8	0	0		5–6	7	0	1
6–7	8	1	0		6–7	6	0	0
7–8	7	0	0		7–8	6	1	1
8–9	7	0	1		8–9	4	0	0
9–10	6	0	0		9–10	4	0	0
Sums:	82	2	2			71	3	4

---

[3] The main purpose here is to illustrate the concept of person-time of exposure, or "population at risk."
[4] Clearly, people do not only die on the last day of a year, but we could have chosen smaller time intervals, for example, days, to make it more realistic.

As the data in Table 19.1 show, among nonsmokers the "population at risk" for experiencing a first AMI or the "total person-time of observation" is equal to 82 person-years: $2 \times 10 + 2 \times 9 + 3 \times 8 + 2 \times 7 + 1 \times 6 = 82$.[5] During that time, we observe two new AMIs. Thus, the 10-year IR for nonsmokers is: IR = new AMIs/person-years at risk = 2/82 = 0.0244. Among smokers the "population at risk" for experiencing a first AMI or "total person-time of observation" is 71 person-years: $1 \times 10 + 2 \times 9 + 2 \times 8 + 1 \times 7 + 2 \times 6 + 2 \times 4 = 71$. During that time, we observe four new AMIs. Thus, the 10-year IR for smokers is: IR = new AMIs/person-years at risk = 4/71 = 0.0563.

If we divide the IR for smokers by the IR for nonsmokers, we get a relative risk (RR) estimate of RR = IR_S/IR_{NS} = 0.0563/0.0244 ≈ 2.3. Note that a simple ratio of the proportions of smokers versus nonsmokers, who experience an AMI, would have given us an estimate of RR = (4/10)/(2/10) = 2. The latter ratio does not take into account that nonsmokers, in the aggregate, were observed for 11 person-years more than smokers. Thus, in a prospective study, *the RR should be computed as the ratio of two IRs*, taking explicitly into account the time dimension of the observations. Only if the average follow-up time is the same in the two groups being compared, will the RR, based on the ratio of two proportions, equal the RR based on the ratio of the two IRs.

THE CONSTRUCTION OF LIFE TABLES

Our discussion of time-to-event and survival analysis continues with the related concept of a **life table**. Life table analysis is used by demographers and health insurance actuaries to get estimates of mortality, survival rates, and life expectancy for the U.S. population as a whole as well as specific population groups defined by gender, ethnicity, state residency, and so forth. Table 19.2 contains an abbreviated version of a life table showing U.S. mortality and life expectancy based on 2008 data.[6] In this table, we only present data for the first 3 years of life, followed by data for every 10th year. What you see here is a so-called "current" life table. It uses Census Bureau data from 2008 about the U.S. population (then approximately 304 million people) and divides the population into 1-year age intervals (the age variable is referred to as "x"). The data in Table 19.2 are standardized to show anticipated deaths and survival per 100,000 persons born in 2008. Of course, the underlying assumption is that the survival pattern of the 2008 cohort can be extrapolated from survival patterns of current older age cohorts. If history is any guide, the resultant life expectancies are almost certainly underestimates of the future survival pattern of the 2008 cohort, but with each year of additional data, these estimates are revised to yield more accurate estimates for this cohort. The table content is read as follows:

- We start with the column labeled "l_x." It is labeled "number surviving to age x"; that is, the column contains the number of persons alive at the beginning of the age interval. Rather than showing us the total number of babies born in the United States in 2008, this column starts in the first row with 100,000 newly born babies (l_0).

---

[5] Alternatively, we can obtain the sum as follows: six persons were observed for 10 years, one for 9, one for 7, one for 4, and one for 2 years. That makes: $6 \times 10 + 1 \times 9 + 1 \times 7 + 1 \times 4 + 1 \times 2 = 82$.

[6] The full data are available from the Centers for Disease Control and Prevention as a pdf file under the heading "United States Life Tables, 2008—Tables updated using revised intercensal populations" at http://www.cdc.gov/nchs/products/life_tables.htm; for a detailed discussion of life table methodology, see http://www.cdc.gov/nchs/data/nvsr/nvsr61/nvsr61_03.pdf

TABLE 19.2 Abbreviated U.S. Life Table Based on 2008 Population Data

Age(x)	PROBABILITY OF DYING BETWEEN AGES X AND X + 1 q_x	NUMBER SURVIVING TO AGE X l_x	NUMBER DYING BETWEEN AGES X AND X + 1 d_x	PERSON-YEARS LIVED BETWEEN AGES X AND X + 1 L_x	TOTAL NUMBER OF PERSON-YEARS LIVED ABOVE AGE X T_x	EXPECTA-TION OF LIFE AT AGE X e_x
0–1	0.006593	100,000	659	99,425	7,816,825	78.2
1–2	0.000479	99,341	48	99,317	7,717,399	77.6
2–3	0.000291	99,293	29	99,279	7,618,083	76.7
.	.	.	.	.	.	.
10–11	0.000080	99,162	8	99,158	6,824,368	68.8
20–21	0.000817	98,811	81	98,771	5,833,863	59.0
30–31	0.001040	97,862	102	97,811	4,850,380	49.6
40–41	0.001789	96,624	173	96,538	3,877,439	40.1
50–51	0.004318	93,974	406	93,771	2,922,590	31.1
60–61	0.008965	88,389	792	87,992	2,007,800	22.7
70–71	0.020298	77,372	1,571	76,587	1,172,767	15.2
80–81	0.052439	55,862	2,929	54,397	495,471	8.9
90–91	0.148357	22,287	3,306	20,634	99,092	4.4
99–100	0.314390	2,419	761	2,039	5,727	2.4
100+	1.00000	1,659	1,659	3,688	3,688	2.2

- The column labeled "d_x" shows us how many of these 100,000 babies die before their first birthday. Those are the deaths occurring during the age interval 0 to 1 (d_0). If we divide the deaths in that age interval by the total number alive at the beginning of the age interval, we get...

- "q_x" or "the probability of dying between the beginning of the age interval (x) and the end of the age interval ($x + 1$)." In the first row, we get the q_0, which refers to the age interval 0 to 1.

- Now, we turn to the column labeled "person-years lived in age interval x to $x + 1$" (L_x). The number there is 99,425. As it turns out, there is one additional piece of information we need to make sense of this number. If you focus on the second row of the column labeled "number surviving to age x," you see the number 99,341. This entry is simply computed as $l_x - d_x$ or the *difference* between the number of persons alive at the beginning of any age interval and the number of persons who died during the age interval. This difference yields the number of persons alive at the beginning of the *next* age interval. Thus, in rows 1 and 2, we get: $100,000 - 659 = 99,341$. Now, we know for sure that these 99,341 babies lived a full year to their first birthday. However, the L_x column ("person-years lived between ages x and $x + 1$") shows the number 99,425. Why the difference? If you subtract 99,341 from 99,425, you get 84. That means that the 659 infants, who died during the first year, lived a *total* of 84 *life-years*. If we divide that total by 659, we get $84/659 = 0.127$. Thus, these 659 infants lived, on average, for only 12.7% of the duration of the first year, which is about 46 days. This 12.7% is also known as the "average fraction of survival during the last year lived." While the table does not show a separate column for the "average fraction of survival," the fraction is implicit and is based on the actual survival data for infants in 2008.

- For older individuals, the average fraction of survival tends toward 50%, as people tend to die relatively evenly across time during any 1-year interval. Babies are an exception, as many neonatal deaths occur in the first month after birth. In sum, L_x tells us how many total years were lived by all the persons, who were alive at the beginning of an age interval (x), until the beginning of the next year ($x + 1$).

- The column labeled "T_x" shows the "total number of person-years lived above age x." In other words, this column shows how many *total* years of living are left among those, who were alive at the beginning of age interval x, *including all subsequent age intervals*. For instance, T_0 shows the number 7,816,825. That means, the initial 100,000 babies born in 2008 are estimated to have a total of 7.82 million life-years left to live. T_0 was calculated simply by adding up all the numbers in the L_x column.[7]

- The final step is the calculation of the "life expectancy" (see the last column labeled "e_x"). Dividing the total number of person-years lived (T_x) by the number of persons alive at the beginning of a particular age interval $x(l_x)$ yields the average number of years lived beyond $x(e_x)$. For instance, in the first row we get: 7,816,825/100,000 = 78.2. That is, in 2008, the average life expectancy of a U.S. resident at birth was 78.2 years, *assuming* that the 2008 age-specific mortality pattern would continue in the future for this population cohort. From the column e_x you can also see that a person, who already reached the 60th birthday was expected to live another 22.7 years. Of course, these are averages for the U.S. population as a whole. If you look at the more detailed life tables in the National Center for Health Statistics (NCHS) pdf file, you will see that life expectancy for women is about 5 years longer than for men, that White men have a 7-year longer life expectancy than Black men, and so forth.

Life tables display the survival (or mortality) patterns in populations or communities, even when the exact survival times of their members are not known. For instance, we mentioned the simplifying assumption that, for most age cohorts, deaths occur at a more or less constant rate within each year. However, while the life table assumes constant mortality rates *within* each age group, mortality (and survival) rates do *change* among *different* age groups. At the same time, life tables use *current* age-specific mortality patterns for the purpose of *extrapolating* to the life expectancy of a particular birth or age cohort.

KAPLAN–MEIER SURVIVAL FUNCTION

As mentioned in the beginning of this chapter, with cohort studies it is often possible to record the exact time (within a day) when a person dies or when a person withdraws for any other reason from the study. Hospitalizations or other events of interest may similarly be recorded for each study participant. This suggests that, rather than relying on some average probability of the occurrence of an adverse outcome within an arbitrary interval, we could construct a

---

[7]This includes, of course, all the years that are NOT shown in this abbreviated table; the full data are shown in the NCHS pdf file labeled "United States Life Tables, 2008—Tables updated using revised intercensal populations" at http://www.cdc.gov/nchs/products/life_tables.htm

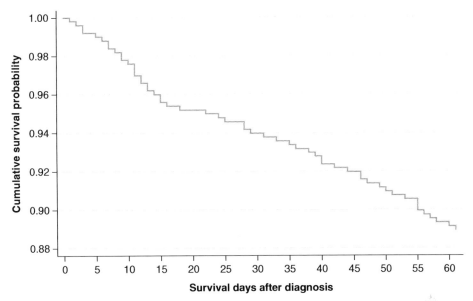

FIGURE 19.2 Kaplan–Meier Survival Estimates to 61 Days After Diagnosis: 500 Lung Cancer Patients Aged 65 to 70.

survival function that is adjusted every time the adverse event occurs or someone is lost to follow-up. Figure 19.2 shows such a survival step-function for 500 newly diagnosed lung cancer patients 65 to 70 years old. Table 19.3 shows the details of survival and mortality probabilities just for the first 12 days after diagnosis. The probability of survival at a particular time t (s_t) is the complement of the probability of mortality, which is also known as the hazard rate (h_t): $s_t = 1 - h_t$. For instance, from the data in Table 19.3, we learn that among the 500 diagnosed lung cancer patients, one person died on the first day after diagnosis, another person on the second day, two on the third, and so forth. Thus the hazard rate on the first day is 1/500 = 0.002; on the second day, it is 1/499 = 0.002004; on the third day it is 2/498 = 0.004016, and so forth. Notice that the denominator of the hazard rate is adjusted each time a person dies or is lost to follow-up, because both events reduce the population at risk for further deaths. An example can be seen in Table 19.3 on Day 5: The "persons at risk for death" are reduced

TABLE 19.3 Six-Day Survival Pattern Among 500 Newly Diagnosed Lung Cancer Patients

Day	Persons At Risk for Death	Loss to Follow-up	Deaths	Probability of Death/Hazard Rate	Probability of Survival (s_t)	Probability (S_t) Cumulative Survival
1	500	0	1	0.002000	0.998000	0.998000
2	499	0	1	0.002004	0.997996	0.996000
3	498	0	2	0.004016	0.995984	0.992000
4	496	1	0	0.000000	1.000000	0.992000
5	495	0	1	0.002020	0.997980	0.989996
6	494	0	1	0.002924	0.997076	0.987101

to 495, even though no one died during the previous day. The relationship among the hazard rate at time t, h_t, the survival probability at time t, s_t, and the *cumulative* survival function, S_t, can thus be summarized as follows:

DEFINITIONS OF HAZARD RATE, SURVIVAL PROBABILITY, AND KAPLAN–MEIER CUMULATIVE SURVIVAL ESTIMATES

Hazard rate at time t, h_t:

$$h_t = \frac{d_t}{n_t},$$

where d_t is the number of persons dying during interval t and n_t is the number of persons at risk for dying at time t.

Survival probability at time t, s_t:

$$s_t = 1 - h_t = \frac{n_t - d_t}{n_t},$$

where $n_t - d_t$ is the number of persons surviving during interval t and n_t is the number of persons at risk for dying at time t.

Cumulative survival probability up to time t, S_t:

$$S_t = \prod_1^k s_{ti} = s_t \times s_t \times \cdots \times s_{tk},$$

where $\prod$ is the product operator indicating that the cumulative survival probability equals the product of each successive survival probability up to time t. This formula is also known as the product-limit formula.

The **Kaplan–Meier cumulative survival function** is also known as the **product-limit survival function**. Cumulative survival probabilities are computed as the products of all time-specific survival probabilities up to the time of interest. For example, based on the data in Table 19.3, we can calculate the cumulative survival probability at Day 3 as follows: $S_3 = 0.998000 \times 0.997996 \times 0.995984 = 0.992000$. If we recompute the survival probabilities every time someone dies—in other words, we are not using broader, predetermined, time intervals like years or weeks—we obtain the Kaplan–Meier survival function.

SUMMARY

In this chapter, we introduced the basic concepts of censoring, IRs, and survival/mortality probabilities we employ in the analysis of time-to-event or survival data. Time-to-event data usually provide partial information about the occurrence of events within the restricted time of observation. The basic approach to handing censored data is to adjust risk estimates based on the time of exposure or observation.

In the next chapter, we will explore ways of *comparing* risks of adverse outcomes in different target populations. As always, as sample data vary from one study sample to the next, we will need statistical tests and confidence intervals for our estimates of survival functions.

LITERATURE APPLICATION

Read: Chan, T. C., Hung, I. F. N., Luk, J. K. H., Shea, Y. F., Chan, F. H. W., Woo, P. C. Y., & Chu, L. W. (2013). Functional status of older nursing home residents can affect the efficacy of influenza vaccination. *Journals of Gerontology. Series A, Biological Sciences and Medical Sciences*, *68*(3), 324–330.

(a) Provide a very brief (three to four sentences) summary of what this study is about.

(b) Define the target population to which the statistical analysis can be generalized. What were the eligibility and exclusion criteria for study participants? Is the study sample a random sample of the target population?

(c) Provide a clear definition of the outcome/dependent variable and a short description of how the outcome event was measured.

(d) Provide a clear definition of all independent/predictor variables and a short description of the instruments used to measure them.

(e) Is this study observational or experimental?

(f) What can the reader learn from Figure 1?

(g) Summarize the main findings in your own words. Are the conclusions of the authors consistent with the evidence presented?

EXERCISES

1. Here are data from a cohort study that compares the risk of lung disease (of any type) among coal miners and truck drivers after the age of 40. A total of 1,000 coal miners and 1,600 truck drivers were followed for up to 10 years:

NO. OF COAL MINERS	FOLLOW-UP PERIOD	PERSON-MONTHS	NO. OF TRUCK DRIVERS	FOLLOW-UP PERIOD	PERSON-MONTHS
600	10 years		1000	10 years	
300	9 years		400	9 years	
200	8 years		200	8 years	
100	7 years		0	7 years	
Total: 1200			Total: 1600		
Incidences of lung disease among coal miners: 55			Incidences of lung disease among truck drivers: 38		

Based on these data, what is the RR of lung disease among coal miners compared to truck drivers?

2. Suppose you read in a study report that the RR of dying within 5 years of a colon cancer diagnosis is 1.6 ($p < .001$) times larger among men than among women. You also learn about the study that 400 of 1,000 men with colon cancer died within 5 years, and 200 of 1,000 women with colon cancer died within 5 years. Are these results necessarily contradictory? Explain.

3. The Kaplan–Meier cumulative survival function is defined as: $S_t = \prod_i^k s_{ti} = s_{t1} \times s_{t2} \times \cdots \times s_{tk}$. Based on this, how can we express the Kaplan–Meier cumulative mortality function? In words, what would the cumulative mortality function tell us?

REFERENCES

Brook, A. D., Ahrens, T. S., Schaiff, R., Prentice, D., Sherman, G., Shannon, W., . . . Kollef, M. H. (1999). Effect of a nursing-implemented sedation protocol on the duration of mechanical ventilation. *Critical Care Medicine*, *27*(12), 2609–2615.

Chan, T. C., Hung, I. F. N., Luk, J. K. H., Shea, Y. F., Chan, F. H. W., Woo, P. C. Y., & Chu, L. W. (2013). Functional status of older nursing home residents can affect the efficacy of influenza vaccination. *Journals of Gerontology. Series A, Biological Sciences and Medical Sciences*, *68*(3), 324–330.

National Center for Health Statistics (NCHS). (2008). *United States life tables*. Retrieved from http://www.cdc.gov/nchs/products/life_tables.htm

CHAPTER 20

Comparing Survival Functions in Different Groups and Hazard Regression

CONFIDENCE INTERVALS FOR SURVIVAL FUNCTION

In the last chapter, we introduced the Kaplan–Meier survival function to describe the cumulative survival probabilities in a single population group. As data are usually sample-based, a familiar statistical question arises: How much variation is there in the point estimates of survival functions from one sample to the next? To answer this question, we need to have a measure of the variance of the estimated survival function at any time t: $\hat{S}_t$. It is provided by Greenwood's formula: $\text{Var}(\hat{S}_t) = \hat{S}_t^2 \times \Sigma \frac{d_t}{n_t(n_t - d_t)}$, summing over all events up to time t. However, the construction of the 95% confidence intervals (CIs) is a bit more complex. Because survival functions are limited to values between zero and one, CIs of survival functions should also not exceed these limits. It is possible to convert the survival function into an unconstrained measure that can take on any positive or negative number using two successive logarithmic transformations, which is known as the log–log survivorship function: $\ln(-\ln(\hat{S}_t^2))$.[1] Then we can obtain a 95% CI for that expression, adding or subtracting 1.96 standard errors: $\ln(-\ln(\hat{S}_t^2)) \pm 1.96\hat{s}e_t$.[2] Finally, we reconvert this expression by taking the antilog twice, and we obtain the desired 95% CI for the original survival function. Figure 20.1 contains the graph of the same Kaplan–Meier survival function as in Figure 19.2, but with the added band showing the 95% CI for the survivor function.

Table 20.1 shows the estimates of the 95% CI for selected days after diagnosis.

THE LOG-RANK TEST

Suppose we compare the survival of lung cancer patients with Stage 1 nonsmall cell lung cancer diagnosis to the survival of Stage 4 (metastatic) nonsmall cell lung cancer patients. Figure 20.2 shows the separate survival graphs for these two groups of lung cancer patients.

---

[1] As the survivor function is a cumulative probability function its values can only range from 0 (no survivors) to 1 (all sample members are still alive). If one takes the logarithm of probabilities between 0 and 1, one obtains negative numbers between $-\infty$ and 0. Multiplying this expression by $(-)$ yields positive numbers between 0 and $+\infty$. Finally, taking another log of positive numbers yields both positive and negative numbers.

[2] The interested reader may consult Hosmer and Lemeshow (2008) for details.

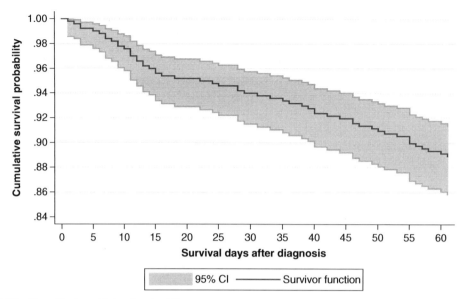

FIGURE 20.1 Kaplan–Meier Survival Estimates to 61 Days After Diagnosis: 500 Lung Cancer Patients Aged 65 to 70.

The fact that the 95% confidence bands, for almost the entire observation period, do not overlap is a graphical indication that the survival curves in the two groups are significantly different. However, we need a formal test that the two survival functions differ over the entire observation period, that is, for all times t. The null hypothesis for this test would be: H_0: $\hat{S}_{s-1,t} = \hat{S}_{s-4,t}$, that is, the survival functions are equal. The test statistic is a chi-squared statistic, known as the log-rank test. Its logic is as follows: Suppose we construct 2×2 frequency tables for each time interval (t), when new deaths are recorded in either comparison group. Then we compare the number of deaths occurring at time t in one of the groups to the number of deaths we would expect, if the null hypothesis is true. Under the null hypothesis, we would expect the *same* proportion of deaths among both population groups at risk

TABLE 20.1 95% Confidence Intervals for Kaplan–Meier Survival Function at Selected Intervals (t)

Day	Persons At Risk for Death	Loss to Follow-up	Deaths	Cumulative Survival Prob.(S_t)	Standard Error	[95% Conf.	Int.]
1	500	0	1	0.9980	0.0020	0.9859	0.9997
2	499	0	1	0.9960	0.0028	0.9841	0.9990
3	498	0	2	0.9920	0.0040	0.9788	0.9970
4	496	1	0	0.9920	0.0040	0.9788	0.9970
5	495	0	1	0.9900	0.0045	0.9761	0.9958
.	.	.	.	.	.	.	.
56	445	0	1	0.8974	0.0136	0.8673	0.9211
57	444	1	1	0.8954	0.0137	0.8650	0.9193
58	442	0	1	0.8934	0.0138	0.8628	0.9175
60	441	0	1	0.8914	0.0140	0.8605	0.9157
61	440	439	1	0.8873	0.0145	0.8554	0.9126

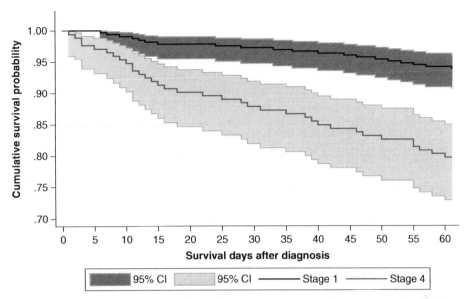

FIGURE 20.2 Comparison of Kaplan–Meier Survival Estimates for Two Groups: Stage 1 Versus Stage 4 Patients Aged 65 to 70.

for dying. To illustrate how to set up a table that compares observed to expected mortality risks at a given observation day, we start with the data in Table 20.1 for Day 3. As the table shows, at the beginning of Day 3, there were $n_3 = 498$ lung cancer patients at risk for dying. There were also $d_3 = 2$ deaths, implying that, at the end of the day there were $n_3 - d_3 = 498 - 2 = 496$ survivors, as nobody was lost to follow-up on the day. Thus, the mortality probability among all lung cancer patients in the sample at Day 3 equals $d_3/(n_3 - d_3) = 2/498 = 0.00402$. As it turns out, at Day 3 there were 327 lung cancer patients at risk for dying in the group with a Stage 1 diagnosis and 171 lung cancer patients at risk for dying in the group with a Stage 4 diagnosis. With this information, we can now construct a 2×2 table as shown in Table 20.2.

Note that at Day 3 we would expect 1.3 deaths in the Stage 1 group and 0.7 deaths in the Stage 2 group, *if* there is no difference in the death rate between the two groups. However, we actually observe zero deaths in the Stage 1 group and two deaths in the Stage 2 group. Now, at each Day t at which a death occurs we construct a similar 2×2 table and compare the observed and expected deaths in each comparison group. Then we add up all the observed

TABLE 20.2 Survival/Mortality Occurrences at Day 3 Among 498 Lung Cancer Patients Still at Risk at $t = 3$

Lung Cancer Diagnostic Group	Persons At Risk for Death	Deaths	Survivors	Expected Deaths:
Stage 1	327	0	327	(2/498) x 327 = 1.3
Stage 2	171	2	169	(2/498) x 171 = 0.7
Total	498	2	496	(2/498) x 498 = 2.0

TABLE 20.3 Log-Rank Test to Compare Survival Distributions Between Two Groups of Lung Cancer Patients (Stage 4 vs. Stage 1 Diagnoses)

failure: mortality = 1, analysis time t: survival days

	Stage 4	Stage 1	Total
Deaths	35	20	55
Person Days Observed	9290	19231	28521
Incidence rate	.0037675	.00104	.0019284 RR = 3.623

Log-rank test for equality of survivor functions

stage	Events observed	Events expected
Stage 1	20	36.99
Stage 4	35	18.01
Total	55	55.00

chi2(1) = 23.87
Pr>chi2 = 0.0000

and expected deaths *over the entire survival distribution* for both the Stage 1 and the Stage 2 groups. This yields a simple chi-square test statistic, as is familiar from Chapter 16:[3]

$$\sum \frac{(O_j - E_j)^2}{E_j} = \frac{(O_{stage\ 1} - E_{stage\ 1})^2}{E_{stage\ 1}} + \frac{(O_{stage\ 2} - E_{stage\ 2})^2}{E_{stage\ 2}}$$

In this formula, O_j refers to the *sum* of all observed deaths over all times (here: days) t in group j, which in this two-group example refers to either the Stage 1 or the Stage 2 lung cancer patients. Similarly, E_j refers to the sum of all expected deaths in either group. With survival distributions being compared in two groups, the associated degrees of freedom (df) of this chi-squared test is $2 - 1 = 1$. Table 20.3 provides summary statistics comparing the relative risk (RR) of mortality in Stage 1 and Stage 4 lung cancer patients as well as the results from the log-rank test. It is easy to see that the log-rank test (chi-square) can be extended to multiple-group comparisons after computing the sums of observed and expected adverse outcomes in each of the groups. One of the attractive features of this test is that it makes no assumptions about the shapes of the survival curves compared.

HAZARD FUNCTIONS AND HAZARD RATIOS

In the last chapter, we defined the probability or *risk* of dying at time t, m_t, as the *proportion* of the individuals dying at time t divided over the number of individuals "at risk for dying" at time t. In Table 19.3 we provided examples of probabilities of dying during one-day intervals.[4] Even though the numbers in the fifth column of Table 19.3 are proportions or probabilities, they refer to populations at risk observed for one day at a time. The recorded deaths actually occur over a time *interval* of 24 hours and the population at "risk for dying" theoretically does not simply refer to everyone alive at the beginning of a day, as some persons may be "lost to

---

[3] This is Bland and Altman's (2004) version of the log-rank test. There is also a modified chi-squared test by Mantel (1966), often referred to as the Mantel–Haenszel test for survival data.

[4] For example, according to the data in Table 19.3, on the third day of following lung cancer patients after diagnosis, 2 out of 498 patients at risk died resulting in a probability of .004016.

DEFINITION OF THE HAZARD RATE

Hazard rate at time t, h_t:

$$h_t = \frac{m_t}{\Delta t} = \left(\frac{d_t}{n_t}\right)/\Delta t$$

where Δt refers to the time interval between $t_k + t_{k+1}$, d_t is the number of persons dying during interval Δt, n_t is the number of persons at risk for dying during the interval Δt, and m_t refers to the probability of death during the time interval Δt, such that $m_t = d_t/n_t$.

If the time interval becomes smaller, $\Delta t \rightarrow 0$, we obtain the "instantaneous" hazard rate.

follow-up" *during* the day before the full 24 hours have expired. Of course, with such a short time interval as a day, it is not worthwhile to record loss to follow-up in hourly intervals; for all practical purposes, the persons alive at the beginning of the day represent the population at risk for dying. It is nonetheless important to reflect on this inherent time dimension. Making the time dimension explicit reminds us that we are actually talking about a death *rate* per day. If t_k refers to the beginning of a time interval of interest and t_{k+1} refers to the beginning of the following time interval, then $t_{k+1} - t_k = \Delta t^5$ refers to the duration of the time interval between t_k and t_{k+1}, which may be measured in weeks, days, hours, seconds, and so forth, as required by the study. Using these shorthand symbols, we can define the **hazard rate** as the risk of an adverse event occurring per time interval Δt. If we shorten the time interval more and more, so that $\Delta t \rightarrow 0$, we get a measure of the "instantaneous" hazard of dying at a particular time t. If the hazard rate $h_t = 0$, this means that no one is at risk for dying at time t. In that case the cumulative survival function would not decline, that is, it would be constant at time t: $S_t = c$. A positive hazard rate (>0) implies a decline in the cumulative survival function, with smaller hazard rates producing more gradual declines and larger hazard rates producing more precipitous declines.[6] Figure 20.3 offers a graphical depiction of two cumulative survival functions over an observation period of 400 days together with their different (and constant) hazard rates: $h_t = 0.01$ and $h_t = 0.005$. Even though the hazard rate for each of the curves is constant, the cumulative survival curve is curvilinear, which means that the slope of each curve becomes less steep. The reason is that with a constant hazard rate, the number of people dying each day declines, as the population at risk, or the remaining survivors, becomes smaller. One feature of constant hazard rates is very attractive when comparing the survival or mortality in two populations: For survival functions with constant hazard rates, the ratio of the hazard rates is the same over the entire time of observation. Thus, this ratio of the two hazard rates would describe the difference in the risk of dying between the two populations. For the survival functions in Figure 20.3, we can summarize the RR of dying by computing the hazard ratio (HR) as follows:

$$HR = \frac{h(t,g1)}{h(t,g2)} = \frac{0.01}{0.005} = 2.0$$

We can say that for these two population groups, the hazard or risk of dying is twice as large among the population with $h(t) = 0.01$ than among the population with $h(t) = 0.005$.

---

[5]The Δ (read: "delta") symbol is the general symbol for *change* between two time points.
[6]Readers familiar with calculus will recognize the survival function as the integral of the hazard function: $S_{(t)} = \exp(-\int_0^t h_{(t)} dx)$.

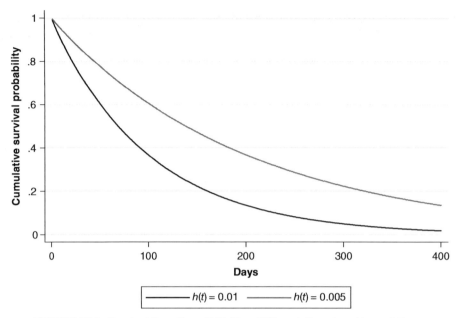

FIGURE 20.3 Survival Functions With Two Different Constant Hazard Rates.

COX PROPORTIONAL HAZARD REGRESSION

As it turns out, constant hazard rates are not all that common in health care studies. For instance, the risk of dying in the initial time period after some surgeries is often greater than the risk a few days later. However, hazard rates do not have to be constant over time for there to be a single HR that describes the RR of dying in the comparison groups. What is required is that the changing hazard rates over time maintain the same proportion between two different comparison groups. This **proportional hazard assumption** can be summarized formally as follows: The ratios of the hazard of dying in groups 1 and 2 do not change between time j and time k:

$$\frac{h(t_j, g1)}{h(t_j, g2)} = \frac{h(t_k, g1)}{h(t_k, g2)}$$

Thus, if the hazard rate in group 1 at time j equals 0.01 and the hazard rate in group 2 at time j equals 0.005, then the HR at time j equals HR = 0.01/0.005 = 2.0. If at time k the hazard rate in group 1 changes to 0.016 and in group 2 it changes to 0.008, then the HR at time k would still be HR = 0.016/0.008 = 2.0. Thus, the crucial point is that hazard rates can change over time, and we may not even be interested in these exact changes, but as long as the hazard rates remain *proportional*, the difference in the hazard or risk of dying, or another adverse event, between different groups of individuals can be expressed in a single number, the hazard ratio (HR).

If we know the hazard rate in one comparison group and we know the HR, which is equivalent to an RR, then we can express the hazard of dying in the other group simply as:

$$h_t(\text{group 1}) = h_t(\text{group 2}) \times \text{HR}$$

This is, of course, a prediction model that is very similar to the logistic regression model, in which we express the odds of an event occurring in one group as the odds of the event occurring in another group times the odds ratio (OR).[7] Just as the OR can be converted to the log-odds (logit), which then are used as the dependent variable in a linear regression model, we can take the logarithm of the HR and convert the multiplicative model above into a linear regression model:

$$\ln[h_1(t)] = \ln[h_0(t)] + bX$$

To see the equivalence to the logistic model, we rewrite the equation by subtracting the intercept term from each side: Then $\ln[h_1(t)] = \ln[h_0(t)] + bX$ becomes $\ln[h_1(t)] - \ln[h_0(t)] = bX$. From Appendix H, we know that we can rewrite the difference between two logarithms to the same base as the logarithm of the ratio of the numbers involved:

$$\ln[h_1(t)] - \ln[h_0(t)] = \ln\left[\frac{h_1(t)}{h_0(t)}\right] = bX$$

If we now exponentiate this equation, we see that the HR is nothing but the antilog of the regression coefficient:

$$\frac{h_1(t)}{h_0(t)} = e^{bX}$$

In a two-group comparison, where $X = 0$ for the "base" group and $X = 1$ for the comparison group, the base hazard rate is set to 1, as $e^{b0} = e^0 = 1$; and the HR is equal to $e^{b1} = e^b$. For a continuous independent variable like age, e^b would represent the HR for a *one-unit change in X*. For instance, comparing a 48- to a 47-year old person would be expressed as follows: $e^{b(48-47)} = e^{b1} = e^b$. In Table 20.4, we revert to the example of comparing the hazard of dying between Stage 1 and Stage 4 lung cancer patients 65 to 70 years old.

BASIC EQUATION FOR PROPORTIONAL HAZARD REGRESSION

$$y = h_1(t) = h_0(t)\mathrm{HR} = h_0(t)e^{bx}$$

In its multiplicative form, the proportional hazard model expresses the hazard or risk of dying in population group 1 as the hazard of dying in population group 0 (baseline hazard) times the HR, which is represented by the exponential expression of e^{bx}.

$$\ln(y) = \ln[h_1(t)] = \ln[h_0(t)] + bX$$

After taking the logarithms on both sides of the equation, the proportional hazard model becomes a linear regression model, with the dependent variable expressed as the logarithm of the hazard rate, an intercept term representing the logarithm of the baseline group hazard and *b* the slope coefficient indicating by how many units the log-hazard changes for a unit change in the independent variable.

When interpreting the output in Table 20.4, observe the formal similarity to the output from a logistic regression model. The overall test of the predictive power of the model is again

---

[7]See the discussion in Chapter 17.

TABLE 20.4 Cox Regression Model Predicting Hazard of Dying Between Two Groups of Lung Cancer Patients (Stage 4 vs. Stage 1 Diagnoses) Aged 65 to 70

```
. stcox stage

                failure _d: mortality == 1   analysis time _t: survdays

Iteration 0:   log likelihood = -338.40897

Cox regression - Breslow method for ties

No. of subjects =        500                    Number of obs =      500
No. of failures =         55
Time at risk    =      28521
                                                LR chi2(1)  =    21.93
Log likelihood  = -327.44512                    Prob > chi2 =   0.0000

-------------------------------------------------------------------------
   _t |  Coeff.   Std. Err.   z    P>|z|   Haz. Ratio   [95% Conf. Interval]
------+------------------------------------------------------------------
stage |  1.2801    .2804    4.57   0.000     3.5970       2.0763    6.2316
-------------------------------------------------------------------------
```

provided by the log-likelihood ratio (LR) test, which is equal to twice the difference between the log-likelihood of the null model (without any independent variable) and the model with stage as the only predictor variable: $2 \times [-327.44512 - (-338.40897)] = 21.93$. The associated p-value for this test yields a very low probability of a Type I error, $p \leq .00005$, if we *reject* the null hypothesis that the independent variable has *no* effect on the hazard outcome. Thus, we can accept, with high confidence, the hypothesis that the stage at diagnosis affects the hazard of dying. The estimate for the regression coefficient associated with the staging variable is 1.2801 and its antilog, $e^{1.2801} = 3.597$ is the HR. Thus, we estimate that individuals with a Stage 4 lung cancer diagnosis have a 3.6 times greater risk of dying than Stage 1 lung cancer patients *at any time during the observation period*. The z-test is based on the assumption of a normal sampling distribution for the regression coefficient; it is the estimated regression coefficient divided by its standard error: $z = 1.2801/0.2804 = 4.57$. To obtain the 95% CI for the HR, we calculate $1.2801 \pm 1.96 (0.2804)$ and exponentiate the results.[8]

It is not surprising that the **Cox Proportional Hazard Model** gives us results that are very similar to those from the log-rank test in Table 20.3, as the underlying survival curves are those in Figure 20.1. However, as always, when we apply statistical models to explain patterns in the data, we need to test whether the assumptions of the model are reasonable, given the data at hand. In particular, for the Cox Regression Model, we need to test whether the data meet the proportionality of hazards assumption. As with previous regression models, we can compare the model predictions to the observations: This allows us to examine the deviations between observations and predictions for any systematic patterns or large outliers. Figure 20.4 shows Kaplan–Meier survival plots, based on predicted and observed survival in both comparison groups. The graph clearly indicates that the predicted survival patterns track the observed patterns quite closely. Alternatively, we can test whether the residuals show any systematic tendency to change in magnitude or direction over the observation period. In the current case, this test, based on so-called scaled Schoenfeld residuals, returns a

---

[8]Here are the results: $e^{1.2801 - 1.96(0.2804)} = 2.0763$; $e^{1.2801 + 1.96(0.2804)} = 6.2316$.

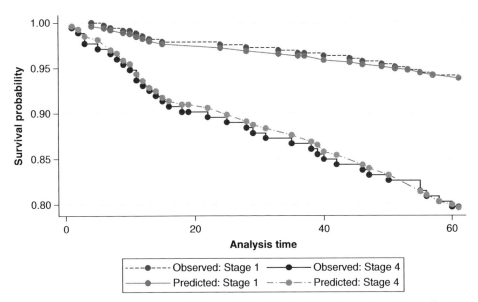

FIGURE 20.4 Predicted and Observed Kaplan–Meier Survival Functions: Predictions Are Based on Cox Proportional Hazard Model With Staging as Only Predictor.

p-value $\geq .297$, meaning, we cannot reject the null hypothesis that there is no systematic change in the residuals over time.

So far, we have only used the Proportional Hazard Regression Model to test for differences in survival patterns of two groups, for which the log-rank test is entirely adequate. However, being a regression model, we can extend the analysis and include more categorical and continuous predictor variables. In Table 20.5, we show the results of a Cox Proportional Hazard Model with age and sex as additional predictors. In the context of focusing on the effects of cancer staging on survival, age, and sex are "control" variables or confounders. As the results show, the overall log-likelihood for this model is -323.31667, with twice the difference from the null model of -338.40897 being equal to 30.18 ($p \leq .00005$). Thus, we conclude that the model as a whole does predict hazards of dying among the lung cancer patients. However, the individual predictor variables show significant effects for the staging (HR = 3.46, $p < .0005$) and the age variable (HR = 1.23, $p \leq .007$), but not for sex (HR = 1.26, $p \geq .397$). Based on this evidence, we can say that, after adjusting for age and sex, the estimate for the HR associated with the different lung cancer stages at diagnosis is slightly reduced to 3.46. With age being a continuous variable representing years of age from 65 to 70, we can say that, independent of the staging of the lung cancer, the average hazard of dying increases by 26% for each additional year of age. However, there are no sex differences in the mortality risk among these newly diagnosed lung cancer patients. In fact, the LR tests, which compare proportional hazard regression models with different configurations of independent or predictor variables,[9] do confirm this pattern: Adding sex to the model, either to stage alone or age and stage, does not improve predictability, as the difference between these models is insignificant, as the p-value is greater than .05. Adding age to the model, either to stage alone or to

---

[9]In Table 20.4, the log-likelihood for the model with stage as the only predictor is -327.44512. In Table 20.5, the log-likelihood for the model with all three predictors (stage, age, and sex) is -323.31667. Computing the difference and multiplying it by 2 yields the LR chi-square of 8.26 with $p \leq .0161$.

TABLE 20.5 Cox Regression Model Predicting Hazard of Dying Between Two Groups of Lung Cancer Patients (Stage 4 vs. Stage 1 Diagnoses) With Age and Sex as Control Variables

```
. stcox stage sex age

                      failure _d: mortality == 1      analysis time _t: survdays

Iteration 0:  log likelihood = -338.40897

Cox regression — Breslow method for ties

No. of subjects  =         500                          Number of obs   =        500
No. of failures  =          55
Time at risk     =       28521
                                                        LR chi2(3)    =      30.18
Log likelihood   =  -323.31667                          Prob > chi2   =     0.0000

---------------------------------------------------------------------------------
   _t  |    Coeff.    Std. Err.     z      P>|z|    Haz. Ratio     [95% Conf. Interval]
-------+-------------------------------------------------------------------------
stage  |    1.2417      .2810     4.42     0.000      3.4617        1.9958   6.0040
 sex   |     .2308      .2722     0.85     0.397      1.2596         .7388   2.1474
 age   |     .2040      .0750     2.72     0.007      1.2263        1.0587   1.4205
---------------------------------------------------------------------------------
                                  Test of proportional-hazards assumption: p≥0.4962

Likelihood-ratio tests:

stage        vs. stage&sex          LR chi2(1) = 0.87       Prob > chi2 = 0.3510

stage        vs. stage&age          LR chi2(1) = 7.55       Prob > chi2 = 0.0060

stage        vs. stage&age&sex      LR chi2(2) = 8.26       Prob > chi2 = 0.0161

stage&age  vs. stage&age&sex        LR chi2(1) = 0.71       Prob > chi2 = 0.3994

stage&sex  vs. stage&age&sex        LR chi2(1) = 7.39       Prob > chi2 = 0.0066
```

stage and sex, does improve the predictability. Overall, the test of proportionality assumption of the model, based on scaled Schoenfeld residuals, is not significant leading us to conclude that the model provides a reasonable description of the survival patterns.

The Cox Proportional Hazard Model is, by far, the most popular regression model used to analyze time-to-event data. As with other regression models, in which multiple predictors are used, the analyst needs to check for possible interactions among the predictors, before accepting a "main-effect" model without interactions. The model can also be modified in some cases, when the proportional hazard assumption does not hold across all comparison groups of interest, by introducing separate strata for such groups. In addition, like other regression models, the Cox Proportional Hazard Model can accommodate time-dependent covariates, that is, independent variables measured at different times. Despite this flexibility, when the proportional hazard assumption is violated across many comparison groups, particularly defined by continuous predictor variables like age or the body mass index, parametric survival regression models, which model survival times explicitly, are called for. These are beyond the scope of this book, but the interested reader may consult Hosmer and Lemeshow (2008).

SUMMARY

This chapter concludes our discussion of statistical models for time-to-event or survival data. Time-to-event data are quite common in clinical data sets, where loss to follow-up and consequently censoring of outcome variables are a regular occurrence. For time-related outcomes, survival models are to be preferred over logistic models, which disregard the time-to-event (for an example, see Cai, Salmon, & Rodgers, 2009). The methods introduced in this and the previous chapter go a long way toward analyzing such data and are commonly encountered in the applied clinical literature. For more complicated analysis models, it is necessary to consult a bio-statistician.

In the final part of this book (Part V), we will turn our attention to statistical models that deal with measurement errors. Clinical data sets often contain quantified scales based on self-report data, repeated physiological measures taken from the same patient, or multiple observations of the same patient by different observers/clinicians. In all of these cases, we observe measurement errors, and we need methods to account for them. We begin in the next chapter discussing commonly used indices of reliability for scale measures and for multiple observations.

LITERATURE APPLICATION

Read: Stommel, M., Olomu, A., Holmes-Rovner, M., Corser, W., & Gardiner, J. C. (2006). Changes in practice patterns affecting in-hospital and post-discharge survival among ACS patients. *BMC Health Services Research*, 6, 140.

(a) Provide a very brief (three to four sentences) summary of what this study is about.

(b) Define the target population to which the statistical analysis can be generalized. What were the eligibility and exclusion criteria for study participants? Is the study sample a random sample of the target population?

(c) What are the shortcomings, if any, in comparing historical cohorts?

(d) Provide a clear definition of the outcome/dependent variable and a short description of how the outcome event was measured.

(e) Provide a clear definition of all independent/predictor variables and a short description of the instruments used to measure them.

(f) Does the Kaplan–Meier survival curve in Figure 2 contradict the results in Table 3. If yes, why, if not, why not?

(g) In Table 2, the model LR χ^2 (df: 16) = 282.51. What does that tell us? Why does this test have 16 dfs?

(h) In your own words, explain the meaning of the HRs for age and beta-blockers in Table 3. What do they tell us?

(i) Are the conclusions of the authors consistent with the evidence presented?

EXERCISES

1. In Table 20.5, the regression coefficient and HR for the variable sex are somewhat larger than the regression coefficient and HR for the variable age, yet the coefficient for age is statistically significant, while the sex coefficient is not. Explain why.

2. As in Table 20.2, construct the relevant 2 × 2 table comparing observed and expected deaths at Day 57 for the data in Table 20.1.

3. The following graph shows the cumulative survival functions for two comparison groups. Do the survival patterns shown here meet the proportional hazard assumption? If yes, why? If no, why not?

Kaplan–Meier Survival Estimates: Men Over the Age of 65

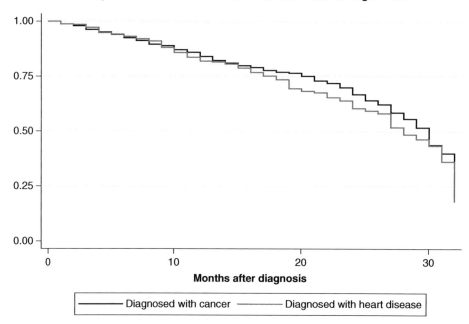

REFERENCES

Bland, J. M., & Altman, D. G. (2004). The logrank test. *British Medical Journal, 328*(7447), 1073.

Cai, Q., Salmon, J. W., & Rodgers, M. E. (2009). Factors associated with long-stay nursing home admissions among the U.S. elderly population: Comparison of logistic regression and the Cox proportional hazards model with policy implications for social work. *Social Work in Health Care, 48*(2), 154–168.

Hosmer, D. W., & Lemeshow, S. (2008). *Applied survival analysis: Regression modeling of time to event data* (2nd ed.). New York, NY: Wiley & Sons.

PART V. MEASUREMENT MODELS

CHAPTER 21

Reliability Coefficients and Medical Test Evaluation

An ever-increasing number of clinical decisions are based on, or are supported by, test scores designed to capture different aspects of a patient's physical and mental health. We use blood pressure (BP) readings, lipid scores, low-density lipoprotein cholesterol, and a host of other routine clinical measurements to supplement more subjective clinical judgments to understand a patient's health status. In many situations, clinicians also use standardized tests based on observations and self-reports, such as physical function measures (SF-36) or depression scores (Center for Epidemiologic Studies-Depression Scale [CES-D]), to screen applicants for nursing homes, make decisions about eligibility for health services, and so forth. Furthermore, outcomes from population-based screening tests for a variety of cancers are often the starting point for more detailed testing and treatments. Given the ubiquity of clinical tests in clinical practice, it is obvious that we must be concerned about the quality of these tests. In general, test results and observations used in clinical practice or research should be "accurate" and should be capable of measuring the intended target, so that they can be useful tools in decision making.

In the psychometric tradition, these twin concerns about the veracity and accuracy of measurement are captured in the key concepts of **validity** and **reliability**. In a way, the concern with validity is the most basic: Are we really measuring what we want to measure? This concern plays a role in both biological and psychological measurement. For instance, the prostate-specific antigen (PSA) test is an example of a test that is used as one factor in deciding about the presence of cancerous cells in the prostate. However, the test does not measure the presence of cancerous cells directly; instead, it measures the presence of aprotein produced by cells of the prostate gland. One problem that has arisen with this test is that higher levels of PSAs in the bloodstream may just be indicators of an enlarged (noncancerous) prostate (NCI, 2013). The presence of such false-positive results leads one to question the validity of the PSA as a screening test for prostate cancer. The test also produces some false-negative results, indicating the absence of prostate cancer when it is present. Again, this leads one to question the validity of the PSA.

Validity is also a substantial concern in psychological measurement. Many psychological concepts of interest to nurses and physicians are measured indirectly: through patients' responses to standardized self-report scales such as the Geriatric Depression Scale (depression), the Self-rating Anxiety Scale (anxiety), or the Patient Health Questionnaire-9 (depression) scales (Kroenke & Spitzer, 2002; Yesavage et al., 1982–1983; Zung, 1971). Measures of depression or anxiety derived from interview responses often include somatic symptoms like loss of appetite and sleeplessness or heart palpitations and sweating.[1] Yet, all of these physical symptoms could also be the results of some extraneous factor like the effects of some medication, or a physical disease such as cancer. Thus, it is difficult to obtain "uncontaminated" measures of psychological states. The problem is not all that different with respect to biophysiological measures. For example, the simple routine of weighing a person on a scale during a primary care visit is fraught with many measurement problems. Assuming that the goal is to get a measure of body weight, there is no question that all sorts of extraneous factors contribute to the actual measurement outcome, including variations in the weight of shoes and clothes as well as a patient's recent eating activities.

While the establishment of measurement validity is an arduous process, it only partially involves statistical methods.[2] On the other hand, the *reliability* of a measurement procedure is primarily established using statistical calculations and estimations.

Reliability of measurement is a characteristic of the *measurement tools or measurement procedures* we use: If reality does not change, that is, if the traits, qualities, and characteristics we are interested in do not change, then the measurement tools we use to measure these traits, qualities, and characteristics should return the same results. Whether different clinicians or researchers apply a measurement tool, whether the measurement occurs at different times, or whether we use multiple indicators of the same underlying quantities being measured, the results should be *consistent*. While it is impossible to compare our measurement results directly against "reality" we can compare the results of multiple measurements. To the extent that such multiple measurement results are consistent, our measurement procedure can be said to be reliable. Thus, reliability in measurement is a precondition of validity[3]; it involves evidence, which shows that the measurement procedures are repeatable and provide similar results, provided that the underlying reality does not change.

SYSTEMATIC VERSUS RANDOM MEASUREMENT ERROR

When we talk about the reliability of measurement, what we mean is that the measurement process should be relatively free of random, that is, unpredictable measurement error.[4] Consider measuring a patient's BP several times within a relatively short time period. There are numerous factors that influence the actual readings: variation in the size of the pressure cuffs, variations in the precise location of the pressure cuffs around the arm, variations in the patient's nervousness, or the patient's calming down after hurrying to the primary care office, variations in background noise, different arms tested, different nurses or physicians taking the measurement, and so forth. Some of these measurement conditions can be standardized through a protocol that may prescribe, for instance, that the same nurse conducts the measurements using the same pressure cuff on the left arm of a patient. However, there are almost infinitely many small variations in the actual measurement procedure from one minute to the next, and there is no way to control all of them. The result is that, even if the

[1] See for instance the CES-D and the Hamilton Anxiety Scale (HAM-A).
[2] For a more extensive discussion of measurement validity, see Stommel and Wills (2004).
[3] A completely unreliable measurement procedure cannot be valid, but a reliable procedure may not be valid either, if it does not measure the intended target characteristic.
[4] There are also systematic measurement errors—as when a wrongly calibrated scale consistently indicates 10% higher weight—but this kind of measurement error does not affect the reliability or repeatability of the measurement results.

TABLE 21.1 Diastolic Blood Pressure (DBP) Readings Obtained From a Single Patient Within 1 Hour

Day	Observed DBP (x_i)	Mean "true" DBP score (t_i)	Deviations of measured from "true" DBP (e_i)	Squared measurement error (e_i)^2
1	86	83	3	9
2	82	83	−1	1
3	81	83	−2	4
4	83	83	0	0
5	86	83	3	9
6	85	83	2	4
7	79	83	−4	16
8	82	83	−1	1
Sums:	$\Sigma(x_i)$: 664	$\Sigma(t_i)$: 664	$\Sigma(e_i)$: 0	$\Sigma(e_i)^2$: 44
Means:	$\Sigma(x_i)/8$: 83	$\Sigma(t_i)/8$: 83	$\Sigma(e_i)/8$: 0	$\Sigma(e_i)^2/(8-1)$: 5.5

patient's underlying BP does not change, the readings are likely to fluctuate *unpredictably* from one measurement instance to the next. Table 21.1 shows eight hypothetical readings of the diastolic blood pressure (DBP) from a single individual obtained within an hour.

The table contains only one column of actual data, which is the column labeled "Observed DBP." At the bottom of the column we see that the mean observed DBP over eight readings equals 83. While we do not know the "true" DBP of this patient, it is reasonable to assume that an average of eight DBP readings comes closer to the true score than any individual reading.[5] If we accept this logic, we can use the mean DBP reading as a "stand-in" estimate of the true score. Furthermore, we can subtract this "true" score from each observed score to obtain a deviation that represents the measurement error at any given measurement instance. In short, we can think of an observed measurement score as consisting of two components: a true score and a measurement error: $O_i = T + e_i$. For instance, the first measurement in Table 21.1 shows the following decomposition of the observed score: 86 = 83 + 3, as 3 = 86 − 83.

The example in Table 21.1 also shows that the sum of all measurement "error terms" equals zero: $\Sigma e_i = 0$. While it is of course true by definition that the sum of all deviations from a mean must be equal to zero, the interpretation of these deviations as measurement errors deviating from the "true" score depends on the reasonableness of the assumption. It is important to note that we refer here to *random* measurement error, which indeed behaves in such a way that some observed scores overestimate the true score and others underestimate it, with the mean *of a long series of scores* approaching the true score. As the mean of many scores comes closer and closer to the true score, measurement errors will cancel each other out, as more measurements are taken. With larger samples of repeated measurements of the same subject's BP, or any other attribute of interest, we can obtain at least an estimate of the true score and, therefore, also an estimate of measurement error. The variance of these error terms gives an indication of how large the average measurement error is. It plays a central part in the notion of measurement reliability, as will be seen shortly.

---

[5]Again, we are assuming here the absence of systematic measurement errors.

THE CONCEPT OF MEASUREMENT RELIABILITY

Suppose now we have several DBP readings from many different patients. We can think of each of these DBP scores as being composed of the true underlying BP of an individual plus or minus some unavoidable measurement error. If the measurement errors are purely random, then the error components are *not* correlated with the true scores. It follows that the variance of the observed scores (V_o) is the sum of the variance of the true scores (V_t) and the variance of the measurement errors (V_e): $V_o = V_t + V_e$.[6] While we cannot observe the true scores and their variance directly, the equation suggests that, if we can get separate estimates of the error variance, we would also get an estimate of the true variance: $V_t = V_o - V_e$.

Before we turn to methods that allow us to estimate true-score variance, we provide this general definition of measurement reliability:

DEFINITION OF MEASUREMENT RELIABILITY
Reliability of measurement is defined as the ratio of true-score variance over observed-score variance.

$$Rel = \frac{V_t}{V_o} = \frac{V_o - V_e}{V_o} = 1 - \frac{V_e}{V_o}$$

Now, let us assume for a moment we obtain three DBP readings on each of 20 individuals within a short time period, say, in less than 10 minutes. For the sake of argument, we further assume that the true DBP readings of these 20 individuals are entirely stable and we are in possession of an error-free measurement procedure. This would mean that the error variance equals zero and the observed score variance (among different individuals) equals the true-score variance:

$$V_o = V_t + V_e = V_t + 0 = V_t$$

If $V_t = V_o$, the ratio of V_t over V_o must be equal to one. Thus, whatever reliability index we use, it should produce the value one in a situation of complete absence of measurement error (perfect reliability). Now assume that all measured individuals have the same true score, so that any observed variance in DBP readings just captures measurement error:

$$V_o = V_t + V_e = 0 + V_e = V_e$$

If $V_o = V_e$ and $V_t = 0$, the ratio of true to observed variance must be equal to zero, implying that this measurement procedure lacks any reliability. In general, when the proportion of the variance of observed scores accounted for by measurement error, V_o/V_t, declines, the proportion of observed variance accounted for by the true scores, V_t/V_o, increases. Thus, a measurement procedure becomes more reliable to the extent that it produces less random measurement errors.

---

[6]The variance of a sum of two *uncorrelated* variables equals the sum of their variances; for a detailed discussion, see the classic text by Nunnally and Bernstein (1994).

NOTE ON THE IMPORTANCE OF MEASUREMENT ERROR

It is not always appreciated how important measurement reliability is in evaluating the magnitude of estimated statistical coefficients. Suppose that two variables (x and y) are perfectly correlated in the real world, with the underlying (unobserved) population Pearson's correlation being $\rho = 1.0$. However, our measurement procedures are less than perfect; thus x may have a measurement reliability of 0.8 and y a reliability of 0.9. As only the true-score portions of the observed measurement scores are correlated, the observed correlation can never be larger than the product of the square roots of the two reliabilities: $\sqrt{0.8} \times \sqrt{0.9} = 0.849$.[7] In short, unreliability can substantially attenuate observed correlations, regression coefficients, and other statistical measures.

THE INTRA-CLASS CORRELATION COEFFICIENT AS AN INDEX OF RELIABILITY

The very definition of reliability as *relative absence of random measurement error* suggests a way of estimating reliability empirically. First of all, if we want to sort out measurement errors from true scores, we need *multiple* measures of the same attribute. If we have only a single DBP reading from a sample of patients, we cannot disentangle true scores from measurement error, as we have no way to determine by how much DBP readings fluctuate from one reading to the next *for a given patient.* In that case, it would be impossible to determine what proportion of the observed score can be attributed to measurement error. But suppose we repeat the DBP measure, in short succession, a second and third time for the same patients. Now we can obtain three correlations from the obtained data (Time 1 and Time 2; Time 1 and Time 3; Time 2 and Time 3). Even on the assumption that each patient's "real" or "true" DBP will not change across these measurement occasions, we would not expect perfect correlations, as some measurement error is to be expected. Given our assumption that the "real" DBP of these 20 subjects is stable, any differences in DBP scores among the three scores of the same individual, that is, *within-subjects variation* of the scores, would then be equated to measurement error. By the same token, any difference in *average* DBP scores among separate individuals, that is, *between-subjects variation,* would then represent true-score variation. We can also use the analysis-of-variance (ANOVA) model to ascertain the amount of "true-score" variance, since we have assumed that mean scores for individuals across the three measurement occasions reflect their true scores.

Consider the data in Table 21.2. There are 20 individuals, represented by the ID variable. We further assume that all of the DBP measures are taken by different health care providers. In this situation, we cannot disentangle the effects that different raters/health care providers have on the DBP readings, and we treat all within-subjects variation in DBP as random error. With 60 observations (DBP scores) as the outcome variable, we could run a one-way ANOVA with the subject ID as the only factor. That way, we can single out between-subjects variance from the within-subjects variance, which in this case equals the error variance. Subtracting from the between-subjects variance the residual variance[8] and dividing the difference by the between-subjects variance gives us an estimate of the **intra-class correlation (ICC)**:[9]

$$ICC = \frac{MS_{ID} - MS_{res}}{MS_{ID}} = \frac{302.53 - 14.35}{302.53} = 0.9526$$

---

[7]See Nunnally and Bernstein (1994).

[8]The 60 outcome scores represent both between- and within-subjects variation.

[9]An ICC is a measure of the degree of similarity among alternative measures of the same characteristics of the target individuals. Being alternative measures of the "same class," we expect them to have the same population variance.

TABLE 21.2 Diastolic Blood Pressure (DBP) Readings Obtained From 20 Different Patients Within 10 Minutes: Test of Reliability (ICC)

Data: 60 DBP Observations from 20 Individuals, each observed 3 times:

ID:	1	1	1	2	2	2	3	3	3	4	4	4	5	5	5	6	6	6	7	7	7	8
OBS:	1	2	3	1	2	3	1	2	3	1	2	3	1	2	3	1	2	3	1	2	3	1
DBP:	60	65	64	79	88	88	77	72	73	66	61	62	86	80	80	82	75	80	84	87	84	90

ID:	8	8	9	9	9	10	10	10	11	11	11	12	12	12	13	13	13	14	14	14	15	15
OBS:	2	3	1	2	3	1	2	3	1	2	3	1	2	3	1	2	3	1	2	3	1	2
DBP:	87	96	69	69	66	70	68	66	59	66	61	72	75	78	77	77	86	62	57	49	72	67

ID:	15	16	16	16	17	17	17	18	18	18	19	19	19	20	20	20
OBS:	3	1	2	3	1	2	3	1	2	3	1	2	3	1	2	3
DBP:	68	48	54	60	80	74	77	62	67	60	70	75	74	75	76	68

Number of obs = 60   R-squared = 0.9092

Source	Seq. SS	df	MS	F	Prob >
Model	5748	19	302.526316	21.08	0.0000
id	5748	19	302.526316	21.08	0.0000
Residual	574	40	14.35		
Total	6322	59	107.152542		

Intra-class correlations one-way random-effects model
Random effects: Number of tested individuals = 20 Number of raters = 3

rating	ICC	[95% Conf. Interval]	
Average	.953	.901	.980

F test that ICC=0.00: $F(19, 40)$ = 21.082 Prob > F = 0.000
Note: ICC estimates reliability of the average measurement made on the same individual.

In this simple one-way model, the ICC estimate is based on only two sources of variation: between-subjects and within-subjects variation. The assumption is that there are no systematic differences in the *average* DBP scores across the 20 individuals obtained at three times within short intervals. This assumption would not be plausible if, say, for all 20 patients, the first measure was taken by nurse Marla, the second by nurse Latisha, and the third by nurse Ashley.

In the latter case, we could reasonably suspect that the individual idiosyncrasies in taking BP measures would show up as systematic differences affecting the average DBP scores obtained by each of the nurses. To demonstrate an observer effect, we modified the data in Table 21.2, subtracting a score of 2 from the first 20 observations ("Marla's readings"), adding a score of 2 to all second 20 observations ("Latisha's readings"), and leaving the third observations ("Ashley's readings") intact. Table 21.3 shows the two-way ANOVA with nurses/measurement occasions added as a second factor.

Note that the *mean* DBP readings for the 20 patients by the three nurses are now different: 70, 74, and 72 instead of a consistent mean of 72 underlying the data in Table 21.2. The systematic differences in mean DBP readings among the three nurses increase the overall variation of DBP scores,[10] while at the same time reducing the *proportion*

---

[10]Compare the total sum of squares in Tables 21.2 and 21.3.

TABLE 21.3 Diastolic Blood Pressure (DBP) Readings Obtained From 20 Different Patients Taken by Three Different Nurses Within 10 Minutes: Test of Reliability (ICC)

```
DBPBY Rater:
 Variable   |  Obs   Mean   Std. Dev.   Min   Max
------------+--------------------------------------
   Marla    |   20    70    10.45794     46    88
   Latisha  |   20    74     9.380832    56    90
   Ashely   |   20    72    11.63479     49    93


        Number of obs =      60        R-squared      = 0.9114
        Root MSE      = 3.88655        Adj R-squared  = 0.8625

      Source  |  Seq. SS   df      MS        F       Prob > F
   -----------+-------------------------------------------------
       Model  |   5908     21   281.333333  18.62     0.0000
  Nurse-rater |    160      2          80    5.30     0.0094
          id  |   5748     19   302.526316  20.03     0.0000
    Residual  |    574     38   15.1052632
   -----------+-------------------------------------------------
       Total  |   6482     59   109.864407
```

Intra-class correlations one-way random-effects model
Random effects: Number of tested individuals = 20 Number of raters = 3

rating	ICC	[95% Conf. Interval]	
Average	.940	.865	.975

F test that ICC=0.00: F(19, 38) = 21.028 Prob > F = 0.000
Note: ICC estimates reliability of the average measurement made on the same individual.

of between-subjects true scores represented by the variance or mean square associated with the ID variable.

At this point, the analyst must make a decision as to how to think about reliability, which can be captured in the juxtaposition of the terms *consistency* versus *absolute agreement*. Recall that we subtracted a constant, namely a score of 2, from each first DBP measure in Table 21.2 and relabeled the result as "Marla's DBP readings"; similarly we added a score of 2 to the second DBP measure in Table 21.2 and named the results as "Latisha's DBP readings." Yet, the correlations between the original first and second observations and the one between the readings of Marla and Latisha are *identical*: In both cases it is 0.8734. This follows directly from the formula for the Pearson's correlation coefficient, which is not affected by shifts in mean scores of a variable.[11] In other words, score *differences between any two measured individuals* are not affected by who conducts the measurement as long as one nurse *consistently* produces DBP readings that are higher by a set margin than those of a second nurse, even though there is disagreement on the absolute level of the DBP readings. Thus, if the issue is that measurement procedure produces consistent rankings regardless of who is measuring, then a reliability index of internal consistency would be sufficient. If, on the other hand, it is important to have absolute agreement among the alternative observers or raters, then a reliability index should be sensitive to differences in the absolute levels of scores, in addition to their relative standing.

---

[11] $r_{xy} = \frac{\Sigma(X_i - \bar{X})(Y_i - \bar{Y})}{(n-1)s_x s_y}$; if we add a constant c to every value of X, then the mean of X, $\bar{X}$ will also be larger by the constant c, resulting in the same difference of $(X_i - \bar{X})$.

The ICC in Table 21.3 based on a two-way mixed-effects ANOVA model shows an estimate of 0.94, slightly lower than the estimate of 0.953 in Table 21.2. This is so, because the second ICC takes into account the additional variation in scores associated with the different nurse raters. For a BP measure, this would certainly be an appropriate approach to measuring reliability. Overall, the results from the repeated DBP readings are quite impressive. If we create a scale score that combines, that is, averages the scores across all three measurement occasions, then the average DBP score will have a *reliability* of 94% true-score variance.

There are a number of different ICCs, depending on the assumption we make about fixed effect versus random effects, for example, comparing a particular nurse versus considering them a random sample of potential measure takers. We may also be interested in the reliability of a single measure taker rather than the reliability of the averaged values, on which we focused here. The interested reader may consult McGraw and Wong (1996) for more information, including the construction of confidence intervals for the ICCs.

CRONBACH'S ALPHA

Cronbach's Alpha is the most widely used reliability coefficient for a summated (or averaged) rating scale consisting of multiple indicator items. Typically, it is applied to responses from standardized rating scales, such as the CES-D depression scale. Such scales contain multiple questions or "items" (the CES-D has 20) designed to capture aspects of a psychological or health-related concept such as depression, anxiety, or physical functioning. Responses to individual items are usually predetermined, using rating scales with fixed numerical scores. Table 21.4 provides an example of response coding for the four "absence of well-being" subscale items of the CES-D depression scale (Radloff, 1977). In this situation, each item is considered more or less an equally good indicator of the underlying trait or psychological state to be measured. To the extent that this is the case, each item captures at least part of the "true" depression state; thus, we would expect respondents' answers to be internally consistent, which means they should correlate positively with each other. For instance, it would be inconceivable for a respondent to state that he or she was happy "most or all of the time" while also checking that he or she enjoyed life "rarely or none of the time." At the bottom of Table 21.4, we see the six bivariate correlations among the four CES-D scale items. These positive correlations do confirm that the responses to these items share common variance. What we need is a single index number that captures the reliability of the averaged scale score consisting of these four items. Cronbach's Alpha is the index of reliability commonly used for such data. The formula for Cronbach's Alpha, using the original, unstandardized scores is as follows:

$$A = \frac{k}{k-1}\left(1 - \frac{\sum_i^k \sigma_{x_i}^2}{\sigma_X^2}\right),$$

where k represents the number of individual items or measures that are part of the summated or averaged score (here: $k = 4$), $\sum_i^k \sigma_{x_i}^2$ refers to the sum of the k individual item variances, and σ_x^2 is the symbol for the variance of the summated scale score. This scale score is the sum of the k individual measures and the variance of a summated score is defined as the sum of the individual variances plus two times the sum of the covariances among the variables:

$$\sigma_X^2 = \sum_i^k \sigma_{x_i}^2 + 2\sum \sigma_{ij}$$

TABLE 21.4 Reliability of Four CES-D Items (Absence of Well-Being Subscale): Cronbach's Alpha

---

Question Stem:During the past two weeks, how often have you felt this way?

RCESD4:   I felt just as good as other people.
RCESD8:   I felt hopeful about the future.
RCESD12:   I was happy.
RCESD17:   I enjoyed life.

Answer categories for the four absence of well-being items are REVERSE coded so that higher numbers indicate greater tendency towards depression:

0 = most or all of the time, 1 = occasionally or a moderate amount of the time, 2 = some or a little of the time, 3 = rarely or none of the time.

Item	Obs	corr.	item-test corr.	item-rest corr.	alpha	Label
RCESD4	468	0.7094	0.4859	0.4856	0.7651	felt as good as others
RCESD8	468	0.7716	0.5705	0.4653	0.7230	hopeful
RCES12	468	0.8204	0.6649	0.4084	0.6745	happy
RCES16	468	0.7880	0.5919	0.4518	0.7117	enjoyed life
Test scale				0.4622	0.7741	

Inter item covariances (obs=468 in all pairs)

	RPCESD4	RPCESD8	RPCES12	RPCES16
RPCESD4	0.7726			
RPCESD8	0.3010	0.8329		
RPCES12	0.3128	0.4464	0.743	
RPCES16	0.3395	0.3689	0.4552	0.8649

Note: Diagonal entries are variances:
0.7726, 0.8329, 0.7430, 0.8649;
Off-diagonal entries are Ocovariances:
0.3010, 0.3128, 0.4464, 0.3395, 0.3689, 0.4552

Inter item correlations (obs=468 in all pairs)

	RPCESD4	RPCESD8	RPCES12	RPCES16	
RPCESD4	1.0000				
RPCESD8	0.3752	1.0000			
RPCES12	0.4128	0.5675	1.0000		
RPCES16	0.4153	0.4346	0.5679	1.0000	Mean Correlation:0.4622

Table 21.4 provides the inter-item covariance matrix for the four CES-D items from a study of 468 middle-aged (40–60) women, with the item variances on the diagonal and the inter-item covariances off the diagonal. With this information, we can compute the sum of the four individual item variances:

$$\sum_{i}^{k}\sigma_{x_i}^2 = 0.7726 + 0.8329 + 0.7430 + 0.8649 = 3.2134$$

Two times the sum of the covariances equals:

$$2\sum\sigma_{ij} = 2(0.3010 + 0.3128 + 0.4464 + 0.3395 + 0.3689 + 0.4552) = 4.4476$$

Thus, the variance of the summated scale score equals:

$$\sigma_X^2 = 3.2134 + 4.4476 = 7.661$$

Substituting into the Cronbach's Alpha formula, we get:

$$A = \frac{k}{k-1}\left(1 - \frac{\sum_i^k \sigma_{x_i}^2}{\sigma_X^2}\right) = \frac{4}{4-1}\left(1 - \frac{3.2134}{7.661}\right) = 0.7741$$

It is instructive to apply the Cronbach's Alpha coefficient to standardized variables or z-scores of the original item responses, as it allows us to see that the magnitude of the alpha coefficient depends only on two values: the number of measures or items (k) and the average correlation among them ($\bar{r}$). The formula for the standardized Cronbach's Alpha becomes[12]:

$$A = \frac{k}{k-1}\left(1 - \frac{k}{k + k(k-1)\bar{r}}\right)$$

This formula contains just two variables: k stands for the number of measures or items to be combined into a scale and stands $\bar{r}$ for the average correlation among them. This means that Cronbach's Alpha is a measure of internal consistency, but not a measure of absolute agreement. For instance, if 10 respondents had shown the following response patterns on two of the CES-D items: 0–0 ($n = 5$), 1–1 ($n = 3$), 2–2 ($n = 2$), then the sample correlation between these two items would be a perfect 1.0 among these 10 subjects; however, the same would be true for the following pairing: 0–1 ($n = 5$), 1–2 ($n = 3$), 2–3 ($n = 2$), even though the mean responses on the second item would be 1.7 instead of 0.7 for the first item. As Cronbach's Alpha is based only on the number of items and the average inter-item correlation, it is insensitive to systematic difference in mean responses across items. For a summated rating scale like the CES-D, which contains different indicator items to capture the underlying concept, this does not matter; in fact, it is often the case that some items (say the somatic indicators of depression) make a bigger or smaller contribution to the total scale score than other items (say the absence of well-being items in Table 21.4). However, for testing the reliability of repeated measures of the same measure, a reliability index like the ICC may be preferable, as it is sensitive to changes in mean scores. That is one reason, why Cronbach's Alpha is rarely used as an index of reliability for such repeated measurements as of the DBP. On the other hand, when mean differences between different measure takers or observers are quite small, Cronbach's Alpha could be used as an index of reliability: For the data in Table 21.2, the alpha coefficient is 0.95, only slightly different from the ICC values of 0.953 and 0.94 in Tables 21.2 and 21.3.

The results in Table 21.4 are quite remarkable. Even though the average correlation among the four CES-D scores is only moderately strong at 0.4622, the magnitude of the Alpha reliability coefficient indicates substantial reliability for the four-item scale score: $A = 0.7741$. Thus, if we create a CES-D subscale score measuring "absence of well-being" that combines,

---

[12] As the variance of a standardized variable is always equal to 1 (see Appendix I), the sum of the individual variances ($\Sigma_i^k \sigma_{x_i}^2$) must be equal to k; covariances between standardized variables are equal to the correlations among them, and thus $2\Sigma \sigma_{ij} = 2\Sigma r_{ij}$; with k variables there are $k(k-1)$ unique correlations, which means that the sum of the correlations equals $k(k-1)$ times the average correlation ($\bar{r}$). Finally, the variance of the summed *standardized* variables σ_{zx}^2 must be equal to $k + k(k-1)(\bar{r})$. Substitution into the original formula for Alpha yields: $A = \frac{k}{k-1}\left(1 - \frac{k}{k+k(k-1)\bar{r}}\right)$.

that is, averages the scores across all four measurement items, then this scale score will reflect an estimated or 77% true-score variance. Why should that be so? We started by assuming that each individual item response is influenced by the person's "true" sense of well-being and all sorts of extraneous, unrelated factors, which we collectively call "measurement error." About these random error components, we can say that sometimes a person overstates his or her sense of well-being; sometimes he or she underestimates it. Thus averaging four responses to similar items[13] will give us a more reliable indication of a person's sense of well-being than a single-item response.

There is an important caveat, when estimating the magnitude of Cronbach's Alpha to gauge the reliability/consistency of responses to multiple questionnaire items: The application of Cronbach's Alpha *assumes* that all the items are indicators of the same underlying concept to be measured. Thus, if indicators of related concepts, such as depression and anxiety, were combined into a single scale, Cronbach's Alpha could not be used to distinguish between them. In addition, the "reliability" of any collection of even marginally correlated items will appear to be quite high, if the number of items is large enough. Let us assume we have 25 items, for which the average inter-item correlation is only 0.15. Substituting these values into the standardized Alpha formula yields:

$$A = \frac{25}{25-1}\left(1 - \frac{25}{25 + 25(25-1)0.15}\right) = 0.815$$

Thus, even if a collection of items does not form a coherent unidimensional scale, but the number of items exceeds 20 or more, it is relatively easy to obtain "impressive" reliability estimates. Thus, before applying Cronbach's Alpha, the dimensionality and scalability of the items must be established first.[14]

COEFFICIENT OF CONCORDANCE *W*

In clinical practice and research, complex judgments must often be made incorporating a wide variety of evidence. One example would be the need to evaluate and grade the quality of the evidence for alternative treatments that the clinician may want to recommend (Guyatt et al., 2008). Another example of complex judgments would be the evaluation of the "medical urgency" for a liver transplant (HRSA, 2013), or the hiring decisions for a new nurse anesthetist concerning the choice among several applicants. In many situations such as these, professional judgments are required involving some kind of rating system. While it may not always be possible to clearly articulate all the implicit criteria used for judgment, it is possible and desirable to have several raters engage in ratings and judge the consistency of this rating process.

Table 21.5 provides a simple example of rating five applicants to a clinical position, with the ratings undertaken by four interviewers. It is important to keep in mind these are unequivocally ordinal ratings, so ICCs in particular, which assume at least interval-level measurement, should not be used. With data like these, Kendall's coefficient of concordance, also known as

---

[13]The term "similar items" is crucial here: It is *assumed*, when estimating the Cronbach's Alpha reliability coefficient that all items involved are designed to measure the same concept. If that is not the case, the alpha coefficient can give highly misleading information. This topic will be taken up in the next chapter on the principles of factor analysis.

[14]In Chapter 22 on factor analysis, we address these issues in more detail.

TABLE 21.5 Ratings of Five Job Applicants by Four Raters: Kendall's Coefficient of Concordance (*W*) as Reliability Test

```
             |            Job Applicants:
    ---------+--------------------------------
    Raters:  |     1     2     3     4     5
    ---------+--------------------------------
        1    |     1     2     3     5     4
        2    |     2     3     1     5     4
        3    |     2     1     3     4     5
        4    |     1     3     2     4     5
    ------------------------------------------
    Average Rank of  |
    Applicant (MRi): |    1.5   2.25  2.25  4.5   4.5
```

Kendall's Coefficient of Concordance:

$W = \Sigma(MR_i - TMR)^2/(N(N^2-1)/12)$,

where MR = mean rank of applicant i, TMR = total mean rank of all applicants

Computation based on Data Example:

$\Sigma[(1.5-3)^2 + (2.25-3)^2 + (2.25-3)^2 + (4.5-3)^2 + (4.5-3)^2]/[5(5^2-1)/12] =$

7.875/10 = 0.7875

Coefficient & p-value (null-hypothesis: complete absence of agreement)

Kendall = 0.7875
P-value = 0.0134

Kendall's *W*, provides a suitable reliability coefficient. One version of the formula for the *W* coefficient is as follows:

$$W = \frac{\sum_i^n (\bar{R}_i - \bar{\bar{R}})^2}{n(n^2 - 1)/12}$$

In Table 21.5, n refers to the number of applicants to be judged.[15] The numerator of this *W* formula shows the sum of squared deviations of each applicant's average rank from the grandtotal rank of all rankings. As the judges rank *n* applicants, each judge's mean rank equals $(n + 1)/2$; for the data in Table 21.5, we have: $(5 + 1)/2 = 3$. By the same token, the *mean* rank across all four judges and applicants, $\bar{\bar{R}}$, must also be 3. The denominator shows an expression, $n(n^2 - 1)/12$, that gives the *maximum possible* sum of squared deviations in the numerator, which would occur, if all raters agreed and the applicants' average ranking simplifies to 1, 2, ... 5. Thus, Kendall's *W* gives us a proportion indicating the ratio observed variation in rankings over the widest possible variation. If all raters agree on the different rankings, $W = 1$, if all applicants get the same average ranking, this means either that the raters cannot agree at all or they "refuse" to rank the applicants by giving everyone the same ranking. In that case $W = 0$, as the sum of squares in the numerator of the formula would be zero. Sample *W*-statistics are approximately distributed like a chi-squared distribution with $n - 1$ degrees of

---

[15]In general, *n* refers to any set of objects that are rank-ordered.

freedom (df).We can use this fact to test the null hypothesis that there is *no* agreement among the raters. For the example in Table 21.5, we have a *p*-value $\leq$.0134; thus we would reject the null hypothesis and conclude that there is substantial agreement among these raters and the rankings can be considered quite reliable ($W = 0.7875$).

COHEN'S KAPPA

Another class of reliability coefficients is kappa-based measures, which are commonly encountered in medical and nursing research and can also be used in clinical judgment situations. Different from the previous reliability coefficients, kappa coefficients can not only be applied to ordinal ratings but also to categorical judgments. A classic example would be the judgments of two or more radiologists who rate the same set of mammograms as indicating either malignancy or non malignancy (Crewson, 2005). Table 21.5 provides two simple examples of 100 mammograms rated by two radiologists. The *first* 2 × 2 frequency table indicates that radiologists A and B each agree that there are 30 images indicating malignant tumors, but they do not fully agree on which ones are indications of malignancy. One simple approach to such data would be to calculate the percentage of agreements: Both radiologists agree that 22 images show malignancies and 62 do not. Thus, for the 100 examined images, we have $(22 + 62)/100 = 0.84$, or 84% agreement between the two radiologists. However, using a mere percentage is a flawed approach, because we could ask: How much agreement would there be by chance if the two radiologists were to throw the dice to decide which of the 30 women have a malignant tumor? In other words, if the judgments about the individual mammograms were completely independent, we could multiply the probability of identifying a malignant tumor (.3) by both radiologists to obtain the joint probability that both radiologists report a malignant tumor: $.3 \times .3 = .09$. We can repeat multiplication to obtain the joint probability that both radiologists rate the images as showing no malignancy: $.7 \times .7 = .49$. So, even if the judgments of the two radiologists about individual cases were completely independent, we would still expect that 58% of the ratings agree ($.09 + .49 = .58$). To account for chance agreement, Cohen (1960) proposed an adjusted measure of agreement as follows:

$$\kappa = \frac{p_o - p_e}{1 - p_e}$$

In the numerator, we have the difference between the proportion of observed agreement, p_o, and the proportion of agreement expected by chance, p_e. Normally, we would expect that $p_o > p_e$ or that the amount of observed agreement exceeds the agreement level expected by chance. The denominator represents the maximum range, by which the proportion of observed agreement can exceed the proportion of expected random agreement, since p_o as cannot exceed 1. For the data in Table 21.6 we have:

$$\kappa = \frac{0.84 - 0.58}{1 - 0.58} = 0.619$$

According to Land is and Koch (1977), kappa values of 0.41 to 0.60 can be considered "moderate," those between 0.61 and 0.80 "substantial," and those between 0.80 and 1.00 "almost perfect." Thus, a classification procedure resulting in a kappa of around 0.62 should be considered to possess a high level of inter-rater reliability. Estimators of standard errors for Cohen's kappa are available for constructing confidence limits and for significance testing (Crewson, 2005; Lee & Tu, 1994). Kappa coefficients can also be computed if judgments are made concerning more than two categories, for example, the radiologists might adopt a rating system with three categories: malignant, suspicious, and nonmalignant. Kappa coefficients are not confined to comparing the rankings of two raters: An extension to the case of multiple raters is also available (Landis & Koch, 1977).

While the idea of judging observed agreement levels relative to agreement levels expected by chance is attractive, kappa coefficients do have some drawbacks. One major issue is the effect that different marginal case distributions have on the magnitude of kappa coefficients.

Table 21.6 provides a second table, which shows the two radiologists again agreeing in their interpretations of 84 out of 100 mammograms, but the marginal percentages indicate far fewer malignant cases (10% vs. 30%). As a result, the magnitude of the kappa estimate drops dramatically from 0.619 to a mere 0.111. This difference is, of course, due to the fact that, in the second case, the expected chance agreement level is much higher. It is not clear whether this should be considered a "problem" in the sense that an 84% agreement should be considered less impressive, if an 82% agreement can be expected by chance. Nonetheless, the

TABLE 21.6 Ratings of 100 Mammograms by Two Radiologists: Comparisons of Two Different Marginal Distributions With Same Percentage of Agreement

Ratings with .7/.3 Split in Marginal Distributions:

Radiologist B	Radiologist A		
	not malignant	malignant	
not malignant	62	8	70
malignant	8	22	30
	70	30	100

Agreement	Expected Agreement	Kappa	Std. Err.	Z	Prob>Z
84.00%	58.00%	0.6190	0.1000	6.190	.0000

Kappa = (0.84 − 0.58)/(1 − 0.58) = 0.619

Ratings with .9/.1 Split in Marginal Distributions:

Radiologist B	Radiologist A		
	not malignant	malignant	
not malignant	82	8	90
malignant	8	2	10
	90	10	100

Agreement	Expected Agreement	Kappa	Std. Err.	Z	Prob>Z
84.00%	82.00%	0.1111	0.1000	1.11	0.1333

Kappa = (0.84 − 0.82)/(1 − 0.82) = 0.111

more lopsided the marginal distributions, the more difficult it becomes for raters to exceed the standard set by the expected chance level of agreement. For a reader to judge the results from rater agreement studies, it is important to obtain information on the absolute level of agreement in addition to the kappa coefficient to provide important context.

EVALUATION OF MEDICAL TESTS

Medical tests are meant to be aids in clinical decision making. As such, they must meet the basic requirements of all measurement instruments: They must be valid and reliable. In the medical literature, the preferred terms are accuracy (validity) and reproducibility (reliability), indicating whether a test measures the intended target (accuracy) and delivers an acceptable level of precision upon repeated measurement (reproducibility). For instance, a blood glucose test may be used in the diagnosis of type 2 diabetes, but blood glucose levels are influenced by many factors, some of which exert transitory effects on the measured glucose levels, such as a patient having had a recent meal, the sampling fluctuations associated with drawing a particular blood sample, the quality control in the laboratory that produces the test results, and so forth. In short, a certain amount of measurement error, and thus unreliability, is endemic to all medical tests.

In most situations, where diagnostic and screening tests are used, the clinical decisions refer to binary outcomes, for example, the ascertainment of the presence or absence of a certain disease or condition. Two index numbers, sensitivity and specificity, are usually employed to indicate how well a diagnostic or screening test performs in identifying whether a person has or does not have an illness or condition of interest. As it turns out however, we cannot compare test results to the "true state of affairs," but only to other test results or diagnostic procedures that we take to be the "gold standard" for diagnosis. Those gold standards are, of course, subject to measurement error as well, even though they may be more reliable. For example, the gold standard in the evaluation of cancer screening tests is usually a biopsy; however, no biopsy procedure is 100% accurate (Kluttig et al., 2007). In the end, we are always comparing one fallible measure to another, even though we may have good reasons to prefer an established diagnostic tool as "better" than a new test. Keeping this in mind, we define **sensitivity** and **specificity** of a diagnostic or screening test as follows:

- The sensitivity of a diagnostic or screening test refers to the proportion of individuals in the target population, who have been—or will be—*diagnosed with a disease and are identified by the test as having the disease.*

- The specificity of a diagnostic or screening test refers to the proportion of individuals in the target population, who have been—or will be—*diagnosed as disease free and are identified by the tests as not having the disease.*

Note, we are not defining sensitivity and specificity in terms of the proportion of a target population who *has* or *does not have* the disease in question, because the only way to know whether they do or do not have the disease is by some other (fallible) methods of diagnosis. Thus, the descriptions in Table 21.7 of "true positives" or "true negatives," while following customary usage, should be taken with a grain of salt: The "truth" of the disease state does depend on diagnostic procedures, which themselves are subject to some error.

In the hypothetical example of Table 21.7, we could have adopted the following criteria as our gold standard for the diagnosis of diabetes mellitus (DM): presence of hyperglycemia symptoms, a fasting plasma glucose value of $FPG \geq 126$ mg/dL, and well-established diabetic retinopathy. Thus, to be diagnosed with DM, individuals would have to meet all of these

TABLE 21.7 Outcomes of a Diagnostic Medical Test of Hemoglobin A1c Levels and Diabetes Diagnosis Among 1,100 Individual Patients (Each Cell Shows the Proportion of Individuals With the Joint Diagnostic and Test Outcome)

		DIABETES DIAGNOSIS		ROW MARGINAL FREQUENCIES
		DIAGNOSED WITH DIABETES	NOT DIAGNOSED WITH DIABETES	
HbA1c	≥6.1%	TP: 0.0573	FP: 0.0236	L: 0.081
	<6.1%	FN: 0.0336	TN: 0.8855	(1− L): 0.919
Column marginal frequencies		P: 0.0909	(1 − P): 0.9091	1.000 (N = 1,100)

FN, false negatives; FP, false positives; L, level of test (percentage of positive test results); N, number of tested individuals; PR, prevalence of disease (percentage of tested individuals diagnosed with the four disease); TN, true negatives; TP, true positives.

criteria; those diagnosed as not having DM may not meet any of the criteria. Suppose now, we have HbA1c test results on 1,100 individuals, collected over 2 years in a large urban hospital, and want to know how good this test is in identifying DM patients. Using as an initial *reference criterion* that any person with a measured HbA1c $\geq 6.1\%$ should be classified as having DM, there are four possible outcomes from the test:

POSSIBLE OUTCOMES OF A DIAGNOSTIC OR SCREENING TEST

True positives (TP): both the HbA1c test and the gold standard are positive
True negatives (TN): both the HbA1c test and the gold standard are negative
False positives (FP): the HbA1c test is positive, but the gold standard is negative
False negatives (FN): the HbA1c test is negative, but the gold standard is positive

---

Before we continue, it is worth pausing here to reflect on the formal similarity of these outcomes to statistical hypothesis testing.

- A **false-positive** result from a diagnostic test is equivalent to the Type I error of a statistical test: That is, the evidence suggests either the effectiveness of an intervention or the presence of a disease, when neither is the case; in fact, the results are due to mere random sampling or measurement error.
- A **false-negative** result from a diagnostic test is equivalent to the Type II error of a statistical test: In these situations, the evidence suggests either the lack of effectiveness of an intervention or the absence of a disease, even though the intervention is effective or the disease is present, but mere random sampling or measurement error obscures this.
- A **true positive** result is equivalent to the power of a test: The test result agrees with the diagnosis about the presence of a disease, and the statistical inference agrees with the true state of affairs about the effectiveness of an intervention.
- Finally, a **true negative** test result leads us to the correct conclusion that the disease is absent, just as the acceptance of the null hypothesis is the correct conclusion, if an intervention is not effective.

When assessing the usefulness of a diagnostic test, a clinician is usually less interested in its sensitivity and specificity and more in the test's ability to predict disease outcomes. The index numbers reflecting the predictive ability of a diagnostic or screening test are known as positive and negative predictive values. Here are the requisite definitions in terms of the four basic test outcomes:

DEFINITIONS OF TEST STATISTICS ASSOCIATED WITH DIAGNOSTIC OR SCREENING TESTS
Sensitivity (SE): $TP/P = TP/(TP + FN)$ Specificity (SP): $TN/(1 - P) = TN/(FP + TN)$ Positive predictive value (PPV): $TP/L = TP/(TP + FP)$ Negative predictive value (NPV): $TN/(1 - L) = TN/(TN + FN)$ The prevalence (PR) of a disease in a target population: $(TP + FN)$ The level (L) of the test: $(TP + FP)$ Efficiency (E): $(TP + TN)$

If we apply these definitions to the data in Table 21.7, we get the following results:

$SE = 0.0573/0.091 = 0.63$; $SP = 0.8855/0.909 = 0.974$; $PPV = 0.0573/0.081 = 0.707$; $NPV = 0.8855/0.919 = 0.964$; $PR = 0.0573+0.0336 = 0.091$; $L = 0.0573+0.0236 = 0.081$; $E = 0.0573+0.8855 = 0.943$.

Based on these data, we see that the HbA1c test with a cut-off point of 6.1% has a sensitivity of 0.63, which means that 63.0% of those diagnosed with DM also have an HbA1c result of equal to or greater than 6.1%. Similarly, specificity for this test is 0.974, or 97.4% of those with a negative diagnosis also fall below the critical test value of 6.1%. Likewise, the PPV of this test is 0.707, meaning that 70.7% of those with a positive test result actually are diagnosed with DM. Among those with a negative test result, 96.4% also have been diagnosed not to have DM (NPV = 0.964). What is perhaps not apparent from the definitions of the PPV and NPV is that their *estimates are dependent on the prevalence of the disease in the target population*. To demonstrate this, we convert the proportions in Table 21.7 to case numbers in Table 21.8, adding a second table with changed prevalence of the diagnostic results.

The data in Table 21.8 show the test results for two different patient populations, one with a 9.09% prevalence of DM according to the gold-standard diagnosis, the other with a 36.36% prevalence of DM. Note that the sensitivity and specificity values of the tests remain the same in the two populations: $SE = 63/100 = 252/400 = 0.63$; $SP = 974/1,000 = 682/700 = 0.974$. However, the PPV in the low-prevalence population is: $PPV_{LPR} = 63/89 = 0.708$; and in the high-prevalence population it is: $PPV_{HPR} = 252/270 = 0.933$. That means that the proportion of false-positive test results is 6.7% $(1 - 0.933)$ in the high-prevalence patient population, but 29.2% $(1 - 0.708)$ in the low-prevalence population. It is this dependency of false-positive rates on the prevalence of a disease that can make the application of screening tests in the general population quite problematic: When the prevalence of a disease is low—for many diseases like various cancer types prevalence is less than 0.5% in the general population—even a test with high levels of sensitivity and specificity returns mostly false-positive results.

TABLE 21.8 Dependence of Positive and Negative Predictive Values on Prevalence of Disease (Based on Gold-Standard Diagnostic Procedure)

TEST RESULTS FROM LOW-PREVALENCE POPULATION			
PREVALENCE OF DIAGNOSIS: 100/1,100 = 9.09%	DIABETES DIAGNOSIS		ROW MARGINAL FREQUENCIES
	DIAGNOSED WITH DIABETES	NOT DIAGNOSED WITH DIABETES	
HbA1c ≥6.1%	63	26	89
HbA1c <6.1%	37	974	1,011
Column marginal frequencies:	100	1,000	1,100
TEST RESULTS FROM HIGH-PREVALENCE POPULATION			
PREVALENCE OF DIAGNOSIS: 400/1,100 = 36.36%	DIABETES DIAGNOSIS		ROW MARGINAL FREQUENCIES
	DIAGNOSED WITH DIABETES	NOT DIAGNOSED WITH DIABETES	
HbA1c ≥6.1%	252	50	279
HbA1c <6.1%	142	650	824
Column marginal frequencies:	400	700	1,100

So far, we have focused on a single cut-off point for the HbA1c test; but we could have chosen many other cut-off points as the critical value for our decision that the patient has the disease in question. Table 21.9 shows the sensitivities and specificities for 13 selected cut-offs or thresholds among the 1,100 patients, 100 of whom are diagnosed with DM (PR = 0.091). A brief look at Table 21.9 reveals the trade-off between sensitivity and specificity: lower

TABLE 21.9 Sensitivities and Specificities for a Range of Referent Values/Cut-Off Points of Hemoglobin A1c Levels to Test for the Presence of Diabetes Mellitus

THRESHOLD FOR CUT-OFF (%)	PREVALENCE	SENSITIVITY (%)	SPECIFICITY (%)	TEST LEVEL (%)	KAPPA-ADJUSTED SENSITIVITY (%)	KAPPA-ADJUSTED SPECIFICITY (%)	EFFICIENCY (%)
≥4.5	0.091	100.0	0.0	100.00		0.00	9.09
≥4.7	0.091	100.0	4.2	85.79	100.00	1.66	12.91
≥4.9	0.091	99.0	8.5	72.88	94.73	3.53	16.73
≥5.1	0.091	98.0	31.6	63.26	84.46	4.90	37.64
≥5.3	0.091	97.0	54.4	50.79	79.68	7.72	58.27
≥5.5	0.091	94.0	71.3	40.46	76.00	11.18	73.36
≥5.7	0.091	89.0	85.4	31.29	68.81	15.11	85.73
≥5.9	0.091	78.0	94.9	21.28	61.89	22.89	93.36
≥6.1	0.091	63.0	97.4	12.10	57.75	41.92	94.27
≥6.3	0.091	47.0	98.1	7.38	46.02	57.73	93.45
≥6.5	0.091	30.0	98.7	3.44	27.51	77.30	92.45
≥6.7	0.091	12.0	99.2	1.04	10.50	100.00	91.27
≥6.9	0.091	0.0	99.8	0.00	0.00		90.73
≥6.9	0.091	0.0	100.0	0.00	0.00		90.91

cut-off points are associated with higher sensitivity values, but lower specificity; higher cut-off points are associated with lower sensitivity values, but higher specificity.[16] Under these circumstances, what is the "right" cut-off point to choose?

The answer is not as straightforward as one might think. In particular, it depends on the purpose of the testing. Suppose, a medical researcher wanted to enroll DM patients in an intervention study designed to improve patient control of DM. In such a study it would be important to have high confidence that all enrolled subjects do have DM. In that situation, one would choose a cut-off point that yields high specificity on the HbA1c tests, as that would ensure that the number of false-positive subjects in the study is minimized. On the other hand, if one intends to screen the general population for DM, it is more important to minimize false-negative results: We would not want to conclude that a tested person does not have DM, if in fact he or she has it. This situation would require us to choose a cut-off point, which results in high sensitivity. In other situations, it may be tempting to choose as a cut-off point the one that produces the highest **efficiency** (percentage of correctly classified individuals, which equals TP plus TN). However, like the predictive values, efficiency changes with the prevalence of a disease or condition in the tested population and does not deliver an unequivocal index of "best" cut-off point.

To complicate matters further, sensitivity and specificity themselves are not unequivocal indices of the quality of a test. So far, we have not asked whether the sensitivity and specificity values of a test exceed the values we would get by chance. Employing kappa-based statistics, we could adjust for the level of *expected* sensitivity or specificity. Going back to the data in Table 21.7, we see that the overall level of the test (L), that is, the probability of getting a positive test result with HbA1c levels greater than or equal to 6.1% is 0.081 or 8.1% *regardless of the actual diagnosis*. Obviously, we anticipate that our test can do better than that among people who are diagnosed with diabetes. Thus, we require at a minimum that the sensitivity exceeds this level. Using the same logic as in the establishment of inter-rater reliability, we can use the results expected from a random test[17] as our benchmark, to construct a kappa-based adjusted sensitivity:

$$\kappa = \frac{SE - L}{1 - L} = \frac{0.632 - 0.081}{1 - 0.081} = 0.600$$

Similarly, we can adjust the specificity values for expected specificities of a random test:

$$\kappa = \frac{SP - (1 - L)}{1 - (1 - L)} = \frac{0.974 - 0.919}{0.081} = 0.679$$

Now it becomes clear that a specificity of 97.4% is less impressive, if 91.9% of all test results are negative, regardless of diagnosis. Table 21.9 shows the test levels and kappa-adjusted sensitivities and specificities for selected cut-off levels of the HbA1c test. The prevalence of diabetes in the target population remains the same, regardless of the cut-off points chosen. On the other hand, the level of the test (L), that is, the percentage of tested individuals with a positive test result, depends on the cut-off point chosen for the HbA1c test: It declines with higher cut-off points. The kappa-*adjusted* sensitivity and specificity values suggest that the HbA1c

---

[16]Again, these trade-offs are analogous to the trade-offs between Type I and Type II errors in statistical hypothesis testing.

[17]A random test would be useless in picking out those who have been diagnosed with DM, because such a test has the same probability of a positive test result among individuals with or without a DM diagnosis.

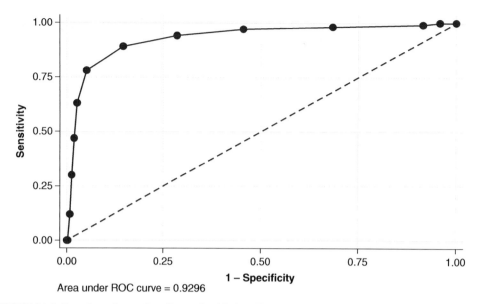

Area under ROC curve = 0.9296

FIGURE 21.1 Receiver-Operating Curve for HbA1c Test to Detect DM, Based on 1,100 Patients of Whom 100 Are Diagnosed With DM.

performs better than a random test at all cut-off points, except if sensitivity and specificity both are either 0% or 100%. However, the test performance is not as good as suggested by the *unadjusted* sensitivity and specificity values (Kraemer, 1992).

So, how should we decide on what is a good test? One way to demonstrate the trade-offs between the sensitivity and specificity of a diagnostic or screening test is to graph a so-called receiver-operating curve (ROC). It shows the trade-off by plotting sensitivity values against the values of 1 − specificity for each test cut-off point contemplated. For example, the ROC plot in Figure 21.1 is based on the 13 cut-off points exhibited in Table 21.9.

The first question we might ask about the quality of the HbA1c test is, whether or not it outperforms a *random test*. A random test has average positive results equal to the level of the test (L), but in a random test, these results are unrelated to the actual diagnosis. Such a test would have the same probability of returning a positive result, regardless of whether a person has been diagnosed with DM or not.

In that case, the expected probability of a TP would be equal to PR × L (the product of prevalence and the level of the test) and the expected probability of a true negative result would be (1 − PR) × (1 − L). It can be shown that, for such a test, SE + SP = 1 and, therefore: SE = 1 − SP. In words, for a random test without any diagnostic capability, sensitivity equals one minus specificity. In Figure 21.1, the trade-off between sensitivity and specificity for a random test is indicated by the dashed diagonal line. For a test that actually contains new information about the patients' disease state, we would expect that TP > PR × L and TN > (1 − PR) × (1 − L). As the data in Table 21.7 show, at the test cut-off point of 6.1%, TP = 0.0573 > PR × L = 0.091 × 0.081 = 0.0074; TN = 0.885 > (1 − PR) × (1 − L) = 0.909 × 0.919 = 0.8354. Thus, the HbA1c test with a cut-off point greater than or equal to 6.1% does perform better than a random test. In fact, as the ROC in Figure 21.1 shows, the sums of sensitivity and specificity values exceed 1 at every cut-off point except at the extremes.[18] Figure 21.1 also indicates that

---

[18]This can also be seen from the results in Table 21.9: there the sums of sensitivity and specificity exceed 100%.

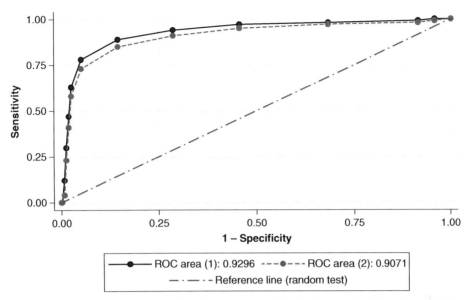

FIGURE 21.2 Comparison of HbA1c Test Results From Two Laboratories, Based on 1,100 Patients of Whom 100 Are Diagnosed With DM.

the area under the ROC curve equals 0.9296. The size of this area can be interpreted as the probability that a person diagnosed with DM will have a higher test score on the HbA1c test than a person not so diagnosed. In general, a greater area under the ROC curve indicates better overall performance of the diagnostic or screening test. From this it follows that we could evaluate the comparative performance of two different test procedures, by comparing the areas under the ROC curves associated with the two different test procedures. Assume we send the blood vials of the 1,100 patients to two different laboratories and then compare the resulting test classifications. Figure 21.2 shows that the area under the ROC curve for the test results from the first laboratory (0.9296) is larger than the area under the ROC curve for the second laboratory (0.9071). DeLong, DeLong, and Clarke-Pearson (1988) developed a chi-squared-based test for the comparison of areas under different ROCs. In this case, we obtain a chi-squared value of 19.84 (df = 1, $p < .0001$) for the null hypothesis that the area under ROC1 − area under ROC2. Estimates of standard errors and confidence limits for the ROC areas are also available. We have established now that the HbA1c test is better than a random or "blind" test,[19] and we have a method for evaluating the comparative performance of different tests or test procedures.

SUMMARY

In this chapter, we have focused on several reliability indices, which are used to gauge the extent to which the measurements are free of random measurement error. This is of great importance for both research and clinical decisions: Unreliable measures reduce our ability to show relationships and they increase errors in clinical decisions. In practice, reliability of

---

[19] We could use the Pearson chi-squared test to establish the appropriate p-values, if we have information on the sample size.

measurement can only be established, if multiple measures or multiple indicators are available: We cannot estimate the amount of reliability or unreliability with a single score measure.

It is important to keep in mind that reliability, even if high, only speaks to the repeatability of a measurement procedure, but not to its validity. Going back to the example of rating mammograms, even if two or more radiologists agree 100% on how to interpret the same radiographs, this is no "guarantee" that the interpretations reflect the "truth": They might both be mistaken. The establishment of validity requires more than showing substantial internal consistency among multiple raters or indicators. Supporting the validity of a measurement tool or procedure may involve the use of external criteria (like biopsy results in the case of mammograms); it also requires a theoretically plausible measurement model that can be tested against data. One large class of statistical models, commonly used in the exploration and testing of measurement models, is factor analysis. The next chapter will provide an outline and some simple examples of factor analytical techniques, as they are often encountered in health-related research articles.

LITERATURE APPLICATION

Read: Monsen, K. A., Lytton, A. B., Ferrari, S., Halder, K. M., Radosevich, D. M., Kerr, M. J., ... Brandt, J. K. (2012). Evaluating reliability of assessments in nursing documentation. *Online Journal of Nursing Informatics, 15*(3).

(a) Provide a very brief (three to four sentences) summary of what this study is about.

(b) Define the target population on which the statistical analysis is based. What were the eligibility and exclusion criteria for study records? Is the study sample a random sample of its target population?

(c) Do the authors explain why they chose their particular measures of reliability?

(d) In your own words, write a short paragraph about the major results.

(e) Are the conclusions of the authors warranted?

EXERCISES

1. The following table shows the correlations among five depression symptoms obtained from a sample of 428 primary care patients. Using a hand calculator and the formula provided in this chapter, compute the sample Cronbach's Alpha coefficient.

```
(obs=428)
          |   sad   nervous restles  shope   less effort
----------+---------------------------------------------
      sad | 1.000
  nervous | 0.567   1.000
 restless | 0.525   0.644   1.000
 hopeless | 0.599   0.513   0.507   1.000
   effort | 0.545   0.524   0.532   0.604   1.000
```

2. If the error variance estimated for a measurement tool equals 15.6 and the total observed variance equals 19.5, what is the estimated reliability of this measurement tool?

3. Compute Kendall's coefficient of concordance (W) for the following ratings of four mammograms by three medical students.

```
                |           Mammograms:
----------------+------------------------------
Student Raters: |  1      2      3      4
----------------+------------------------------
        1       |  1      2      2      3
        2       |  2      1      1      2
        3       |  2      3      3      2
----------------+------------------------------
1 = probably cancer-free
2 = uncertain
3 = probable cancer
```

4. The following table shows the distribution of the test results from a screening test among 10,000 tested individuals. Compute the following statistics: prevalence, sensitivity, specificity, positive and negative predictive values, efficiency, level of the test, kappa-adjusted sensitivity and specificity.

```
              |        True Disease State:
--------------+-----------------+-------------
Test Results: |   has disease   |  no disease
--------------+-----------------+-------------
  positive    |      215        |     780
  negative    |       35        |    8970
--------------+-----------------+-------------
              |      250        |    9750
```

5. Using the statistical models discussed in this chapter, evaluate the reliability of one or two clinical tests used in your clinical practice.

REFERENCES

Cohen, J. (1960). A coefficient of agreement for nominal scales. *Educational and Psychological Measurement, 20*(1), 37–46.

Crewson, P. E. (2005). Fundamentals of clinical research for radiologists: Reader agreement studies. *American Journal of Roentgenology, 184*(5), 1391–1397.

DeLong, E. R., DeLong, D. M., & Clarke-Pearson, D. L. (1998). Comparing the areas under two or more correlated receiver operating characteristic curves: A nonparametric approach. *Biometrics, 44*(3), 837–845.

Guyatt, G. H., Oxman, A. D., Vist, G. E., Kunz, R., Falck-Ytter, Y., Alonso-Coello, P., . . . Schünemann, H. J.; for the GRADE Working Group. (2008). GRADE: An emerging consensus on rating quality of evidence and strength of recommendations. *British Medical Journal, 336*(7650), 924–926.

HRSA. (2013). Organ procurement and transplantation network. Retrieved from http://optn.transplant.hrsa.gov

Kluttig, A., Trocchi, P., Heinig, A., Holzhausen, H. J., Taege, C., Hauptmann, S., . . . Stang, A. (2007). Reliability and validity of needle biopsy evaluation of breast-abnormalities using the B-categorization—Design and objectives of the Diagnosis Optimisation Study (DIOS). *BMC Cancer, 7*, 100. doi:10.1186/1471-2407-7-100

Kroenke, K., & Spitzer, R. L. (2002). The PHQ-9: A new depression and diagnostic severity measure. *Psychiatric Annals, 32*(9), 509–521.

Landis, J. R., & Koch, G. G. (1977). The measurement of observer agreement for categorical data. *Biometrics, 33*(1), 159–174.

Lee, J. J., & Tu, Z. N. (1994). A better confidence interval for kappa on measuring agreement between two raters with binary outcomes. *Journal of Computational and Graphical Statistics, 3*(3), 301–321.

McGraw, K. O., & Wong, S. P. (1996). Forming inferences about some intra class correlation coefficients. *Psychological Methods, 1*(1), 30–46.

National Cancer Institute (NCI): Prostate-specific antigen (PSA) test. Retrieved from http://www.cancer.gov /cancertopics/factsheet/detection/PSA (accessed 1 October 2013).

Nunnally, J. C., & Bernstein, I. H. (1994). *Psychometric theory* (3rd ed.). New York, NY: McGraw-Hill.

Radloff, L. S. (1977). The CES-D scale: A self report depression scale for research in the general population. *Applied Psychological Measurements, 1*(3), 385–401.

Yesavage, J. A., Brink, T. L., Rose, T. L., Lum, O., Huang, V., Adey, M., . . . Leirer, V. O. (1982–1983). Development and validation of a geriatric depression screening scale: A preliminary report. *Journal of Psychiatric Research, 17*(1), 37–49.

Zung, W. W. (1971). A rating instrument for anxiety disorders. *Psychosomatics, 12*(6), 371–379.

CHAPTER 22

Factor Analysis

In the last chapter, we addressed reliability in measurement, but skirted issues of validity. As stated previously, reliability is essentially a matter of reproducibility and repeatability of measurement results, which implies the relative absence of random measurement error. To address validity in measurement is not just a statistical matter, but also a conceptual and theoretical problem. For instance, nurses have developed pain and symptom scales, are interested in psychological constructs such as self-efficacy, patient resiliency, depression and anxiety, and so forth, because of their well-documented relationship to patient coping behavior, speed of recovery from illness, or adherence to a medication regimen. In addition, concepts such as physical and social functioning and the very concept of health itself are indispensable for judging the effectiveness of clinical interventions. At the same time, such constructs are exceedingly abstract and are not easy to measure. Still, measurement of the key concepts in an investigation is the most basic requirement for progress in science: without valid and reliable measurement, we do not have an empirical basis, beyond the level of personal impression, for documenting advances in clinical treatment. As psychology has been the first discipline to operationalize, that is, to develop, empirical indicators for concepts representing attitudes, behaviors, and emotions, the statistical models to test the appropriate measurement models have been developed in a specialized branch of statistic known as psychometrics.

Most of the psycho-social concepts mentioned—for example, pain, resiliency, depression—cannot be measured directly, but their presence must be inferred from empirical indicators, which often consist of observations of patient behavior or self-reports by patients. The most common approach to measuring such concepts is to use questionnaire responses to multiple questions, which are designed to cover the concept of interest. The development of such items is an arduous process, which takes many iterations. It is discussed in several research method texts (Polit & Beck, 2011; Stommel & Wills, 2004; Trochim & Donnelly, 2008), but our focus here is on the main statistical tool employed in the development and confirmation of such multiple-item instruments: factor analysis.

At its most basic, factor analysis is a set of statistical techniques that can be used to either find variable groupings or clusters (exploratory factor analysis [EFA]) or test for the existence of predetermined variable groupings or clusters (confirmatory factor analysis [CFA]). Many factor analysis models are based on the *assumption* that observed variables are expressions of some underlying *latent* variables, which are not directly observable.

TABLE 22.1 Hypothetical Correlations Among the Responses to Six CES-D Question Items Designed as Indicators of Depression

X1: I felt depressed; X2: I felt hopeful about the future; X3: I was happy; X4: I enjoyed life; X5: I had crying spells; X6: I felt sad.

Answer categories (with reverse coding for positively worded items 2, 3, 4): "rarely or none of the time" (0 or 3); "some or little of the time" (1 or 2); "occasionally or a moderate amount" (2 or 1);"most or all of the time" (3 or 0)

	X1	X2	X3	X4	X5	X6
X1	1.00					
X2	0.21	1.00				
X3	0.34	0.40	1.00			
X4	0.34	0.40	0.64	1.00		
X5	0.56	0.24	0.38	0.38	1.00	
X6	0.63	0.27	0.43	0.43	0.72	1.00

Thus, if the factor model is a correct description of reality, these latent variables, also called *common factors*, would account for most if not all of the covariances or correlations among the observed variables.

To get a handle on the basic principles of factor analysis, we will start with a simple model. Suppose we want to measure clinical depression among a sample of patients. According to the *Diagnostic and Statistical Manual of Mental Disorders,* 5th edition (*DSM-5*),[1] clinical depression involves multidimensional symptoms; among them are depressed mood and anhedonia, which refers to the inability to experience pleasure, including a lack of positive affect. Many of the standardized depression scales, such as the Beck Depression Inventory (BDI), Hamilton Depression Scale (HDS), and Center for Epidemiologic Studies-Depression Scale (CES-D) have individual indicators of both depressed mood and anhedonia.[2] Table 22.1 shows six question items from among the 20 items of the CES-D self-report scale (Radloff, 1977), together with the response formats and the codes in parentheses. The table also shows a hypothetical correlation matrix among these six items. The correlations are similar to what one might observe in a real data set, but they were constructed so as to fit a theoretical factor model *exactly*. When we analyze the responses to questions such as these depression items, we make the basic assumption that it is the underlying, unobservable depression, or its absence, that gives rise to the particular answers chosen by a respondent. For instance, an individual, who suffers from depression at the time when he or she is asked to fill out the questionnaire, is unlikely to choose the answer "most or all of the time" in response to the statement "I was happy." Similarly, this respondent is likely to check "most or all of the time" or at least "occasionally or a moderate amount of time" following the statement "I feel sad." Thus, we would expect that responses to these six questions all correlate positively with each other, as depressed individuals are likely to choose higher-scoring responses and non depressed individuals are likely to choose lower-scoring responses.

At the same time, we do not expect the responses to be perfectly correlated, because not all symptoms addressed in these six question items need to be present in a depressed person.

[1]Fifth edition of the *Diagnostic and Statistical Manual of Mental Disorders,* 5th edition (*DSM-5*), published by the American Psychiatric Association (www.dsm5.org/Pages/Default.aspx).
[2]Beck Depression Inventory (BDI), Hamilton Depression Scale (HDS), Center for Epidemiologic Studies-Depression Scale.

In addition, there are random measurement errors[3] and individuals may differ in their understanding of the unique wording of a particular item.[4]

We can formalize these assumptions into a model. Earlier we stated that depression is a multidimensional concept that includes the dimensions of "depressed mood" and "lack of positive affect." The six question items displayed in Table 21.1 are intended to capture these two distinct aspects of the depression concept, with three indicators for each subconcept. It may not be hard to discern, based on the contents of the items, which three question items are intended to capture a respondent's depressed mood and which three are intended to capture a lack of positive affect. But a purely conceptual analysis of concepts and their question indicators is not enough, because the important empirical question remains: Do the *respondents* actually make this distinction between depressed mood and absence of positive affect? Thus we have to use the empirical information contained in the correlation pattern to see whether the theoretical distinction we draw actually reflects how members of the target population think about depression.[5] As for Table 22.1 the correlations were constructed that way on the basis of hypothetical data, a factor model is available that explains the observed correlations *perfectly* and comports with the theoretical assumptions. Figure 22.1 provides a graphical depiction of that model. It shows two (common) factors, with F_1 referring to "Depressed Mood" and F_2 referring to "Lack of Positive Affect." The curved two-sided arrow on the left side indicates that we assume that these two factors are correlated, as they are subsumed under the broader concept of "Depression." The gray boxes represent the measured variables, that is, the responses to the six CES-D items. According to the graph, they are being influenced by the two latent common factors, each of which affects the responses of three indicator variables directly. In addition, the responses to the six items are also influenced by "unique" factors (U), which may include reactions to the particular wording of an item as well as the effects of random measurement errors.

The following equations capture the main features of the factor model in Figure 22.1:

$$Z_1 = 0.7F_1 + 0.71U_1; \quad Z_5 = 0.8F_1 + 0.6U_5; \quad Z_6 = 0.9F_1 + 0.44U_6$$

$$Z_2 = 0.5F_2 + 0.87U_2; \quad Z_3 = 0.8F_2 + 0.6U_3; \quad Z_4 = 0.8F_2 + 0.6U_4$$

The dependent variables in these equations are standardized versions (z_i-scores) of the observed indicator variables: They have means equal to zero and variances equal to one.[6] The coefficients associated with the factors, which are also standardized, are known as factor loadings (l). These factor loadings can be thought of as standardized regression coefficients

---

[3] Again, measurement error is ubiquitous; for instance, a particular respondent may have poor eyesight leading him to make the check mark on a response category that does not reflect his true feelings, or there may be data entry errors, and so forth.

[4] Some questions may provoke responses that are unique to them, because the language used in them is misunderstood, for instance.

[5] Depression is a well-developed psychological concept, but many concepts used in nursing research such as "perceptions of critical incidents" (O'Connor & Jeavons, 2003) or "student satisfaction with nursing education" (Espeland & Indrehus, 2003) are in an exploratory stage, whose value remains to be determined. Certainly during the scale development phase for such concepts, the researcher cannot know in advance how the responses to the proposed indicator items actually relate to each other in a particular target population.

[6] $z_i = \dfrac{X_i - \overline{X}_i}{SD_i}.$

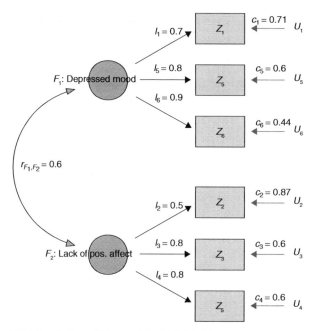

FIGURE 22.1 Graphical Depiction of Factor Model With Six Indicators and Two Correlated Factors.

or betas.[7] Finally, the unique factors (U_i) represent all idiosyncratic influences on individual item responses (including measurement error). They are standardized as well with variances of one, and the standardized coefficients (c_i) associated with the U_i reflect the strength of these unique influences on an observed indicator variable.

The graph in Figure 22.1 also incorporates additional features and assumptions:

1. The two latent factors are correlated, with $r_{F1,F2} = 0.6$.

2. All correlations between unique factors equal zero: $r_{Ui,Uj} = 0.0$.

3. All correlations between latent factors and unique factors equal zero: $r_{Fi,Uj} = 0.0$.

4. The amount of variance, which each observed indicator variable shares with the other variables through the common factor, equals the square of its factor loading (l_i^2).[8] This shared variance is also known as *communality*, which is usually indicated by h_i^2. The amount of variance that is *unique* to each observed indicator variable is represented by the square of the coefficient representing the influence of U_i (c_i^2). As the source of variance of an observed variable is either shared with the common factors (common variance) or unique, we get: communality = 1 − uniqueness, or $l_i^2 = 1 - c_i^2 = h_i^2$. Thus communality and uniqueness make up the total variance of the observed indicator variable.

---

[7]See Chapter 12. In a simple regression, with one independent variable, or factor as in this case, the betas are equal to the correlation between the factor and the indicator variable. The reason for standardizing all the variables in these equations is that it simplifies the presentation: Covariances of standardized variables reduce to correlations and variances are all equal to 1. See Appendix I for more details.
[8]This is true, because each observed variable in this model loads only on a single factor. With multiple factor loadings, the expression for shared variance is a bit more complicated.

With these equations and assumptions in place, we can now reconstruct the correlation matrix in Table 22.1. For instance, correlations between indicator variables of the *same* factor simplify to the product of the two factor loadings involved, for example, $r_{Z1,Z2} = 0.7 \times 0.8 = 0.56$. Correlations between indicator variables of different factors are equal to the product of the factor loadings and the correlation between the two factors, for example, $r_{Z6,Z3} = 0.9 \times 0.6 \times 0.8 = 0.43$. Using the equations and the inter-factor correlations, we can reconstruct all correlations among the indicator variables in Table 22.1. When a factor model provides a good description of the inter-item correlation pattern, it represents a substantial empirical (and conceptual) simplification of the data: After all, in the example we showed that the six indicator variables can be reduced to two factor variables, which capture the entire correlational pattern among the original six variables.

Of course, the factor model presented in Figure 22.1 reproduces the correlation matrix in Table 22.1 perfectly, because the latter was *constructed* on the basis of the predetermined factor model. However, in a typical research situation, we would have sample data and could compute the correlations among the relevant variables, but we would not know for sure what the underlying factor model should be; rather, in EFA we start with the data, which are subject to sampling fluctuations, and try to "extract" a factor model from the data that is both consistent with the data and theoretically plausible.[9] As it turns out, this is not always an easy task, because factor solutions are fundamentally indeterminate, that is, they have multiple solutions.

STEPS IN EFA

Initial Factor Extraction

While we have emphasized that factors are latent variables, which are not directly observable, in Figure 21.1 we treated them like any other observable variable, referring to standardized regression coefficients or "loadings" linking the observed variables to the factors. However, we have not yet answered the questions (a) how to obtain scores that represent these factors, and (b) how to determine how many factors are needed to represent the correlation pattern well enough. As EFA is a data reduction technique, the whole point of the technique is to find fewer factors than the number of original variables, which nonetheless capture most of the important variation in the data. For instance, in the factor model presented in Figure 22.1 we have two factors, labeled "Depressed Mood" and "Lack of Positive Affect" that account for the common variance among six variables. If we can find a way of substituting factor scores for the original scores from the six variables, we would still capture all the essential information in the data, but would have simplified the analysis both from a conceptual and an empirical point of view.

There are entire books devoted to the ins and outs of factor-analytic techniques, but these are for the specialist to study. A full technical understanding requires knowledge of matrix algebra, because a major part of factor analysis revolves around the problems of solving simultaneous equations.[10] Still, given that factor-analytic applications are widespread in the nursing and medical literature (Watson & Thompson, 2006), it is important to gain a thorough conceptual understanding of this technique.

---

[9] In some EFA, the underlying "theory" or conceptual framework is not yet well developed and researchers let themselves be guided to some degree by the patterns discovered in the data. Such analyses are preliminary and require confirmation with new data sets. For a nontechnical discussion of what is involved in scale development, see Chapter 16, Stommel and Wills (2004).

[10] A classic text is Harman (1976); a nontechnical introduction is provided by Child (2006).

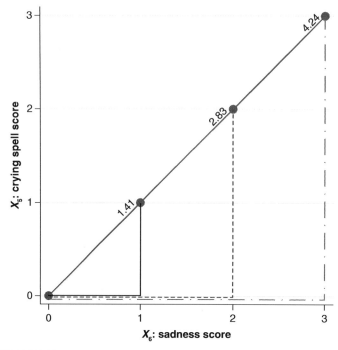

FIGURE 22.2 Principal Axis Representing Scores of Two Variables.

Among the techniques for the initial extraction of factors are principal component analysis (PCA),[11] principal axis factoring, maximum likelihood factoring (MLF), least squares factoring (LQF) and a few others. Here, we will not discuss all the details and differences among them, in part, because different extraction methods tend to give very similar results, *if* the data really can be represented by a few factors. Instead, we aim at clarifying the underlying ideas of what "factor extraction" represents, followed by an example of how to interpret the output from an EFA performed on actual data.

Suppose we have the scores of four respondents to two of the CES-D items shown in Table 22.1: X_5: "I had crying spells" and X_6: "I felt sad." Now suppose further that, while each respondent experiences a different level of depressed mood, he or she is consistent in answering both questions. Thus we get the following pairs of scores: 0–0, 1–1, 2–2, and 3–3. Figure 22.2 provides a graphical representation of the four scores on each of the variables.

As the paired scores on both variables are the same, the line connecting the scores is a 45° diagonal. Given this perfect alignment of the scores on the two variables, we can simplify the description of each individual's responses. Rather than describing each respondent's position using two scores from two variables, we could, without loss of information, transform the two scores of each individual into a single score on a new variable. Using the Pythagorean theorem about the length of the sides of a rectangular triangle, we can convert the two X_5 and X_6 scores into a new single score on the diagonal "depressed mood" line: $DM = \sqrt{X_5^2 + X_6^2}$. For instance, a respondent, who checked "occasionally or a moderate amount" (=2) on both of the original variables, would now get a score of $DM = \sqrt{2^2 + 2^2} = \sqrt{8} = 2.83$. In short, we have come up with a new single variable or "factor" that represents the responses of the study

---

[11] PCA is not exactly a factor-analytic tool, as it aims to decompose variance and not to account for covariance or correlation patterns; however, as a practical matter, both methods often yield similar results.

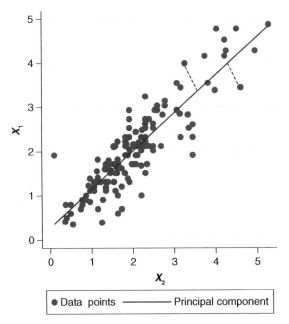

FIGURE 22.3 Principal Component for Scores on Two Variables: Pearson's *r* Correlation 0.85.

participants on two variables. In fact, we have collapsed a two-dimensional space defined by two coordinates into a one-dimensional space, defined by a single coordinate. While in this example the two item scores are perfectly correlated ($r = 1.0$), with real data, this is almost never the case. Figure 22.3 shows data for two variables (X_1 and X_2) that are highly, but not perfectly, correlated. Again, we could represent an individual's score on the newly formed principal axis drawn to capture the maximum variation of individual scores in a single score. As it turns out, in this case, the scores of individuals on the newly formed principal axis capture more than 80% of total score variation of both original variables. Given the extraction method used here (PCA), we call this first "factor" a first "principal component." An important point about this (initial) factor extraction is that the remaining variation is shown as perpendicular distances of data points from the principal axis line. With only two original variables, we could locate the precise location of all data points using a second axis perpendicular to the first one, but then we would not have reduced the complexity of the data: We would have just replaced the coordinates of the scores on the original two observed variables by coordinates on the newly transformed factor variables.

As a matter of fact, it is always possible to replace the original variables with an equal number of transformed factor variables or principal components, which are weighted linear combinations of the original variables. If we have as many factors as original variables, we can predict the locations of all individual data points in *n*-dimensional space precisely.[12] Still, there is a point to this: We have reexpressed the scores on the original variables as scores on

---

[12]The term "*n*-dimensional space" refers to the geometric representation of the data. With two indicator variables, we need *maximally* two dimensions to represent the data points graphically, but as Figure 22.2 shows, if the two variables are perfectly correlated, all the data points lie on a single line, and we can use a one-dimensional depiction (i.e., a single straight line) to represent all data. With three original variables, we maximally need three dimensions to plot all data points exactly; this can be generalized to *n*-dimensional space, if *n* variables are involved.

two new factor variables, but we have shown that one of these new factor variables captures most of the variation in scores among the original two variables. This is only possible if and when the two original variables are correlated. In Figure 22.3, we see that the scatter of data points depicting scores on the two original variables is confined to a fairly narrow band along a single straight line: It is for this reason that we can replace the original scores on two variables with a single score on one factor variable or principal component and still capture most of the individual variation. If the two variables had not been correlated ($r = 0$), no simplification would have been possible, as no linearly transformed factor variable would exist that explains more variance than the original observed variables. This is as it should be: Two variables that are uncorrelated cannot possibly be indicators of the same underlying and unobserved latent variable.

Table 22.2 shows output from a factor analysis performed on actual data, using the same six CES-D variables as in Table 22.1. The analysis was performed on data from a sample of 371 women between the ages of 21 and 60, who responded to all 20 CES-D questionnaire items, but for simplicity's sake, we confine ourselves to just these six variables. The extraction method chosen here is PCA, which starts by extracting a first component or "factor," which is a weighted sum of the six observed depression indicator variables; the weights are chosen in such a way that the first extracted component accounts for a maximum amount of variance among the individual

TABLE 22.2 EFA of Responses to Six CES-D Question Items Designed as Indicators of Depression

X1: I felt depressed; X2: I felt hopeful about the future;
X3: I was happy; X4: I enjoyed life; X5: I had crying spells;
X6: I felt sad.

Factor analysis/Extraction			Number of obs	= 371
Method: principal-component factors			Retained factors	= 2
Rotation: (unrotated)			Number of params =	11

Factor		Eigenvalue	Difference	Proportion	Cumulative
Factor1		3.4167	2.4072	0.5694	0.5694
Factor2		1.0095	0.3849	0.1682	0.7377
Factor3		0.6246	0.2258	0.1041	0.8418
Factor4		0.3988	0.0628	0.0665	0.9083
Factor5		0.3360	0.1215	0.0560	0.9642
Factor6		0.2145	.	0.0358	1.0000

LR test: independent vs. saturated: chi2(15) = 1024.26 Prob>chi2 = 0.0000

Initial Factor loadings (pattern matrix) and unique variances

Variable		Factor1	Factor2		Uniqueness	Communality
X1		0.7867	−0.3485		0.2597	0.7407
X2		0.5346	0.6247		0.3239	0.6761
X3		0.7886	0.3178		0.2772	0.7228
X4		0.7404	0.3661		0.3177	0.6823
X5		0.7714	−0.4117		0.2355	0.7645
X6		0.8643	−0.3054		0.1598	0.8402

scores, which are located in the original six-dimensional space. (The solid line in Figure 22.3 is an example of such an extracted component, albeit from a two-dimensional space.). In a second step, we extract another component, which is orthogonal, that is, uncorrelated, to the first component, and its weights are chosen so as to explain the maximum proportion of the variance in the data *remaining* after the variance associated with the first component is removed. We continue this process until we have as many components or factors as we have variables, at which point we will be guaranteed that all variation in the data can be explained by our factors.

Important information about the extraction results is contained in the column in Table 22.2 labeled "Eigenvalue."[13] In the current context, the eigenvalues represent the amount of variance that is accounted for by the extracted components or factors. Recall that the variance of standardized variables is always equal to one. With six (standardized) variables, we need to account for a total variance of 6. The first factor extracted has an associated eigenvalue of 3.4167. When divided by the sum of the six standardized variables, 3.4167/6 = 0.5694, we see that the first factor accounts for 56.94% of the total variance among these six variables.

Successive orthogonal components or factors account for additional parts or all of the remaining variance. For instance, the second factor has an eigenvalue of 1.0095, which translates into 16.82% additional variance accounted for. The overall cumulative proportion of variance accounted for by the first two factors is 0.7377, which is the sum of 0.5694 and 0.1682, except for a small rounding error. In an analysis involving standardized variables, the sum of the eigenvalues equals the number of variables, each of which has variance one. Many statistical software programs use an eigenvalue of one as a default criterion for determining when to stop the extraction of additional factors. This is by no means a rule of thumb that should always be followed—sometimes it makes sense to use different eigenvalue criteria or use a predetermined number of factors, if the researcher already has experience with and information about the observed variables from prior studies—but as a criterion to limit the maximum number of factors extracted, it often makes sense. Remember, that a standardized variable has a variance of one. Replacing an observed variable with a factor that explains less variance than the observed variable would not be terribly helpful, as the goal here is to simplify and come up with fewer variables containing much of the information contained in the original observed variables. In addition, recall from the last chapter on reliability that observed variables usually contain a good deal of measurement error and the ultimate goal of factor analysis is to account for the *common* variance, that is, covariance among the observed variables. In short, in this case we extract two factors, which account for almost 74% of total variance.

Table 22.2 also shows the initial factor loadings as well as the communalities and uniqueness values associated with each original variable (uniqueness = 1 – communality). The communality value indicates what proportion of the variance of a variable is shared with the common factors and, thus, the other variables correlated with the common factors. As we can see, the communalities vary between 0.6761 and 0.8402, thus showing that the two-factor model accounts for substantial proportions of variances in each of the observed variable. If one or more communalities are very low, let us say less than 0.2, this would either indicate that the variable may not be correlated well with any of the other indicator variables or that more factors would need to be extracted to account for common variance. Incidentally, for a factor model with orthogonal or uncorrelated factors, there is a simple relationship between the factor loadings and the communalities: the sum of the squared loadings equal the communality.

---

[13]Eigenvalue is a term used in linear algebra. For a short description, see the Wikipedia entry by the same name. In this chapter, we have avoided using matrix algebra notation, which underlies much of the factor-analytic methods.

For instance, the factor loadings of variable X_6, "I felt sad," can be used to compute the communality value as follows: $0.8643^2 + (-0.3054)^2 = 0.8402$. As it turns out, the initial factor loadings are often difficult to interpret; we must take one additional step in the analysis and "rotate" the factors to obtain more interpretable factor loadings.

Factor Rotation

We emphasized earlier that factor solutions are indeterminate: There is not only one solution, but multiple solutions. Each is an equally valid representation of the correlation pattern in the data. To see this point, we first take a look at the factor loadings in Table 22.3 and their graphical depiction in the two-dimensional graphs of Figures 22.3 and 22.4.

TABLE 22.3 Factor Loadings After Orthogonal and Oblique Rotations

X1: I felt depressed; X2: I felt hopeful about the future; X3: I was happy;
X4: I enjoyed life; X5: I had crying spells; X6: I felt sad.

Factor analysis: No. of obs = 371; Retained factors = 2; No. of params = 11;
    Initial Factor loadings (pattern matrix) and unique variances

Variable	Factor1	Factor2	Uniqueness	Communality
X1	0.7867	−0.3485	0.2597	0.7407
X2	0.5346	0.6247	0.3239	0.6761
X3	0.7886	0.3178	0.2772	0.7228
X4	0.7404	0.3661	0.3177	0.6823
X5	0.7714	−0.4117	0.2355	0.7645
X6	0.8643	−0.3054	0.1598	0.8402

Rotation: orthogonal varimax (Kaiser normalization)
Rotated factor loadings (pattern matrix) and unique variances

Variable	Factor1	Factor2	Uniqueness
X1	0.8327	0.2163	0.2597
X2	0.0302	0.8217	0.3239
X3	0.4199	0.7392	0.2772
X4	0.3521	0.7472	0.3177
X5	0.8601	0.1574	0.2355
X6	0.8667	0.2983	0.1598

Rotation: oblique oblim in (Kaiser normalization)
Rotated factor loadings (pattern matrix) and unique variances

Variable	Factor1	Factor2	Uniqueness
X1	0.8520	0.0186	0.2597
X2	−0.1698	0.8831	0.3239
X3	0.2743	0.6926	0.2772
X4	0.1986	0.7188	0.3177
X5	0.8963	−0.0524	0.2355
X6	0.8688	0.0987	0.1598

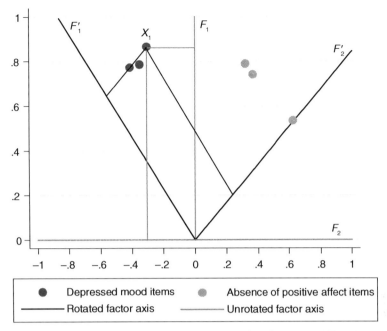

FIGURE 22.4 Change in Factor Loadings After Orthogonal Rotation.

Table 22.3 shows three sets of factor loadings ("pattern matrix") for six CES-D items and two factors. The first pattern matrix again shows the results from the initial extraction in Table 22.2.

Based on the size and distribution of the 12 loadings after the initial extraction of two factors, it is not immediately obvious that these two factors represent clearly distinct dimensions. The different signs of the loadings for Factor 2 do hint at the existence of separate dimensions, but often enough, the loadings of the initial factor solutions do not provide clarifying information concerning the underlying grouping or clusters of variables, even if there is such a grouping. This is often the case when a large number of variables and their loadings on several factors are examined. For maximum clarity about factor loading patterns, the ideal outcome would be that each variable has high loadings on only one factor, with the loadings on the other factors being close to zero. As it turns out, if the observed variables do fall into well-defined clusters that are separable, one can obtain such factor pattern matrices[14] revealing the simple structure through the rotation of the coordinate axes.

To clarify the meaning of the previous statements, let us look at the graph in Figure 22.4. It shows that the six CES-D items do, in fact, form two distinct clusters based on their initial factor loadings: The variables belonging to the "depressive mood" cluster (X_1, X_5, X_6) are closer to each other than the variables forming the "absence of positive affect" cluster (X_2, X_3, X_4) and vice versa. Concerning the coordinate system, we first ignore the dark gray lines and focus on the (light gray line) horizontal and vertical axes in the graph: They represent the *initial* factors (F_1, F_2). The graph also shows six small circles, representing the six variables, whose location in the plane is determined by coordinates equal to their factor loadings. For

---

[14]A pattern matrix contains the factor loadings of the observed variables on the factors. Table 22.3 provides three examples.

example, X_1 ("I felt sad") has a loading of 0.8643 on the initial Factor 1 (F_1) and a loading of -0.3054 on F_2. These values are the coordinates for X_1, indicated by the perpendicular solid lines. It is obvious that the initial Factor 1 provides little discrimination between the variables belonging to the "depressive mood" cluster (X_1, X_5, X_6) and the "absence of positive affect" cluster (X_2, X_3, X_4): All of these loadings are fairly high. Only the loadings on Factor 2, which are negative for the first and positive for the second variable cluster, help to separate the clusters.

The dark gray lines in Figure 22.4 represent an orthogonal rotation, which produces another right-angled coordinate system.[15] Here we used the popular *varimax* procedure for orthogonal rotation. This procedure maximizes the *variance* of the squared loadings of each factor, subject to the constraint that the rotated factors remain orthogonal or uncorrelated. Of course, maximizing the variance of the loadings means to make them as different from each other as possible. In short, this procedure would entail rotating the axes until a position is found, in which some loadings have large values and others relatively small values. Details of the calculations involved can be found elsewhere,[16] but Figure 22.4 provides the results of the rotation, with the dark gray lines representing the rotated factors. There are several important observations to be made about this rotation: (a) we rotated the *coordinate system*, but left the original data untouched.[17] That means that the relationships among the original variables and their clustering remain completely unaffected by the rotation. (b) As the second panel in Table 22.3 shows, the uniqueness, and thus the communality of shared variance, is unaffected by the rotation of the factor axes. (c) As with all orthogonal rotations, the sums of the squared factor loadings remain the same and equal the communality index for a variable. For instance, variable X_1 has the following sums of squared factor loadings from the unrotated and rotated factor solutions: $0.7867^2 + (-0.3485)^2 = 0.8327^2 + 0.2163^2$. Both expressions are equal to the communality: 0.7407.

After rotation of the coordinate axes by 38°, we get new factors (F_1', F_2') and greater clarity with respect to the factor loadings. Drawing perpendicular (dashed) lines for the variable X_1 onto the rotated (dashed lines) factor axes, we can see that X_1 now has a high loading on F_1' (0.8327) and a low loading on F_2' (0.2163), as do the other depressed mood items. Conversely, the three variables representing "absence of positive affect" have relatively high loadings on F_2' and much lower loadings on F_1'. The important point here is that we made no changes in the original variables and their relative position to each other, but after rotation, the factor pattern matrix containing the factor loadings offers a clearer picture of the variable clusters.

With these data, we can improve on the clarity and separation of the factor loadings even further, if we relax the assumption that the factors are uncorrelated and perform an "oblique" rotation. As the items were originally all designed to be indicators of depression, we can assume that the factors extracted here represent sub-dimensions of depression. This would mean that the assumption of uncorrelated, orthogonal factors is somewhat suspect. There is every reason to expect that different clusters of depression indicators, which form separate subscales, are correlated at the level of the subscales. Figure 22.5 offers a visual representation of an oblique rotation, using a technique called *oblimin*. This procedure minimizes the covariance of the squared loadings for distinct factors.[18] At the bottom of Table 22.3, we show

---

[15]Harman (1976) is a classic, comprehensive treatment of this subject.

[16]An older but useful nontechnical treatment can be found in Kim and Mueller (1978).

[17]We can express the location of each variable on the new coordinate system employing the following trigonometric equations: $l_1' = l_1\cos\theta + l_2\sin\theta$ and $l_2' = l_1\sin\theta + l_2\cos\theta$, where l_1 and l_2 are the loadings on the initial factors F_1 and F_2 and l_1' and l_2' are the loadings on the orthogonally rotated factors F_1' and F_2'.

[18]Detailed explanations can be found in Haman (1976).

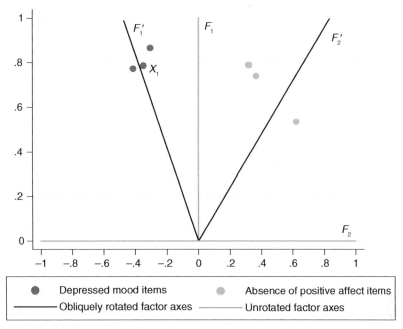

FIGURE 22.5 Factor Loadings After Oblique Rotation.

the pattern matrix with factor loadings after the oblique rotation. In terms of separating the factor loadings on the two factors, such that each variable has a high loading on only one of the factors and a low loading on the other, the oblique rotation results in the clearest, that is, most easily interpretable pattern matrix. Figure 22.5 provides a graphical depiction of the obliquely rotated factor axes. It is apparent that the oblique rotation tracks the two clusters of variables better than the orthogonal rotation. In fact, the two obliquely rotated factors in Figure 22.5 correlate at a level of $r = 0.4419$. This implies that they share 19.53% of common variance ($r^2 = 0.4419^2 = 0.1953$), enough to prefer oblique over orthogonal rotation as a better description of the data pattern. However, oblique rotations lead to more complex relationships between the factor loadings in the pattern matrix and the communality of the variables. This is so because, after oblique rotations, the factor loadings in the pattern matrix no longer equal in size the correlations between the variables and the factors, which are now shown in a separate "structure matrix" (see Table 22.4).

EFA and Scale Development

Even though factor analysis can be used as a data reduction technique to identify any highly correlated clusters of variables, in the nursing and health care research literature, EFA is most of the time used for scale development. Researchers usually start with a conceptual exploration of a construct of interest, such as job satisfaction or patient coping skills. After further exploration of the construct with a few members of the target population, perhaps using focus groups, scale developers then write question items they hope will capture the main aspects of the construct. At this stage, the researcher cannot know yet, which of the items will produce interpretable responses, so it is necessary to write many items in order to retain a sufficient number of usable items in the final scale. If a 10-item scale is the goal, one would typically develop 30 to 40 questionnaire items, many of which will turn out to be of little value.

TABLE 22.4 Pattern and Structure Matrices After Oblique Rotation

X1: I felt depressed; X2: I felt hopeful about the future; X3: I was happy; X4: I enjoyed life; X5: I had crying spells; X6: I felt sad.

Variable-Factor Loadings (Pattern Matrix) and Variable-Factor Correlations (Structure Matrix) after Oblimin Rotation

	Pattern Matrix		Structure Matrix	
Variable	Factor1	Factor2	Factor1	Factor2
X1	0.8520	0.0186	0.8602	0.3951
X2	−0.1698	0.8831	0.2205	0.8080
X3	0.2743	0.6926	0.5803	0.8138
X4	0.1986	0.7188	0.5163	0.8065
X5	0.8963	−0.0524	0.8731	0.3437
X6	0.8688	0.0987	0.9124	0.4826

If the construct of interest is conceptually subdivided (as in the example in this chapter of "depressed mood" and "absence of positive affect"), then there must be a sufficient number of items which represent these "subscales" or factors. For the latter, a minimum of three items per subscale is absolutely essential, but four or five items are advisable. After deciding on a desirable number of items, the researcher must then determine how large a sample is needed to submit the new items to an exploratory analysis. As a rule of thumb, the study sample should be representative of the target population of interest and should contain at least 10 subjects per item in the instrument (Watson & Thompson, 2005).

EFA performed on data from small samples is unlikely to yield results that can be replicated in another study. The reader of this chapter may perhaps have noted that we did not mention any significance testing or confidence intervals (CIs). That means we did not employ the usual apparatus of statistical inference and hypothesis testing. The main reason for this is that EFA is, well, exploratory. That is, we often start with some sample data and explore correlation patterns within these data, but when we are developing an instrument, we rarely have well-developed hypotheses about which variables measure which concepts. In other words, to some degree, we use the data to determine which items "go together" with other items and form an interpretable scale. From a statistical point of view, we are taking advantage (if you can call it that) of sampling chance. As factor analysis is based on the analysis of correlation (or covariance) tables, which are computed from sample data. Sample data are subject to sampling fluctuations, thus it should not be surprising that any particular factor structure "discovered" in a particular data set may not be reproducible with another data set. In order to reduce the chances of that happening, one should use fairly large samples with hundreds of subjects, if one plans to perform EFAs, as larger samples are less likely to be subject to sampling fluctuations.

We have described some criteria for how many factors to extract, for example, eigenvalues greater than 1, and what rotation methods to employ (orthogonal or oblique). Other criteria used to achieve "simple structure" include the decision to discard items that load on multiple factors, as such items are difficult to interpret. For many of these decisions during an EFA there are no simple rules that can be applied regardless of context. For instance, a rule to discard items that show no factor loadings larger than 0.3 is eminently reasonable, but even then we should not forget that factor loadings, like all statistical measures computed from sample data, are subject to sampling chance. Furthermore, once variables are discarded, the data need to be reanalyzed with the remaining items to see whether the factors extracted in the prior analysis are still the same. In the final analysis, EFA is a very valuable tool in the development of scales, but a single exploratory analysis, even when performed on a large data set, is just the beginning and not the end of scale development.

Finally, once the exploratory analysis reveals that variables form consistent uni-dimensional clusters, that is, the variables in a cluster have large loadings on a single factor and close to zero loadings (<0.2) on the other factors, the scale developer needs to decide whether the variable clusters represent meaningful and interpretable subscales on their own. This is, of course not a statistical criterion, but one of conceptual validity. The point here is that, with EFA, one cannot mechanically use a set of formal rules to decide which variables form scales, as the underlying mathematics ultimately group variables based on their correlations with each other. The question as to why two or more variables correlate is not a mathematical question: It is a substantive and theoretical question. For instance, two variables may correlate for reasons other than that they are indicators of the same underlying latent variable. For instance, an indicator of depression may correlate with an indicator of anxiety, because depression and anxiety are often linked in the same person; thus, the decision about which items to retain in a depression or anxiety instrument rests on nonstatistical criteria as well. In short, we need to keep in mind a fundamental asymmetry in inferences concerning the scalability of several indicators: The lack of a correlation between two items designed to be indicators of the same concept would lead us to reject the hypothesis that they are measuring the same concept, but the presence of such a correlation is not proof that they are measuring the same concept.

REQUIREMENTS AND ASSUMPTIONS FOR SUCCESSFUL EFA

1. In principle, one can subject any set of correlated variables to a factor analysis, but to be successful in obtaining a scalable multiitem instrument potential indicators must be vetted conceptually and pretested with members of the target population.

2. Factor analysis generally assumes interval-level observed variables and linear relationships among the observed variables and latent factors.

3. Final factor solutions should at least contain three observed variables per factor; four or more per factor are preferable.

4. Sample sizes should be "large" to reduce sampling variability in the correlations and covariances that are the basis for factor analysis. Ideally the sample size for exploratory analysis should exceed 10 times the number of observed indicator variables involved; but n must be larger than the number of estimated parameters (e.g., the number of factor loadings, variances, and covariances to be estimated).

5. To achieve "simple structure," only items that load on a single factor should be retained. As a practical matter, loadings on the reference factor should differ in magnitude from the loadings on nonreference factor(s) by at least 0.3.

6. Obliquely rotated factors that correlate well above 0.7 may not be sustainable as separate factors with new data; a simpler factor structure combining highly correlated factors may fit the data reasonably well.

COMMENTS ON CFA

In this section, we confine ourselves to a few statements about CFA, as there are many excellent treatments available now.[19] Concerning the discussion of EFA so far, the reader may in fact have been wondering, why we did not mention any significance testing or CIs; in short, we did not engage the usual apparatus of statistical inference and hypothesis testing. The main reason for this is that EFA is exploratory. That is, we often start with some sample data and explore correlation patterns within these data, but when we are developing an instrument, we rarely have already well-developed hypotheses, which variables measure which concepts. This makes hypothesis testing difficult, because our hypotheses would be rather ad hoc, that is, formulated based on momentary hunches. In addition, if we are using data as a guide to formulating our measurement hypotheses, for example, which variables "go together" and measure a common concept, or what the size of the factor loadings are likely to be, we are not really engaging in statistical hypothesis testing, because we are taking advantage of sampling chance. In EFA, the raw data are the covariances or correlations among the variables, which we subject to the EFA. These are, of course, subject to the usual sampling chance, which means that the size of these correlations may vary from one sample to the next, making the factors extracted subject to sampling chance as well. Thus, the first rule of thumb, when performing EFA for the purpose of developing scalable instruments is that the EFA be based on large study samples representative of the target population; and to obtain stable solutions, the sample size should, at a minimum, involve five cases per indicator item.

By contrast to EFA, CFA is oriented toward hypothesis testing. The fundamental idea is to construct a factor model *a priori* and test for its compatibility with the data at hand. Of course, the construction of the factor model, like the one in Figure 22.1, is based on prior theory and the results of prior EFA. In particular, we employ CFA to validate the results from EFA with entirely different study samples. In fact, a major strength of CFA is that we can test, whether a particular measurement (factor) model holds for subjects of *different target populations* or whether the model is stable upon *repeated measurement occasions* of the same subjects. Furthermore, we can specify more precisely the specific features of a factor model. Going back to the graph in Figure 22.1, you see for instance that the model does not include direct factor loadings of the three depressed mood items on the lack of positive affect factor and no direct factor loadings of the lack of positive affect items on the depressed mood factor. In short, these (potential) factor loadings have been set to zero. If we impose this factor model on actual data and get estimates for the factor loadings and inter factor correlations, we can reconstruct a correlation matrix based on this factor model, as was shown for the correlation matrix in Table 22.1. However, this correlation matrix was *generated* by the factor model; so it is no wonder that there is a perfect fit.

With correlation matrices based on observed sample data, there will generally not be a perfect fit between the observed correlation matrix and the one generated by the factor model. Even if the factor model holds true in the target population, mere sampling fluctuations would prevent a perfect fit. However, how well our factor model does in explaining the observed correlation matrix can now be tested by constructing a residual matrix as shown in the simple four-variable example of Table 22.5. This residual correlation matrix contains the differences between the parallel elements of the observed correlation matrix and the one predicted on the basis of the hypothesized factor model. A perfect fit of the factor model would mean that all the elements of the residual matrix are equal to zero.

---

[19] A short introduction may be found in Stommel and colleagues (1994), and an excellent nontechnical introduction is Byrne (2010).

TABLE 22.5 Comparison of Observed, Predicted, and Residual Correlation Matrices After CFA

```
                           Correlation Matrices:
     ------------------------------------------------------------------

         Observed Matrix:     |   Predicted Matrix:    |  Residual Matrix:
         X1   X2   X3   X4     |   X1   X2   X3   X4    |  X1     X2    X3    X4
     ---------------------------+------------------------+----------------------
 X1  |  1.00                   |  1.00                  |  0.00
 X2  |  0.55 1.00              |  0.49 1.00             |  0.06  0.00
 X3  |  0.47 0.69 1.00         |  0.53 0.62 1.00        | -0.06  0.07  0.00
 X4  |  0.54 0.66 0.73 1.00    |  0.57 0.66 0.72 1.00   | -0.03  0.00  0.01  0.00
     -----------------------------------------------------------------------

 Chi-squared test (df.=6):   7.64;   p>0.266;   N=134
```

As the chi-squared test shows, the deviations from this research hypothesis are well within expected sampling chance for a sample of $N = 134$. Thus we accept the hypothesis that the factor model can reproduce the observed correlation matrix and is consistent with the data. Hypothesis testing in modern CFA is usually done comparing observed and expected covariance matrices instead of the standardized correlation matrices. There are numerous fit indices having different advantages or disadvantages; however, the basic logic remains the same. CFA has become an indispensible tool for evaluating scaling models. Published measurement scales/instruments based solely on a few exploratory factor models should be treated with considerable caution without confirmatory evidence tested on independent samples. CFA is a subtle analysis tool, which allows the researcher great flexibility in specifying a model, but a fuller treatment of CFA and its relation to structural equation modeling is beyond the scope of this book. The interested reader may start with a good, nontechnical introduction by Byrne (2010).[20]

SUMMARY

In this chapter, we provided an introduction to the main principles underlying factor analysis. Factor analysis is a tool for data reduction, and as such it is indispensable to the researcher and analyst. For readers of health care and nursing research journals, the technical details of factor analysis are less important than a conceptual grasp of the main principles underlying this technique.

While factor analysis is explicitly used to find variable combinations, which represent common concepts, in a broader sense, it could be argued that all of statistics can be considered a tool for data reduction: It serves to discover or confirm patterns in the data, which are not "visible" in any other way. We hope that the reader, who made it this far, has come to appreciate the power and subtlety of statistical analysis. Statistics has become a vast field, which is expanding rapidly. This is especially true in the health care field, where methods of "mining" the ever-increasing number of data sets can help identify, address, and sometimes solve problems concerning the distribution of diseases in the population, access to health care services or the effectiveness of clinical interventions.

---

[20]The reference is to a book with applications for a specific software program, but this author has also published other monographs related to EQS and M-plus. Further general software packages that perform CFA and structural equation modeling include SAS and STATA.

LITERATURE APPLICATION

Read: Poghosyan, L., Aiken, L. H., & Sloane, D. M. (2009). Factor structure of the Maslach Burnout Inventory: An analysis of data from large scale cross-sectional surveys of nurses from eight countries. *International Journal of Nursing Studies, 46*(7), 894–902.

(a) Provide a very brief (three to four sentences) summary of what this study is about.

(b) Define the target population to which the statistical analysis can be generalized. What were the eligibility and exclusion criteria for study participants? Is the study sample a random sample of the target population?

(c) What was the purpose of employing both EFA and CFA?

(d) Why was EFA employed after CFA? What does that say about how much trust we can have in the final factor solution?

(e) The authors employed EFA to each country's data separately. Argue for and against this decision.

(f) The authors wrote: "The fact that one other item failed to exhibit a substantial loading in Germany… and another item failed to exhibit a substantial loading in Armenia… is largely ignorable. This is suggested by the fact that all three … scales yield Cronbach Alphas, which exceed the critical value of .70." Do you agree? Are similar magnitudes of Alpha values across countries evidence of a similar factor structure across countries?

(g) What additional information might a second CFA yield beyond the EFA presented?

EXERCISES

1. In your own words, distinguish exploratory from confirmatory factor analysis.

2. Suppose you have four indicators of anxiety, and a single common factor model explains all the joint variation among these variables. With factor loadings of $Z_1 - F = 0.6$, $Z_2 - F = 0.4$, $Z_3 - F = 0.5$, and $Z_4 - F = 0.6$, what are the correlations among the observed variables?

3. If the number of factors accounting for 100% of the variance among the observed variables is smaller than the number of observed variables, what must be true about the correlations among the observed variables?

4. List reasons why an observed correlation matrix might differ significantly from a predicted correlation matrix based on a factor model.

REFERENCES

Byrne, B. M. (2010). *Structural equation modeling with AMOS: Basic concepts, applications and programming* (2nd ed.). New York, NY: Routledge, Taylor & Francis.

Child, D. (2006). *Essentials of factor analysis* (2nd ed.). New York, NY: Bloomsbury Academic.

Espeland, V., & Indrehus, O. (2003). Evaluation of students' satisfaction with nursing education in Norway. *Journal of Advanced Nursing, 42*(3), 226–236.

Harman, H. H. (1976). *Modern factor analysis* (3rd ed.). Chicago, IL: University of Chicago Press.

Kim, J.-O., & Mueller, C. W. (1978). *An introduction to factor analysis: What it is and how to do it* (Quantitative applications in the social sciences 13). Newbury Park, CA: Sage.

O'Connor, J., & Jeavons, S. (2003). Nurses' perceptions of critical incidents. *Journal of Advanced Nursing, 41*(1), 53–62.

Polit, D. F., & Beck, C. T. (2009). *Nursing research* (9th ed.). Philadelphia, PA: Lippincott, Williams & Wilkins.

Radloff, L. S. (1977). The CES-D scale: A self report depression scale for research in the general population. *Applied Psychological Measurements, 1*(3), 385–401.

Stommel, M., Wang, S., Given, C. W., & Given, B. A. (1992). Confirmatory factor analysis (CFA) as a method to assess measurement equivalence. *Research in Nursing & Health, 15*(5), 352–360.

Stommel, M., & Wills, C. (2004). *Clinical research: Concepts and principles for advanced practice nurses.* Philadelphia, PA: Lippincott Williams & Wilkins.

Trochim, W. M. K. (2006). *The research methods knowledge base.* Retrieved April 2013, from Andover: Cengage Publishing: http://www.socialresearchmethods.net/kb/index.php

Watson, R., & Thompson, D. R. (2006). Use of factor analysis in Journal of Advanced Nursing: literature review. *Journal of Advanced Nursing, 55*(3), 330–341.

PART VI. ISSUES IN DATA MANAGEMENT

CHAPTER   23

Data Management and Privacy Concerns

In the Preface of this book, we emphasized that our goal was to prepare graduates from Doctor of Nursing Practice (DNP) programs and other advanced health care professionals to become more sophisticated users of the best research evidence available to facilitate both clinical practice and health system changes. In short, we envisioned that the readers would become clinical experts who could understand and evaluate current and future health care research, which offers more and more examples of sophisticated statistical analyses. Likewise, future administrative leaders must become familiar with the literature on program evaluation, which also has become more sophisticated with regard to the statistical analysis models used for evaluation. However, beyond being a more sophisticated reader of research literature, both health care providers and administrators work in environments in which electronic data records are proliferating at accelerating rates. Such data often contain valuable information about patient care problems, medical diagnoses, as well as billing and insurance information. They may also provide insights for administrators concerned with improving organizational efficiency, quality of care, and compliance with organizational rules as well as state and federal laws. To the extent that such data contain personal identifiable information, they are subject to the Health Insurance Portability and Accountability Act (HIPAA) of 1996 and its amendments, as well as the 2009 Health Information Technology for Economic and Clinical Health Act (HITECH; see USDHHS, 2013a).

The basic privacy rule of HIPAA involves the prohibition of using and disclosing personal health information without authorization of the patient. There are a few exceptions, listed under the heading of Treatment, Payment, and Health Care Operations (TPO), which involve sharing of information with other providers and insurance plans for treatment and payment purposes. In addition, there are various public health exceptions, for instance, when HIPAA-covered entities may report to relevant public agencies information pertinent to epidemics and so on. In the following sections, we will discuss the main issues involved in using this information for research and quality improvement purposes.

RESEARCH USING DATA IN CLINICAL SETTINGS

Existing data sources in clinical settings are assembled for a variety of purposes and involve several sources: (a) patient self-report data obtained through clinical interviews or written questionnaires; (b) patient health histories and histories of medication use; (c) results from laboratory tests and other biophysiological measures; (d) provider observations and evaluation of patients available in patient records; (e) records of diagnostic and treatment histories; (f) billing and coding information and insurance records. As all such information is tied to individual patients, access to this information is principally restricted to personnel involved in the treatment or financial billing of particular patients. It is important to realize that, even if a clinician or administrator has legitimate access to such information about patients in treatment, such information cannot be used for *research* purposes unless a formal research proposal has been submitted and approved by the relevant institutional review board (IRB).

All data collection and analysis, whose main purpose is to enhance knowledge rather than treat individual patients or address internal organizational issues, are classified as research. More specifically, according to the Code of Federal Regulation (see Title 45 CFR 46.102; USDHHS, 2013b), research is defined as "a systematic investigation, including research development, testing, and evaluation, designed to develop or contribute to generalizable knowledge." Such activities are subject to review by local and other relevant IRBs, whose main function is to protect the rights of the research subjects and to weigh the potential benefits and risks of a research undertaking. Data sets collected or assembled as part of a research project must meet the confidentiality requirements of the IRB, which may include reviews by the Data and Safety Monitoring Boards (DSMBs).

A HIPAA-covered entity may use or disclose health information for research purposes, if it has been de-identified (in accordance with 45 CFR 164.502(d), and 164.514(a)–(c) of the Rule). Thus, whenever possible, clinical data sets that, in their original form, contain private health information should be stripped of all identifiable information (see Box 23.1 for more information on de-identification), if they are to be used in secondary data analysis for research purposes.

In addition to the approval of the analysis plan by the IRB, clinical and administrative data sets may be made available for secondary analysis to researchers only after the signing of a "data use agreement" between the researchers and the "covered entity" (health care organization). Such agreements would (a) specify the particular uses of the data sets, (b) identify all persons with access to the data, (c) list provisions for safeguarding the data, and (d) detail procedures for destroying the data after a specified period for analysis.

If personally identifiable information is to be accessed for research purposes, it is important to remember that HIPAA privacy rules require that patients must have given prior authorization that their data can be used for such purposes. Many hospitals nowadays ask patients to sign consent forms that include such provisions, but if signed consent forms do not exist, it is principally the responsibility of the researcher to obtain such consent. Even when general written consents have been obtained, IRBs may require the researcher to go back to the patients, if any *identifiable* data are used.

In some research situations, contacting former patients and obtaining consent after the fact may involve an undue burden or be impossible, if patient records go back for several years. In such cases, the IRB may provide a *waiver* of the consent requirement, but only after making a determination that "the use or disclosure of protected health information involves no more than a minimal risk to the privacy of individuals" (see OCR HIPAA Privacy; USDHHS, 2013c). In addition, such waivers require IRB-approved plans to guard against improper disclosure and to delete all personally identifiable information as soon as it is no longer necessary for the research. In these instances, the researchers are required to submit the reasons detailing why access to personally identifiable information is vital. In all such cases, it is the prerogative of the IRB to determine whether researchers/data users follow adequate procedures, and data access may be revoked, if violations occur. It is important to remember that researchers must obtain waivers, even in the case of deceased subjects: the determination of what constitutes adequate protection of privacy is never to be made by the researchers themselves.

BOX 23.1	EXAMPLES OF PERSONAL IDENTIFIERS THAT NEED TO BE EXCLUDED FROM "DE-IDENTIFIED" DATA SETS

- Names
- Address information, except for township, census tract, state or zip code[1]
- Telephone numbers
- Fax numbers
- E-mail addresses
- Social security numbers
- Medical record numbers
- Biometric identifiers, including finger and voice prints
- Full face photographic images and comparable image
- Health plan beneficiary numbers
- Credit card numbers
- Bank and other organizational account numbers
- Certificate/license numbers
- Vehicle identifiers and serial numbers, including license plate numbers
- Device identifiers and serial numbers
- Web universal resource locators (URLs) for personal websites
- Internet protocol (IP) address numbers

PRINCIPLES FOR STORING AND ARCHIVING DATA SETS

A few simple rules can go a long way to ensure confidentiality and anonymity of patients, and assist researchers, in case a study or evaluation project is audited.

First, as a basic principle, the analyst should distinguish between the original data set as received from a HIPAA-covered entity and the analytical file. A copy of the original data without any additions or alterations should be retained on a secure server or an encrypted medium like a CD or jump drive, which would be stored in a secure file location. If the original data are not de-identified, but contain information that allows for personal identification, it is highly advisable to separate this information from the remaining data and substitute a new study ID, while retaining the identification information in a separate file with the study ID. The latter file is preferably stored in a different, secure location. Access to such information needs to be highly restricted, involving no one other than the principal investigator or the project data manager.

Second, analytical files to be used in daily work should always be in de-identified format, only containing the study ID for reference. Especially for projects that involve several

---

[1]*Note*: Indicators of smaller geographic units should be suppressed, if a combination with other information in the file (e.g., age of subject > 100) would allow individual identification. Public use data released by the National Center for Health Statistics have long followed such rigorous procedures to protect the confidentiality of survey respondents.

analysts and users of the data, it is advisable to create a "master data file," that contains—where applicable—missing value imputations for variables with nonresponse, new scale variables, and other transformed variables to be used in the analysis. This step ensures consistency among several analysts of the same data set and facilitates the audit trail, if questions about data veracity were to be raised.

Third, analytical data sets need to be accompanied by a codebook that specifies the list of all variables in the data set; variables and value labels associated with the codes; information on all newly created transformed variables (e.g., computation formulas for scale variables); information on missing value imputations, using flags to identify imputed values. Software commands that incorporate the data transformations contained in the data file (recoding, scale computations, missing value imputations, and so on) are necessary for both audit trails and future analysts, if the data were to be used again in secondary analysis.

Fourth, the study documentation should contain analytical notes accompanying the data, providing information on the purpose of the original research project that led to the assembly of the data set, the source of the data, and the sampling procedures used. The latter would include the identification of weighting variables or variables identifying primary sampling units, if complex sampling designs were involved.

Finally, research activities are usually subject to requirements imposed by a grant agency or other sponsors of the research, and these requirements may involve rules about keeping the data for a specified period of time. Often such rules stipulate which, if any, personal identification information should be kept. Thus, it is important to be aware of the distinction between confidentiality and anonymity. When researchers promise confidentiality in a consent form, they promise not to divulge any information that links analysis reports to the persons, whose information was used. Likewise, they promise that no unauthorized person gains access to personal identification information. However, as long as the researcher is in possession of a key that links the study ID to specific identifiable individuals, these study individuals remain traceable in a study audit. Thus, anonymity cannot be guaranteed. To minimize the risks of inadvertent disclosure of personal information, good data management demands that any and all information that allows for personal identification be destroyed, as soon as the study protocol no longer requires recontacting individuals (as in longitudinal studies) and stipulations in the contract with the sponsoring agency are fulfilled. Careless handling of data, including the use of unencrypted files containing personal identification information, and the copying of data files onto a large number of computers or data storage media, has no place in this electronic age.

SUMMARY

At the end of this brief overview of data management and privacy issues, we want to stress again that handling data, collected on individual patients in a health care setting, requires the utmost diligence and care. The principle of "do no harm" does not only apply to patient care itself, but also to the data we collect about these patients. It may be tempting to use one's access to confidential information as a data source for answering an interesting research question, but there is a clear demarcation line between data accessed for reasons of patient care or internal organizational issues and data acquired for research purposes. The latter always requires IRB approval of a proposed research project, even if it is small and unfunded; and it goes without saying that publications based on data accessed without IRB approval violate the spirit, if not the letter of HIPAA and the Title 45 Code of Federal Regulation 46.

REFERENCES

U.S. Department of Health and Human Services (USDHHS). (2013a). *Health Information Privacy.* Retrieved March 12, 2014, from http://www.hhs.gov/ocr/privacy/

U.S. Department of Health and Human Services (USDHHS). (2013b). *Title 45 Code of Federal Regulation (CFR 46.102).* Retrieved March 12, 2014, from http://www.hhs.gov/ohrp/humansubjects/guidance/45cfr46.html

U.S. Department of Health and Human Services (USDHHS). (2013c). *OCR HIPAA Privacy: Research, 2003.* Retrieved from http://www.hhs.gov/ocr/privacy/hipaa/understanding/special/research/

Estimating Population Variance From Sample Variance

We want to show that the sample variance with $n-1$ in the denominator (s_x^2) is an unbiased estimator $\hat{\sigma}_x^2$ of the population variance (σ_x^2):

$$s_x^2 = \sum \frac{(x_i - \bar{x})^2}{n-1} = \hat{\sigma}_x^2$$

We start by noting that the population variance can be decomposed into two components: the variance of individual values around the sample means and the variance of sample means around the true, usually unknown, population mean.[1]

$$\sigma_x^2 = \sum \frac{(x_i - \mu)^2}{n} = \sum \frac{(x_i - \bar{x})^2}{n} + \sum \frac{(\bar{x} - \mu)^2}{n}$$

If we rearrange these terms, we get:

$$\sum \frac{(x_i - \bar{x})^2}{n} = \sum \frac{(x_i - \mu)^2}{n} - \sum \frac{(\bar{x} - \mu)^2}{n}$$

But $\sum \frac{(x_i-\mu)^2}{n} = \sigma_x^2$ and $\sum \frac{(\bar{x}-\mu)^2}{n} = \frac{\sigma_x^2}{n};$ [2] thus we get:

$$\sum \frac{(x_i - \bar{x})^2}{n} = \sigma_x^2 - \frac{\sigma_x^2}{n} = \frac{n\sigma_x^2 - \sigma_x^2}{n} = \frac{(n-1)\sigma_x^2}{n}$$

---

[1] When we take random samples of size n from a target population, the sample means fluctuate around the true population mean; thus the distance of each individual value from the population mean can be decomposed into the difference of that individual value from a sample mean and the difference of the sample mean from the population mean.

[2] Sample means vary around the population mean, but as sample means are averages of n values, they vary less than the individual values around the population mean. In fact, the variance of sample means around the population mean equals the variance of individual values around the population mean divided by the sample size of n: σ_x^2/n.

As, $\frac{n-1}{n} < 1$, the expression $\sum \frac{(x_i-\bar{x})^2}{n}$ *underestimates* the population variance (although in large samples, the bias becomes negligible). To correct for this bias, we multiply the expression by $n/(n-1)$ and get:

$$\left(\frac{n}{n-1}\right)\sum\frac{\left(x_i-\bar{x}\right)^2}{n} = \sum\frac{\left(x_i-\bar{x}\right)^2}{n-1} = s_x^2$$

APPENDIX B

One-Sided Probabilities for z-Scores of the Standard Normal Distribution

z	.00	.01	.02	.03	.04	.05	.06	.07	.08	.09
0.0	.5000	.5034	.5080	.5120	.5160	.5200	.5239	.5279	.5319	.5359
0.1	.5398	.5438	.5478	.5517	.5557	.5596	.5636	.5675	.5714	.5754
0.2	.5793	.5832	.5871	.5910	.5948	.5987	.6026	.6064	.6103	.6141
0.3	.6179	.6217	.6255	.6293	.6331	.6368	.6406	.6443	.6480	.6517
0.4	.6554	.6591	.6628	.6664	.6700	.6736	.6772	.6808	.6844	.6879
0.5	.6915	.6950	.6985	.7019	.7054	.7088	.7123	.7157	.7190	.7224
0.6	.7258	.7291	.7324	.7357	.7389	.7422	.7454	.7486	.7518	.7549
0.7	.7580	.7612	.7642	.7673	.7704	.7734	.7764	.7794	.7823	.7852
0.8	.7881	.7910	.7939	.7967	.7996	.8023	.8051	.8079	.8106	.8133
0.9	.8159	.8186	.8212	.8238	.8264	.8289	.8315	.8340	.8365	.8389
1.0	.8413	.8438	.8461	.8485	.8508	.8531	.8554	.8577	.8599	.8621
1.1	.8643	.8665	.8686	.8708	.8729	.8749	.8771	.8790	.8810	.8830
1.2	.8849	.8869	.8888	.8907	.8925	.8944	.8962	.8980	.8997	.9015
1.3	.9032	.9049	.9066	.9082	.9099	.9115	.9131	.9147	.9162	.9177
1.4	.9192	.9207	.9222	.9236	.9251	.9265	.9279	.9292	.9306	.9319
1.5	.9332	.9345	.9357	.9370	.9382	.9394	.9406	.9418	.9430	.9441
1.6	.9452	.9463	.9474	.9485	.9495	.9505	.9515	.9525	.9535	.9545
1.7	.9554	.9564	.9573	.9582	.9591	.9599	.9608	.9616	.9625	.9633
1.8	.9641	.9649	.9656	.9664	.9671	.9678	.9686	.9693	.9700	.9706
1.9	.9713	.9719	.9726	.9732	.9738	.9744	.9750	.9756	.9762	.9767
2.0	.9773	.9778	.9783	.9788	.9793	.9798	.9803	.9808	.9812	.9817
2.1	.9821	.9826	.9830	.9834	.9838	.9842	.9846	.9850	.9854	.9857
2.2	.9861	.9865	.9868	.9871	.9875	.9878	.9881	.9884	.9887	.9890
2.3	.9893	.9896	.9898	.9901	.9904	.9906	.9909	.9911	.9913	.9916
2.4	.9918	.9920	.9922	.9925	.9927	.9929	.9931	.9932	.9934	.9936
2.5	.9938	.9940	.9941	.9943	.9945	.9946	.9948	.9949	.9951	.9952
2.6	.9953	.9955	.9956	.9957	.9959	.9960	.9961	.9962	.9963	.9964
2.7	.9965	.9966	.9967	.9968	.9969	.9970	.9971	.9972	.9973	.9974
2.8	.9974	.9975	.9976	.9977	.9977	.9978	.9979	.9980	.9980	.9981
2.9	.9981	.9982	.9983	.9983	.9984	.9984	.9985	.9985	.9986	.9986
3.0	.9987	.9987	.9987	.9988	.9988	.9989	.9989	.9989	.9990	.9990
3.1	.9990	.9991	.9991	.9991	.9992	.9992	.9992	.9992	.9993	.9993
3.2	.9993	.9993	.9994	.9994	.9994	.9994	.9994	.9995	.9995	.9995
3.3	.9995	.9995	.9996	.9996	.9996	.9996	.9996	.9996	.9996	.9997
3.4	.9997	.9997	.9997	.9997	.9997	.9997	.9997	.9997	.9998	.9998
3.5	.9998	.9998	.9998	.9998	.9998	.9998	.9998	.9998	.9998	.9998

The numbers in the body of the table represent the area under the normal curve to the left of the standardized z-value. As the standard normal curve is symmetric around the mean of zero, 50% of the area under the normal curve lies to the left of the z-value of zero.

Steps in determining probability values associated with specific z-values of a normally distributed test-statistic:

- Convert the (normally distributed) test statistic into a standardized z-score: $z = \dfrac{x - \mu}{\sigma}$.

- Truncate the obtained z-score to the nearest lower z-value in the table. For example, a z-value of 2.432 can be approximated by the value 2.43 in the table.

- Locate the area under the curve to the left of this z-value in the body of the table at the intersection of the row value representing z-increment of 0.1 and the column value representing z-increments of 0.01. For example, the area under the curve associated with a z-value of 2.43 can be found at the intersection of the row labeled "2.4" and the column labeled ".03": it is 0.9925.

- As the table shows the area under the normal curve *below* the indicated z-value, the probability of obtaining a z-score of 2.43 or *larger* for a normally distributed test statistic is $p \le .0075$ (1 − .9925).

- For *negative z-scores*, the table entries indicate the area under the normal curve to the right of the z-score. For example, with a z-score of −2.43, the area under the curve to the right of this z-score covers 0.9925.

- To obtain the *two-sided probability* that a test statistic differs from the null-hypothesis value of zero by the *absolute value* of the z-score in either direction, we multiply the one-sided probability by 2, as the normal distribution is symmetric. For example, the probability of obtaining a z-score of +2.43 or larger or −2.43 or smaller equals $p \le .015$ (.0075 × 2).

APPENDIX C

Table of Critical *t*-Values for Several Significance Levels of *t*-Distributions With Different Degrees of Freedom (df)

Probabilities (Significance Levels):

(One-Tailed):	.10	.05	.025	.02	.01	.005	.0025	.001	.0005
(Two-Tailed):	.20	.10	.05	.04	.02	.01	.005	.002	.001
df									
1	3.078	6.314	12.71	15.89	31.82	63.66	127.3	318.3	636.6
2	1.886	2.920	4.303	4.849	6.965	9.925	14.09	22.33	31.60
3	1.638	2.353	3.182	3.482	4.541	5.841	7.453	10.21	12.92
4	1.533	2.132	2.776	2.999	3.747	4.604	5.598	7.173	8.610
5	1.476	2.015	2.571	2.757	3.365	4.032	4.773	5.893	6.869
6	1.440	1.943	2.447	2.612	3.143	3.707	4.317	5.208	5.959
7	1.415	1.895	2.365	2.517	2.998	3.499	4.029	4.785	5.408
8	1.397	1.860	2.306	2.449	2.896	3.355	3.833	4.501	5.041
9	1.383	1.833	2.262	2.398	2.821	3.250	3.690	4.297	4.781
10	1.372	1.812	2.228	2.359	2.764	3.169	3.581	4.144	4.587
11	1.363	1.796	2.201	2.328	2.718	3.106	3.497	4.025	4.437
12	1.356	1.782	2.179	2.303	2.681	3.055	3.428	3.930	4.318
13	1.350	1.771	2.160	2.282	2.650	3.012	3.372	3.852	4.221
14	1.345	1.761	2.145	2.264	2.624	2.977	3.326	3.787	4.140
15	1.341	1.753	2.131	2.249	2.602	2.947	3.286	3.733	4.073
16	1.337	1.746	2.120	2.235	2.583	2.921	3.252	3.686	4.015
17	1.333	1.740	2.110	2.224	2.567	2.898	3.222	3.646	3.965
18	1.330	1.734	2.101	2.214	2.552	2.878	3.197	3.611	3.922
19	1.328	1.729	2.093	2.205	2.539	2.861	3.174	3.579	3.883
20	1.325	1.725	2.086	2.197	2.528	2.845	3.153	3.552	3.850
21	1.323	1.721	2.080	2.189	2.518	2.831	3.135	3.527	3.819
22	1.321	1.717	2.074	2.183	2.508	2.819	3.119	3.505	3.792
23	1.319	1.714	2.069	2.177	2.500	2.807	3.104	3.485	3.768
24	1.318	1.711	2.064	2.172	2.492	2.797	3.091	3.467	3.745
25	1.316	1.708	2.060	2.167	2.485	2.787	3.078	3.450	3.725
26	1.315	1.706	2.056	2.162	2.479	2.779	3.067	3.435	3.707
27	1.314	1.703	2.052	2.158	2.473	2.771	3.057	3.421	3.690
28	1.313	1.701	2.048	2.154	2.467	2.763	3.047	3.408	3.674
29	1.311	1.699	2.045	2.150	2.462	2.756	3.038	3.396	3.659
30	1.310	1.697	2.042	2.147	2.457	2.750	3.030	3.385	3.646

(*continued*)

Probabilities (Significance Levels):

(One-Tailed):	.10	.05	.025	.02	.01	.005	.0025	.001	.0005
(Two-Tailed):	.20	.10	.05	.04	.02	.01	.005	.002	.001
df									
40	1.303	1.684	2.021	2.123	2.423	2.704	2.971	3.307	3.551
50	1.299	1.676	2.009	2.109	2.403	2.678	2.937	3.261	3.496
60	1.296	1.671	2.000	2.099	2.390	2.660	2.915	3.232	3.460
80	1.292	1.664	1.990	2.088	2.374	2.639	2.887	3.195	3.416
100	1.290	1.660	1.984	2.081	2.364	2.626	2.871	3.174	3.390
1000	1.282	1.646	1.962	2.056	2.330	2.581	2.813	3.098	3.300
z	1.282	1.645	1.960	2.054	2.326	2.576	2.807	3.091	3.291

The numbers in each column of the body of the table represent the *t*-threshold values associated with the probability values at the top of the column. Example (see the graph below):

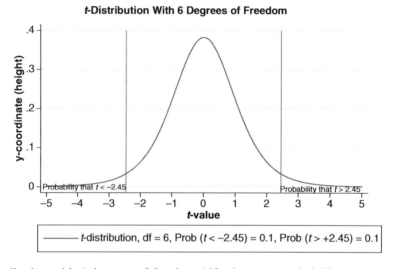

t-Distribution With 6 Degrees of Freedom

For a *t*-distribution with 6 degrees of freedom (df), the area (probability) under the curve *to the right* of the *t*-value of 2.447 comprises 0.025 of the total area. Being symmetric, the area under the curve to the left of the *t*-value of −2.447 also comprises 0.025 of the total area. The joint probability of exceeding the absolute value of ($t > |\pm 2.447|$) on both sides equals 0.05. At the bottom of the table (see row labeled "*z*"), there are the threshold values for the standard normal distribution. For larger samples ($n > 120$) the differences between the *t*-distribution and the normal distribution are negligible.

Steps in determining appropriate threshold *t*-values associated with selected probabilities for a test statistic following a *t*-distribution:

- Determine the df, which equal *n* minus the number of free population parameters to be estimated: df = *n* − no. of parameters; for example, with a sample size of 8, an independent sample *t*-test comparing two group means has df = 8 − 2 = 6.
- Locate the *t*-value corresponding to the chosen significance level. For instance, if a two-tailed significance level of $\alpha = 0.05$ is chosen as the decision criterion for rejecting the null hypothesis, a *t*-distribution with 28 df has a threshold value of $t = 2.447$.
- Compute the *t*-value from the sample data; for example, *t*-value = a mean difference divided by its standard error.
- If the computed *t*-value is greater than the threshold value of 2.447, then the null hypothesis can be rejected at the $p < .05$ level.

Normalizing a Nonnormal Distribution

Normalizing the distribution of a variable can have several related meanings. In preparation for data analysis, analysts often transform a nonnormal distribution into an approximately normal one, so as to better meet the assumptions of normal distribution tests about the shape of the sampling distribution. Not every nonnormal distribution can be transformed into an approximately normal one, but frequently uni-modal and skewed distributions can be transformed into normal distributions as the following graph for the body mass index (BMI) distribution shows.

Distribution of BMI Before and After Lognormal Transformation

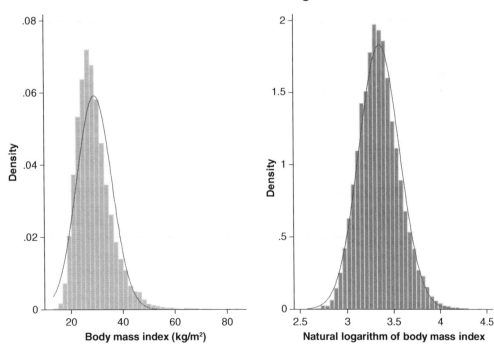

Researchers often use other transformations, such as the square root transformation ($\sqrt{x}$) or $1/x$.

Note: Normalization of a variable should not be confused with its *standardization*: converting a variable into a z-score leaves the *shape* of the distribution unchanged.

Table of Critical *f*-Values at the Significance Level of α = 0.05 of *f*-Distributions With Different Degrees of Freedom (df)

DF₁	1	2	3	4	5	6	7	8	9	10	15	20	30	40	60	120	∞
DF₂																	
1	161.5	199.5	215.7	224.6	230.2	234.0	236.8	238.9	240.5	241.9	246.0	248.0	250.1	251.1	252.2	253.3	254.3
2	18.51	19.00	19.16	19.26	19.30	19.33	19.35	19.37	19.39	19.40	19.43	19.45	19.46	19.47	19.48	19.49	19.50
3	10.13	9.552	9.277	9.117	9.014	8.941	8.887	8.845	8.812	8.786	8.703	8.660	8.617	8.594	8.572	8.549	8.526
4	7.709	6.944	6.591	6.388	6.256	6.163	6.094	6.041	5.999	5.964	5.858	5.803	5.746	5.717	5.688	5.658	5.628
5	6.608	5.786	5.410	5.192	5.050	4.950	4.876	4.818	4.773	4.735	4.619	4.558	4.496	4.464	4.431	4.399	4.365
6	5.987	5.143	4.757	4.534	4.387	4.284	4.207	4.147	4.099	4.060	3.938	3.874	3.808	3.774	3.740	3.705	3.669
7	5.591	4.737	4.347	4.120	3.972	3.866	3.787	3.726	3.677	3.637	3.511	3.445	3.376	3.340	3.304	3.267	3.230
8	5.318	4.459	4.066	3.838	3.688	3.581	3.501	3.438	3.388	3.347	3.218	3.150	3.079	3.043	3.005	2.967	2.928
9	5.117	4.257	3.863	3.633	3.482	3.374	3.293	3.230	3.179	3.137	3.006	2.937	2.864	2.826	2.787	2.748	2.707
10	4.965	4.103	3.708	3.478	3.326	3.217	3.136	3.072	3.020	2.978	2.845	2.774	2.700	2.661	2.621	2.580	2.538
11	4.844	3.982	3.587	3.357	3.204	3.095	3.012	2.948	2.896	2.854	2.719	2.646	2.571	2.531	2.490	2.448	2.405
12	4.747	3.885	3.490	3.259	3.106	2.996	2.913	2.849	2.796	2.753	2.617	2.544	2.466	2.426	2.384	2.341	2.296
13	4.667	3.806	3.411	3.179	3.025	2.915	2.832	2.767	2.714	2.671	2.533	2.459	2.380	2.339	2.297	2.252	2.206
14	4.600	3.739	3.344	3.112	2.958	2.848	2.764	2.699	2.646	2.602	2.463	2.388	2.308	2.266	2.223	2.178	2.131
15	4.543	3.682	3.287	3.056	2.901	2.791	2.707	2.641	2.588	2.544	2.403	2.328	2.247	2.204	2.160	2.114	2.066
16	4.494	3.634	3.239	3.007	2.852	2.741	2.657	2.591	2.538	2.494	2.352	2.276	2.194	2.151	2.106	2.059	2.010
17	4.451	3.592	3.197	2.965	2.810	2.699	2.614	2.548	2.494	2.450	2.308	2.230	2.148	2.104	2.058	2.011	1.960
18	4.414	3.555	3.160	2.928	2.773	2.661	2.577	2.510	2.456	2.412	2.269	2.191	2.107	2.063	2.017	1.968	1.917
19	4.381	3.522	3.127	2.895	2.740	2.628	2.544	2.477	2.423	2.378	2.234	2.156	2.071	2.026	1.980	1.930	1.878
20	4.351	3.493	3.098	2.866	2.711	2.599	2.514	2.447	2.393	2.348	2.203	2.124	2.039	1.994	1.946	1.896	1.843
21	4.325	3.467	3.073	2.840	2.685	2.573	2.488	2.421	2.366	2.321	2.176	2.096	2.010	1.965	1.917	1.866	1.812
22	4.301	3.443	3.049	2.817	2.661	2.549	2.464	2.397	2.342	2.297	2.151	2.071	1.984	1.938	1.889	1.838	1.783
23	4.279	3.422	3.028	2.796	2.640	2.528	2.442	2.375	2.320	2.275	2.128	2.048	1.961	1.914	1.865	1.813	1.757
24	4.260	3.403	3.009	2.776	2.621	2.508	2.423	2.355	2.300	2.255	2.108	2.027	1.939	1.892	1.842	1.790	1.733

(continued)

(*continued*)

DF$_1$	1	2	3	4	5	6	7	8	9	10	15	20	30	40	60	120	∞
DF$_2$																	
25	4.242	3.385	2.991	2.759	2.603	2.490	2.405	2.337	2.282	2.237	2.089	2.008	1.919	1.872	1.822	1.768	1.711
26	4.225	3.369	2.975	2.743	2.587	2.474	2.388	2.321	2.266	2.220	2.072	1.990	1.901	1.853	1.803	1.749	1.691
27	4.210	3.354	2.960	2.728	2.572	2.459	2.373	2.305	2.250	2.204	2.056	1.974	1.884	1.836	1.785	1.731	1.672
28	4.196	3.340	2.947	2.714	2.558	2.445	2.359	2.291	2.236	2.190	2.041	1.958	1.869	1.820	1.769	1.714	1.654
29	4.183	3.328	2.934	2.701	2.545	2.432	2.346	2.278	2.223	2.177	2.028	1.945	1.854	1.806	1.754	1.698	1.638
30	4.171	3.316	2.922	2.690	2.534	2.421	2.334	2.266	2.211	2.165	2.015	1.932	1.841	1.792	1.740	1.684	1.622
40	4.085	3.232	2.839	2.606	2.450	2.336	2.249	2.180	2.124	2.077	1.925	1.839	1.745	1.693	1.637	1.577	1.508
60	4.001	3.150	2.758	2.525	2.368	2.254	2.167	2.097	2.040	1.993	1.836	1.748	1.649	1.594	1.534	1.467	1.389
120	3.920	3.072	2.680	2.447	2.290	2.175	2.087	2.016	1.959	1.911	1.751	1.659	1.554	1.495	1.429	1.352	1.254
∞	3.842	2.996	2.605	2.372	2.214	2.099	2.010	1.938	1.880	1.831	1.666	1.571	1.459	1.394	1.318	1.221	1.000

The *f*-distribution or probability density function (PDF) comprises a "family" of functions. The functions differ depending on two parameters: the degrees of freedom (df) in the numerator of the *f*-ratio (df$_1$) and the degrees of freedom in the denominator (df$_2$) of the *f*-ratio. The graph below shows just one *f*-distribution with df$_1$ = 10 and df$_2$ = 10. The distribution is skewed to the right and the blackened area under the curve corresponds to 5% of the total area under the curve. This area lies to the right of the critical *f*-value of 2.978.

The graph indicates that any test statistic, which has the shape of the *f*-distribution with df$_1$ = 10 and df$_2$ = 10, would produce a sample *f*-value of 2.978 or larger by chance only 5% of the time, if the null hypothesis of no effect is true. Thus, for this *f*-distribution, an *f*-value obtained from the sample data larger than 2.978 would be considered "statistically significant."

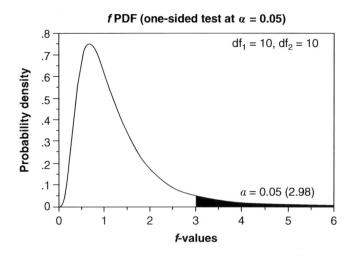

We use *f*-values in the table to determine whether a sample *f*-ratio occurs by chance in less than 5% of all possible samples drawn randomly from the same target population:

1. Compute the *f*-ratio with the appropriate df in the numerator and the denominator from the sample data.

2. Read off the critical f-value at which $\alpha = 0.05$ located at the intersection of df_1 (numerator) and df_2 (denominator) for the distribution with the appropriate df. (Use nearest df for approximations.)

3. Compare the magnitude of the sample value of the f-ratio to the critical f-value; if the former is larger than the latter, the result is "statistically significant" at the 0.05 level.

Example: The critical f-value for an f-distribution ($df_1 = 4$, $df_2 = 120$) equals $f(4,129) = 2.447$. Thus, any observed sample f-ratio >2.447 would lead to the rejection of the null hypothesis with at least 95% confidence that the inference is true. Exact f-values for different α-values are usually obtained from software applications.

Proof That Phi = Pearson's *r*

Here are the formulas for the correlation coefficients Phi and Pearson's *r*:

$$\text{Phi}(\Phi) = \frac{(AD - BC)}{\sqrt{EFGH}}$$

$$r_{xy} = Cov(z_x z_y) = \frac{\Sigma(X_i - \bar{X})(Y_i - \bar{Y})}{(n-1)s_x s_y} = \frac{\Sigma z_x z_y}{(n-1)}$$

Because the proof using the formula equivalence involves exceedingly tedious algebra, we use example data to show the equivalence. The data table is similar to Table 16.3, but in order to simplify the calculations, we chose smaller numbers:

2 × 2 Table Showing Joint Distribution of Study Subjects Across Two Variables: Gender and Diabetes Status (Numerical Example)

		DIABETES STATUS (=Y)		ROW MARGINAL FREQUENCIES
		HAS DIABETES (1)	NO DIABETES (0)	
Gender (=X)	Women (1)	3 (=A)	9 (=B)	12 (=G)
	Men (0)	3 (=C)	5 (=D)	8 (=H)
Column marginal frequencies		6 (=E)	14 (=F)	20 (=A+B+C+D)

1. Using the Phi formula, we get: $\text{Phi}(\Phi) = \dfrac{(3 \times 5 - 3 \times 9)}{\sqrt{6 \times 14 \times 12 \times 8}} = \dfrac{(15 - 27)}{\sqrt{8064}} = \dfrac{-12}{89.7998} = -0.13363$

2. Using the Pearson's *r* formula, we first compute the covariance and variances:

As $\bar{X} = \dfrac{G}{(A+B+C+D)} = \dfrac{12}{20} = 0.6$ and $\bar{Y} = \dfrac{E}{(A+B+C+D)} = \dfrac{6}{20} = 0.3$, and X_i and Y_i can only take on the value 1 or 0, we can express the covariance and variances of X and Y as follows:

$$Cov(XY) = \frac{\sum (X_i - \bar{X})(Y_i - \bar{Y})}{n-1}$$

$$= \frac{1}{19}[(1-0.3)(1-0.6)\times 3 + (1-0.3)(0-0.6)\times 3 + (0-0.3)(1-0.6)\times 9$$

$$+(0-0.3)(0-0.6)\times 5] = -0.03158$$

$$Var(X) = \frac{\sum (X_i - \bar{X})^2}{n-1} = \frac{1}{19}[(1-0.6)^2 \times 12 + (0-0.6)^2 \times 8] = 0.252632;$$

$$Var(Y) = \frac{\sum (Y_i - \bar{Y})^2}{n-1} = \frac{1}{19}[(1-0.3)^2 \times 6 + (0-0.3)^2 \times 14] = 0.221053;$$

Finally, we express the Pearson's r as standardized covariance:

$$r_{xy} = \frac{Cov(XY)}{SD_x SD_y} = \frac{-0.03158}{\sqrt{0.252632} \times \sqrt{0.221053}} = \frac{-0.03158}{0.50265 \times 0.47016} = -0.13363$$

Table of Critical Chi-Square Values for Several Significance Levels of Chi-Square Distributions With Different Degrees of Freedom (df)

Probabilities (Significance Levels)

df	0.10	0.05	0.025	0.01	0.005
1	2.706	3.841	5.024	6.635	7.879
2	4.605	5.991	7.378	9.210	10.597
3	6.251	7.815	9.348	11.345	12.838
4	7.779	9.488	11.143	13.277	14.860
5	9.236	11.070	12.833	15.086	16.750
6	10.645	12.592	14.449	16.812	18.548
7	12.017	14.067	16.013	18.475	20.278
8	13.362	15.507	17.535	20.090	21.955
9	14.684	16.919	19.023	21.666	23.589
10	15.987	18.307	20.483	23.209	25.188
11	17.275	19.675	21.920	24.725	26.757
12	18.549	21.026	23.337	26.217	28.300
13	10.812	22.362	24.730	27.688	29.819
14	21.064	23.685	26.119	29.141	31.319
15	22.307	24.996	27.488	30.578	32.801
16	23.542	26.296	28.845	32.000	34.267
17	24.769	27.587	30.191	33.409	35.718
18	25.989	28.869	31.526	34.805	37.156
19	27.204	30.144	32.852	36.191	38.582
20	28.412	31.410	34.170	37.566	39.997
25	34.382	37.652	40.646	44.314	46.928
30	40.256	43.773	46.979	50.892	53.672
40	51.805	55.758	59.342	63.691	66.766
50	63.167	67.505	71.420	76.154	79.490
60	74.397	79.082	83.298	88.379	91.952
70	85.527	90.531	95.023	100.43	104.22
80	96.578	101.88	106.63	112.33	116.32
90	107.57	113.15	118.14	124.12	128.30
100	118.50	124.34	129.56	135.81	140.17

The table shows critical threshold chi-square (χ^2) values for five probabilities. The χ^2-values in the body of the table indicate the threshold values, beyond which the area under the χ^2-curve equals the proportion of the area indicated at the top of a column as the probability or significance level. Example (see the graph below): The probability that a test statistic following the χ^2-distribution with 2 degrees of freedom (df) exceeds the value 5.991, even though the null hypothesis is true, equals $p = .05$.

Steps in determining appropriate χ^2-values associated with selected probabilities for a test statistic following a chi-square distribution:

- Determine the df; for a frequency tabulation, df = (no. of rows − 1) × (no. of columns − 1).
- Locate the chi-square value corresponding to the chosen significance level. For instance, if the significance level of $\alpha = 0.01$ is chosen as the decision criterion for rejecting the null hypothesis, a chi-square-distribution with 2 df has a threshold value of $\chi^2 = 9.21$.
- Compute the χ^2-value from the sample data.
- If the computed χ^2-value is greater than the threshold value of 9.21, then the null hypothesis can be rejected at the $p < .01$ level.

Chi-Square Distribution With 2 Degrees of Freedom

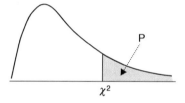

Refresher on Exponential and Logarithmic Transformations

Even though exponential and logarithmic functions are part of College Algebra, some readers may want to review this appendix to refresh their familiarity with these transformations, as they are essential in understanding the output from logistic and survival regression models. The aim here is to provide an informal introduction; the use of a hand-held calculator may be advisable as you read through this appendix.

EXPONENTIALS

Consider the following sequence of numbers:

$$32, 16, 8, 4, 2, 1, \frac{1}{2}, \frac{1}{4}, \frac{1}{8}, \frac{1}{16}, \frac{1}{32}$$

We can rewrite this sequence of numbers using power expressions to the base 2:

$$2^5, 2^4, 2^3, 2^2, 2^1, 2^0, \frac{1}{2^1}, \frac{1}{2^2}, \frac{1}{2^3}, \frac{1}{2^4}, \frac{1}{2^5}$$

In case you have forgotten, another way of writing the fractions is as follows: $\frac{1}{2^2} = 2^{-2}$, so that the whole sequence can also be written as:

$$2^5, 2^4, 2^3, 2^2, 2^1, 2^0, 2^{-1}, 2^{-2}, 2^{-3}, 2^{-4}, 2^{-5}$$

Note: The original number sequence shows as its highest value 32 and as its lowest value 1/32, which can also be expressed as a decimal: 0.03125. In short, the original number sequence only contains positive (>0) numbers. By contrast, the exponents for the rewritten number sequence of 2^5 to 2^{-5} range from +5 to −5. In addition, they contain the value 0.

As you can see from the example sequence, $2^0 = 1$; in fact, *any* number raised to the power of zero equals one. This follows directly from the basic rules of multiplication and division of the original numbers.

Addition/Subtraction Rules for Exponents

Suppose you want to multiply 8×4; it is quite obvious that $8 \times 4 = 32$. Now, using our previous examples, we can substitute 2^3 for the number 8, as $8 = 2 \times 2 \times 2 = 2^3$; likewise we can substitute 2^2 for the number 4, as $4 = 2 \times 2 = 2^2$. From this, it follows that the product 8×4 could be rewritten as $2^3 \times 2^2$, which can also be written as: $2 \times 2 \times 2 \times 2 \times 2 = 2^5 = 32$. Thus we note that while the base numbers are multiplied, the exponents are *added*: $2^3 \times 2^2 = 2^{(3+2)} = 2^5$.

This principle works in the same way for the division of base numbers and the subtraction of exponents: Suppose you want to divide 32 by 4; again, it is obvious that $32/4 = 8$. Substituting the exponential expressions to the base 2 for the original numbers, we get $32 = 2^5$, $4 = 2^2$, and $8 = 2^3$. Thus, the division of the base numbers, $32/4 = 8$, can be rewritten as $2^5/2^2 = 2^3$. Note that the division of the base numbers is expressed as a *subtraction* of the exponent numbers: $2^5/2^2 = 2^{(5-2)} = 2^3$. You can also show this after rewriting $2^5/2^2$ as a ratio of two products of 2s:

$$\frac{32}{4} = \frac{2^5}{2^2} = \frac{2 \times 2 \times 2 \times 2 \times 2}{2 \times 2} = \frac{2 \times 2 \times 2}{1} = 2^3$$

Now let us see what happens, if we divide a number by itself. For instance, 8/8 is obviously equal to 1. Expressed as exponential numbers to the base 2, we get:

$$\frac{8}{8} = \frac{2^3}{2^3} = \frac{2 \times 2 \times 2}{2 \times 2 \times 2} = 2^{(3-3)} = 2^0 = 1$$

In short, dividing any number by itself will result in one; when replacing the number in the ratio by an equal-valued exponential number, the difference in the associated exponents will be equal to zero, regardless of what base is chosen. Another example of this principle would be the division of 27 by itself: $27/27 = 1$ and $3^3/3^3 = 3^{(3-3)} = 3^0 = 1$.

Finally, we see why we can rewrite the fraction 1/4 as 2^{-2}: $1/4 = 2^0/2^2 = 2^{(0-2)} = 2^{-2} = 1/2^2 = 1/4$.

Fractional Exponents

As $2^4 = 16$, we call 2 the fourth root of 16. This is written as $\sqrt[4]{16} = 16^{1/4} = 2$. From this, it follows that $25^{1/2} = \sqrt[2]{25} = 5$, as $5^2 = 25$ and $27^{1/3} = 3$, as $3^3 = 27$, and so on. We can also solve $27^{2/3} = 9$, as $27^{2/3} = (27^{1/3})^2 = 3^2 = (27^2)^{1/3} = 729^{1/3} = 9$.

LOGARITHMS

Consider the equation: $2^x = 32$. It shows the number 32 as equivalent to the base number raised to the power of x. Thus, if the number 32 is given to us, we are asking: To what power must we raise the (base) number 2, in order to get the (yield) number 32? The number x to which 2 must be raised to yield the number 32 is called the logarithm to the base 2. In this case, it is easy to solve the equation for x in our head: $2^x = 32$ implies that x must be equal to 5, as $2^5 = 32$. We write the logarithmic equation as follows:

$$\log_2 32 = 5 \text{ ("the logarithm of 32 to the base 2 equals 5").}$$

In principle, we can express *any* number y as the logarithm to the base 2: $2^x = y$. We can also express any number y as the logarithm to the base 10. For instance, if $y = 100$, the logarithm to the base 10 is 2, as $10^x = 100$ implies that x must be equal to 2: $10^2 = 100$. We write this logarithmic equation as follows:

$$\log_{10} 100 = 2 \text{ ("the logarithm of 100 to the base 10 equals 2")}.$$

Finally, we already saw that we are not just limited to whole numbers in the exponents. In addition to fractions, exponents can take on any real number, such as 0.153. Even if the number is "irrational" (which means it cannot be written as a finite fraction), it can always be approximated with a fraction to any level of precision, and we already saw how to solve an equation with a fractional exponent. For instance, raising 2 to the power of 153/1,000 yields the following equation: $2^{0.153} = 1.1119$. As we can represent 0.153 as the fraction, 153/1,000, we can solve $2^{0.153} = y$ in this way: $2^{0.153} (2^{153})^{\frac{1}{1000}} = 1.1119$.

The same applies to logarithms. We can find the exponent to the base 10 (or any other base) that will yield any number we like with sufficient precision: for instance, $y = 10^{2.301} \approx 200$, as $10^{2.301} = 199.98$. We say that the logarithm to the base 10, which yields 200, equals approximately 2.301.

Conversions to Logarithms

The conversion of positive fractional numbers (like odds ratios [ORs] and relative-risk ratios [RRRs]) to logarithms yields numbers that encompass the whole range (positive and negative) of the numbers. For instance, we can convert the sequence listed earlier:

$$32, 16, 8, 4, 2, 1, \frac{1}{2}, \frac{1}{4}, \frac{1}{8}, \frac{1}{16}, \frac{1}{32}$$

into the following sequence of *logarithms to the base 2*:

$$5, 4, 3, 2, 1, 0, -1, -2, -3, -4, -5,$$

as $2^5 = 32$, $2^4 = 16$, ... $2^0 = 1$, $2^{-1} = 1/2$, and so on.

We now see that the first sequence of only positive numbers pivots around the value one, with the fractions being the reciprocals of the whole number, for example, 1/16 = inverse of 16. The resulting distribution of values tends to be highly skewed, as is the case for ORs and RRRs. However, after converting this sequence to logarithms to base 2, we obtain a second sequence that is symmetric around the pivot of zero.

Logarithms to the Base *e*

In most statistical applications of logarithms, we use a seemingly weird base number called "*e*" ($e = 2.718281828$; the "*e*" stands for the 18th-century Swiss mathematician Euler). The reason for using "*e*" as a base number (instead of 2 or 10) is that it actually simplifies many calculations in calculus. The number is also the basis for compound interest calculations.

Here, we treat "*e*" just like any other number. Thus, instead of using the base 2 or the base 10 to find the logarithm, we use the base e: $e^x = y$. This expression is also known as the exponential function.

The logarithm associated with the base number e, $\log_e$, is also known as the "natural logarithm." It is symbolized as "ln." If you have a hand-held calculator, you should have buttons for both the symbols "e^x" (the exponential function) and the symbol "ln" or "ln$x$" for the logarithm to the base e. For instance, if you type in the number 5 for x and then press "e^x," you should get $e^5 = 2.718281828^5 = 148.41316$. If you then take the natural logarithm of this number, you should get back to 5, as that is the number to which e was raised to obtain 148.41316.

Algebraic Rules for Logarithms

We already know that $\log_2 16 = 4$, as $2^4 = 16$. We could rewrite $\log_2 16 = \log_2(4^2) = 4$; but $\log_2 4 = 2$, so $2 \log_2 4 = 4$. As a general rule, we have that the logarithm of a number raised to the nth power equals n times the logarithm of the number: $\log_2(4^2) = 2 \log_2 4$ or, in general:

$$\log(a^n) = n \log(a)$$

Other important relations are:

$$\log(ab) = \log(a) + \log(b)$$

$$\log(a/b) = \log(a) - \log(b)$$

These rules follow directly from the rules for exponentials:

Using the base 2, we have $2^x = y$. Suppose $x = 3 + 2 = 5$; then $2^5 = 2^{3+2} = 2^3 2^2$.

Now, let us take the logarithm of the expression 2^x: $\log_2 2^x = x \log_2 2$;

if $x = (3 + 2)$, we have: $\log_2 2^{3+2} = \log_2(2^3 2^2)$;

but also: $\log_2 2^{3+2} = (3 + 2)\log_2 2 = 3\log_2(2) + 2\log_2(2)$;

thus: $\log_2(2^3 2^2) = 3\log_2(2) + 2\log_2(2)$.

Likewise: $\log_2(2^3/2^2) = \log_2 2^{3-2} = 3\log_2(2) - 2\log_2(2)$.

Standardization of Interval-Level Variables

- Standardizing an interval-level variable (x_i) means converting it into a z-score:

$$z_i = \frac{(x_i - \bar{x})}{s_x}$$

- The mean of a z-score always equals 0:

$$\bar{z}_x = \frac{\Sigma z_i}{n} = \frac{\Sigma(x_i - \bar{x})}{n} = \frac{\Sigma x_i}{n} - \frac{\Sigma \bar{x}}{n} = \frac{n\bar{x}}{n} - \frac{n\bar{x}}{n} = 0$$

- The variance of a z-score always equals one:

$$s_z^2 = \frac{\Sigma(z_i - \bar{z})^2}{(n-1)} = \frac{\Sigma(z_i - 0)^2}{(n-1)} = \frac{\Sigma z_i^2}{(n-1)} = \frac{1}{(n-1)}\Sigma\left(\frac{(x_i - \bar{x})}{s_x}\right)^2$$

$$= \frac{1}{(n-1)}\Sigma\frac{(x_i - \bar{x})^2}{s_x^2} = \frac{1}{s_x^2}\Sigma\frac{(x_i - \bar{x})^2}{(n-1)} = \frac{1}{s_x^2}s_x^2 = 1$$

- The standard deviation of a z-score always equals 1, since the square root of one equals one:

$$s_z = \sqrt{\frac{\Sigma(z_i - \bar{z})^2}{n-1}} = 1$$

- The covariance between two standardized variables z_x and z_y equals the Pearson's r correlation:

$$Cov(z_x z_y) = s_{z_x z_y}^2 = \frac{\Sigma(z_{xi} - \bar{z}_x)(z_{yi} - \bar{z}_y)}{(n-1)} = \frac{\Sigma(z_{xi} - 0)(z_{yi} - 0)}{(n-1)} = \frac{\Sigma z_{xi} z_{yi}}{(n-1)}$$

$$= \frac{1}{(n-1)}\Sigma z_{xi} z_{yi} = \frac{1}{(n-1)}\Sigma\frac{(x_i - \bar{x})}{s_x}\frac{(y_i - \bar{y})}{s_y} = \frac{1}{s_x s_y}\frac{\Sigma(x_i - \bar{x})(y_i - \bar{y})}{(n-1)}$$

$$= \frac{Cov(xy)}{s_x s_y} = r_{xy}$$

APPENDIX J

Answers to Selected Exercises

CHAPTER 2

1. (a) Pap smear results (interval)
   (b) Body mass index (interval/ratio)
   (c) Food groups (nominal)
   (d) Biopsy results from breast tissue (ordinal)
   (e) Food preferences (ordinal)
   (f) Religious affiliation (nominal)

2. Mean rank for men (sex = 2): 4; mean rank for women (sex = 1): 6.5. Mean DBP score for men (sex = 2): 92.5; mean BDP score for women (sex = 1): 83.33. Since ranks were assigned such that lower number = higher score, both ways of scoring lead to the conclusion that men in this sample have higher average DBP.

CHAPTER 3

1. (a) Mean = 12.1.
   (b) Median = (10 + 1)/2 = 5.5th value, thus: (11 + 12)/2 = 11.5.
   (c) Standard deviation = 5.3.
   (d) The IQR is bounded by the 2.75th value [$(n + 1)/4 = 2.75$] and the 8.25th value {$[(n + 1) \times 3]/4 = 8.25$}, thus the IQR ranges from 7.75 to 16.5, a difference of 8.75.
   (e) (a) Mean = 13.7.
       (b) Median = 11.5.
       (c) Standard deviation = 9.43.
       (d) IQR = 7.75–16.5.
   (f) Changing the outlier value changed the mean and the standard deviation, but had no effect on the median and the IQR.

2. (a) Distribution C has the largest SD, followed by distribution B and then distribution A. Notice that the extreme values in distribution C are farther apart than in distribution B, which are farther apart than in distribution A. All the values in distribution A differ by 2, but in distribution B there is a "jump" in the middle, where the two values differ by 6. Distribution C shows increments of 1 between the values at either extreme, but a difference of 16 between the fifth and sixth value.

   (b) Distribution C is skewed to the *right* (mean > median), while the other two distributions are symmetric around the mean.

CHAPTER 4

1. (a) With replacement: $P(5 \text{ red balls}) = (3/5)^5 = .078$.
   (b) Without replacement: $P(5 \text{ red balls}) = (30/50)(29/49)(28/48)(27/47)(26/46) = .067$.

4. No. The probability of catching the flu and the probability of experiencing pollen allergies are unlikely to be independent.

6. $P = .192$; this probability is also known as the "positive predictive value" or PPV.

CHAPTER 5

3. (a) $6!/(3!3!) = 20$.

5. (a) Given the sample size, we assume the sampling distribution of the mean has a normal shape. Thus the 95% CI for the mean is: $148 \pm 1.96 \times 1.25 = 149 \pm 2.45$. Since 150 mg/dL lies within the 95% CI, the sample evidence is consistent with the hypothesis.
   (b) No. 145 mg/dL lies outside the 95% CI of 149 ± 2.45.
   (c) No. The *sampling distribution of the mean* is not to be confused with the distribution of individual values/scores within a particular sample. While the sampling distribution of sample means may well be normally distributed, we cannot assume that the actual sample values within the sample of 256 nursing home residents are normally distributed. Thus, we cannot assume that 10% of the residents have LDL cholesterol levels above 181, even though that value is 1.65 sample standard deviations above the sample mean $(181-148)/20 = 1.65$.

CHAPTER 6

1. (a) $80 \times 10^8/L \pm 1.96 \times 0.746 \times 10^8/L = 80 \times 10^8/L \pm 1.462 \times 10^8/L$.
   $\left(\text{SEM} \times \text{FPC} = \frac{20}{\sqrt{400}} \times \sqrt{\frac{900-400}{900-1}} = 0.746\right)$.

   (b) No. The 95% CI covers the range of $78.538 \times 10^8/L$ to $81.462 \times 10^8/L$.

4. The standard errors of sample statistics are smaller in larger study samples, indicating less sampling fluctuation and greater ability to discover smaller differences.

CHAPTER 7

1. No. If the nursing home residents are not randomly assigned to the mattress brands, there may be many confounding factors, such as the average weight of residents in wing A being higher than in wing B.

CHAPTER 8

1. (a) Yes.
   (b) No, we can.
   (c) No. The standard error of the test statistic is $26/\sqrt{169} = 26/13 = 2$.
   (d) Yes. The t-value equals $-4.0 = (86 - 94)/2$.
   (e) The 95% CI for the test statistic does not include the null value of 0:
       $-8.0 \pm 1.96 \times 2$.

2. Answer (c) is correct: 145 ± 1.372.
   [SD $= \sqrt{441} = 21$; SEM $= 21/\sqrt{900} = 0.7$; SE $= 1.96 \times 0.7$].

4. (a) $-2.807; p < .023$
   (b) $-3.1034; p < .015$
   (c) $-5.6569; p < .005$
   (d) $-2.7456; p > .05$
   (e) $-5.4995; p < .001$

CHAPTER 9

1. (a) $f = (15{,}000/3)/(45{,}000/300) = 33.33$.
   (b) Variance attributable to the independent factor: $15{,}000/(15{,}000 + 45{,}000) = 0.25$ or 25%.
   (c) Error variance? $45{,}000/300 = 150$.
   (d) The exact f-value at the cut-off point of $\alpha = 0.05$ (significance level) for an f-distribution with 3 df in the numerator and 300 df in the denominator equals 2.635. Using the table in Appendix E, we can get an approximate f-value, since df2 $= 300 > 120$ and df2 $= 300 < \infty$. The table indicates that the f-value must be less than 2.68 at the 0.05 cut-off point. Since the observed $f = 33.33$ far exceeds the 0.05 cut-off point, the association is significant.

3. (a) No. The overall f-test results in a p-value $> .14$; thus, we have no firm grounds to conclude that depression scores differ in the target population groups of nonsmokers, former smokers and current smokers.
   (b) Error variance $= 17{,}750 \times (1 - \eta^2) = 17{,}750 \times 0.8 = 14{,}200$.
   (c) No, this is an observational study. It involves random selection of a sample from a specified target population, but not random assignment of subjects to different smoking patterns.
   (d) To adjust the risk of a Type I error in multiple t-tests, we can use a significance level of $\alpha = 0.05/3 = 0.0167$.

CHAPTER 10

1. $r_{xy} = 8/(3 \times 4) = 0.067$.

2. $b_1 = \sum(X_i - X)(Y_i - Y)/\sum(X_i - X)^2 = \text{Cov}(XY)/\text{Var}(X) = 8/9 = 0.89$.

4. (a) Among adults, each additional inch of height, on average, translates into 4.9 pounds of additional weight.
   (b) 6 foot 1 inch $= 73$ inches; thus $= -149 + 4.9(73) = 208.7$. A 6 foot 1 inch tall adult is expected to weigh 208.7 pounds on average.

    (c) The intercept of -149 has no meaning in itself, since there are no adults with zero height.

    (d) Yes. If the standard error had been 4.0, the t-value for the regression coefficient would have been $4.9/4.0 = 1.225$. We would have to conclude that the true population regression coefficient is likely to be zero, since $t < 1.96$, the conventional cut-off point for a 0.05 significance level. Such a finding would not make any sense, since it implies that the average weight of taller persons is not greater than the average weight of shorter persons.

8. $Cov(XY) = 0.5 \times 8 \times 10 = 40$.

CHAPTER 11

4. (a) SS (intervention vs. control group): 50; SS (sex): 8; SS (sex–group interaction): 12.5; BGSS: $50 + 8 + 12.5 = 70.5$; WGSS: 5; TSS: $70.5 + 5 = 75.5$.

    (b) df (intervention vs. control group): 1; df (sex): 1; df (interaction): 1; df model: $1 + 1 + 1 = 3$; df error: 4; df total: $3 + 4 = 8 - 1 = 7$.

    (c) Model f-ratio: $(70.5/3)/(5/4) = 23.5/1.25 = 18.8$; this is larger than the critical f-value of 6.591 ($\alpha = 0.05$) for the f-distribution with 3 df1 and 4 df2. The f-ratio for the group factor is $50/1.25 = 40$; the f-ratio for the sex factor is $8/1.25 = 6.4$, and the f-ratio for the interaction is $12.5/1.25 = 10$.

    (d) The intervention improves adherence scores in general, but is more effective among women than among men as indicated by the significant interaction term.

CHAPTER 12

1. $R^2 = $ Model SS/TSS $= 717.689/1059.511 = 0.6774$.

2. (a) Turnover rates among hospital nurses are lower in hospitals that pay more: for each $1,000 in average nurses' salaries above the national median earnings, turnover rates in hospitals decline by 0.7%. Turnover rates among hospital nurses are higher among hospitals with older nursing staff: for each additional year in average age of the nursing staff, turnover rates increase by 0.5%. Finally, turnover rates are lower in rural hospitals (-0.85%) and urban hospitals (-2.23%), when compared to suburban hospitals.

    (b) $\hat{Y} = 17.70 - 0.70(3) + 0.50(0) - 2.23(0) = 17.7 - 2.1 = 15.6$. Thus, the expected annual turnover rate among nurses in a suburban hospital that pays its nurses $3,000 more than the U.S. median earnings is 15.6%.

    (c) Yes. If we compute the ratios of the sample regression coefficients to their respective standard errors, we get the t-values: $17.7/1.82 = 9.73$; $0.7/0.25 = 2.8$; $0.5/0.18 = 2.78$; $0.85/0.38 = 2.24$; $2.23/0.76 = 2.93$. In all of these cases, the estimated t-value based on the sample data exceeds the critical t-value of ± 1.96, which would indicate statistical significance at the α-level of 0.05. Since the study sample comprises $n = 450$ hospitals, we can safely assume that the sample estimates of the regression coefficients are normally distributed, and we would reject the null hypothesis that a regression coefficient equals zero in the population, when a sample regression coefficient exceeds ± 1.96 standard errors.

(d) The intercept shows the value of the predicted dependent variable ($\hat{Y}$), if all the independent variables (X_i) are set to zero. In this example, the intercept indicates that suburban hospitals with a nursing staff of U.S. median age and median wages will have a predicted average turnover rate of 17.7%.

3. The first equation predicts that African Americans in the urban area have 3.6 [= 2.7 + 0.9(1)] emergency department (ED) visits per person, while members of other ethnic groups have, on average, 2.7 [= 2.7 + 0.9(0)] ED visits per person. However, when taking into account family income, the differences between African Americans and other ethnic groups decline from 0.9 annual ED visits to 0.5 annual ER visits. Finally, after also accounting for differences in health insurance, there are no longer significant differences in the frequency of annual ED visits between African Americans and other ethnic groups in this urban area. In other words, if we were to compare African American and other ethnic families with the same family income and the same health insurance coverage (that is what "accounting for the effects of the other variables" means), then we would no longer find any differences in the frequency of ED visits per person.

CHAPTER 13

2. Changes in the outcome variable are the same/do not differ for intervention and control groups.

3. No. Changes in the outcome variable are the same for intervention and control groups; that all comparison groups (including the control group) change at the same rate cannot be attributed to the intervention.

CHAPTER 15

2. (a) Spearman's rho correlation tests whether the two rankings of the same hospitals are correlated.
   (b) The two teams report rankings that are independent of each other.
   (c) $r_s = 0.912, p < .001$.

3. (a) Wilcoxons's rank-sum test for independent samples.
   (b) The mean ratings/rank sums are the same for both states.
   (c) No. The rank sum for State A equals 140.5, for State B 159.5. This difference is not significant ($p > .55$).

CHAPTER 16

1. (a) Comparing seniors to juniors, we have: OR = (100/350)/(80/520) = 1.86; RR = (100/450)/(80/600) = 1.67.
   (b) 95% CI of OR: SE of ln(OR) = 0.165; ln(OR) ± 1.96 × SE = 0.62 ± 0.165; lower limit: $e^{0.455} = 1.576$; upper limit: $e^{0.785} = 2.192$; thus, 1.576 < OR < 2.192. 95% CI of RR: SE of ln(RR) = 0.136; ln(RR) ± 1.96 × SE = 0.513 ± 0.136; lower limit: $e^{0.377} = 1.458$; upper limit: $e^{0.649} = 1.94$; thus, 1.458 < RR < 1.94.

(c) Neither the OR nor the RR differs from the value 1 in the target population. $\chi^2 = 14.31$ with 1 df; $p < .005$.
(d) Phi $= (100 \times 520 - 80 \times 350)/\sqrt{180 \times 870 \times 450 \times 600} = 0.117$.
(e) If the sample is representative of seniors and juniors in the school, we can state that seniors are 1.67 times more likely to smoke than juniors.

3. If RR > 1, OR > 1. Since RR $= p_1/p_2$, RR > 1 implies $p_1 > p_2$; then $p_1/(1 - p_1) > p_2/(1 - p_2)$ and OR > 1.

5. $\chi^2 = 34.03$ with 1 df; $p < .005$.

CHAPTER 17

2. (a) What are the odds of nonsmokers experiencing pneumonia? $e^{-3.6889} = 0.025$.
(b) What are the odds of smokers experiencing pneumonia? $e^{-3.6889+1.609} = 0.125$.
(c) How many nonsmokers experienced pneumonia? The probability of pneumonia among nonsmokers can be obtained from the odds: $p = $ odds$/(1 + $ odds$) = 0.025/1.025 = 0.0244$; $205 \times 0.0244 = 5$.
(d) $p = $ odds$/(1 + $ odds$) = 0.125/1.125 = 0.1111$; $135 \times 0.1111 = 15$.

3. $\hat{Y} = \ln(p/(1 - p)) = -2.3 + 0.47\,(1) + 0.01\,(50) = -1.33$; odds: $e^{-1.33} = 0.264$ to 1.

CHAPTER 18

3. Log odds among men: $\ln(p/(1 - p)) = -2.996 + 0.0198(60) - 0.0513(12) - 0.1054(0) = -2.4236$.
Log odds among women: $\ln(p/(1 - p)) = -2.996 + 0.0198(45) - 0.0513(16) - 0.1054(1) = -3.0312$.
Difference in log odds: $-2.4236 - (-3.0312) = 0.6076$; thus OR $= e^{0.6076} = 1.836$.
Alternatively, OR $= e^{-2.4236}/e^{-3.0312} = 0.0886/0.04826 = 1.836$.

4. (a) The odds of suffering a serious functional limitation increase by 4.2% with each year of age.
(b) Compared to a person with 10 years of formal education, the odds of a serious functional limitation are predicted to be 37.2% higher [OR associated with education years is 0.9; thus, $0.9^{(7-10)} = 0.9^{-3} = 1/0.9^3 = 1.372$].
(c) Yes. Even though the odds ratios in the table compare each marital status group to the reference category of "married" people—and thus, we do not have a direct formal test of the difference between separated and widowed persons—the wide gap between the upper limit of the 95% CI for widowed persons and the lower limit of the 95% CI for separated persons would make it likely that the odds ratios in the two groups are significantly different.

CHAPTER 19

1. RR $= (55/11,000)/(38/15,200) = 2$.

3. The Kaplan–Meier cumulative mortality function equals 1 – the survival function: $M_t = 1 - S_t$. The cumulative mortality function gives us the proportion of a target population having died at time t.

CHAPTER 20

1. The magnitudes of the regression coefficient and HR for the variables sex and age are not comparable, since these variables are measured in different units. To test for statistical significance, we use the ratio of a regression coefficient to its associated standard error, which in this example is larger for age than for sex.

3. The graphs of the cumulative survival functions appear to cross, thus the survival patterns shown do not meet the proportional hazard assumption.

CHAPTER 21

1. Cronbach's Alpha: $A = (5/4)[1 - 5/(5 + 5 \times 4 \times 0.556)] = 0.86$.

4. Prevalence: 0.025; sensitivity: 0.86; specificity: 0.92; PPV: 0.216; NPV: 0.996; efficiency: 0.9185; level of test: 0.0995; kappa-adjusted sensitivity: 0.845; kappa-adjusted specificity: 0.196.

CHAPTER 22

2. $r_{12} = 0.6 \times 0.4 = 0.24$; $r_{13} = 0.6 \times 0.5 = 0.3$; $r_{14} = 0.6 \times 0.6 = 0.36$; $r_{23} = 0.4 \times 0.5 = 0.2$; $r_{24} = 0.4 \times 0.6 = 0.24$; $r_{34} = 0.5 \times 0.6 = 0.3$.

3. Some of the variables are perfectly correlated with other variable(s) or a linear combination of other variables.

Index

Made in the USA
Lexington, KY
25 August 2017